McRae's

# ELECTIVE
# ORTHOPAEDICS

Seventh Edition

# McRae's
# ELECTIVE
# ORTHOPAEDICS

**Paul J Jenkins**
MBChB, FRCSEd (Tr & Orth), MD, MFSTEd
Consultant Orthopaedic Surgeon,
Glasgow Royal Infirmary,
Honorary Clinical Associate Professor,
University of Glasgow
Glasgow, Scotland

**David W Shields**
MBChB, MSc, DipMedEd, FRCS (Tr & Orth), PhD
Consultant Orthopaedic Surgeon,
Queen Elizabeth University Hospital;
Honorary Senior Clinical Lecturer,
University of Glasgow
Glasgow, Scotland

**Timothy O White**
BMedSci, MBChB, FRCSEd (Tr & Orth), MD, FFTEd
Consultant Orthopaedic Trauma Surgeon,
Royal Infirmary of Edinburgh;
Honorary Reader in Orthopaedic and Trauma Surgery,
University of Edinburgh
Edinburgh, Scotland

ELSEVIER

**ISBN:** 9780702081255
9780702081040

*Content Strategist:* Trinity Hutton
*Project Manager:* Shruti Raj
*Design:* Patrick Ferguson
*Illustration Manager:* Muthukumaran Thangaraj
*Marketing Manager:* Belinda Tudin

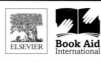

Working together
to grow libraries in
developing countries

www.elsevier.com • www.bookaid.org

Printed in Scotland
Last digit is the print number:  9  8  7  6  5  4  3  2  1

# Contents

The McRae series of textbooks has long delivered clear, concise, and accessible information about Trauma and Orthopaedic Surgery. Their unique combination of text and instructive illustrations have ensured their place as regular reference handbooks for the Orthopaedic and Emergency Medicine communities. The publication of the third edition of *McRae's Orthopaedic Trauma and Emergency Fracture Management* led an evolution of this concept through completely revised text and illustrations. The success of the Trauma edition has highlighted the unmet need for a companion textbook that covers Elective Orthopaedics and Clinical Examination.

This book is written for a wide audience that includes: orthopaedic trainees, physiotherapists, nurse practitioners, and physician assistants. It will also be of assistance to medical students encountering patients with musculoskeletal conditions for the first time. Consultant Orthopaedic Surgeons will also find it of interest to refresh their knowledge.

This book is organised into two parts. The first part covers the relevant applied clinical sciences. The second part adopts an approach based on anatomical regions. Within each region, individual conditions are described along with nonoperative and operative management. There are special boxes highlighting important clinical examination pearls and surgical techniques. This is followed by the relevant clinical history and examination techniques.

We hope that this book will continue the McRae tradition of providing an instructive textbook of unrivalled clarity, using concise text and high-quality illustrations.

PJJ

DWS

TOW

# Contributors

**Emily J Baird**

MBChB, FRCS (Tr & Orth), FFSTEd

Consultant Paediatric Orthopaedic Surgeon,
Royal Hospital for Children and Young People,
Edinburgh, Scotland

*Chapter 10—Paediatric Orthopaedics*

**Michael JC Brown**

MBChB, FRCS (Tr & Orth)

Consultant Orthopaedic Surgeon,
Queen Elizabeth University Hospital,
Glasgow, Scotland

*Chapter 3—The Knee*

**Eoghan Donnelly**

MBChB

Specialty Registrar,
West of Scotland Orthopaedic Training Scheme,
Glasgow, Scotland

*Chapter 8—Spine*

**Sanjay Gupta**

MBBS, MRCS (Glasg), MSC (Orth), MPhil, FRCS
(Tr & Orth)

Consultant Orthopaedic Surgeon and
Musculoskeletal Oncologist,
Glasgow Royal Infirmary
Glasgow, Scotland

*Chapter 9—Oncology*

**Ignatius Liew**

MBChB

Specialty Registrar,
North West Anglia Training Scheme,
Norfolk, England

*Chapter 8—Spine*

**Alistair Macey**

BA (Mod) Microbiology, MBChB, FRCS (Tr & Orth)

Specialty Registrar,
West of Scotland Orthopaedic Training Scheme,
Glasgow, Scotland

*Chapter 2—Hip*

**Jane Madeley**

MBChB FRCS (Tr & Orth)

Consultant Orthopaedic Surgeon,
Glasgow Royal Infirmary,
Glasgow, Scotland

*Chapter 4—Foot & Ankle*

**Alastair Murray**

BSc, MD, FRCS (Tr & Orth), FFST

Consultant Paediatric Orthopaedic Surgeon,
NHS Lanarkshire, Scotland;
Associate Postgraduate Dean,
NHS Education Scotland,
Edinburgh, Scotland

*Chapter 10—Paediatric Orthopaedics*

**Odhrán Murray**

MBChB, FRCS (Tr & Orth)

Consultant Orthopaedic Spinal Surgeon,
Galway Clinic,
Galway, Ireland

*Chapter 8—Spine*

**Chloe EH Scott**

MD MSc FRCSEd(Tr & Orth)

Consultant Orthopaedic Surgeon,
NHS Research Scotland Clinician,
Royal Infirmary of Edinburgh
Edinburgh, Scotland

*Chapter 3—The Knee*

## OSTEOARTHRITIS

## Background

Osteoarthritis (OA) is a degenerative condition of articular cartilage within synovial joints (which form the vast majority of large and small joints within the body). It is characterised by progressive cartilage loss and subchondral bone remodeling (osteophytes).

OA is the most common joint disease worldwide; it affects approximately 15% of those above 60 years of age and 50% of those above age 75. In the United Kingdom, the knee is most commonly affected (20%), followed by the hip (15%) and then the hands and wrists (6%). varies depending on the expected force transmission (6 mm in the patella versus 1 mm in the carpal bones), the microscopic architecture remains similar.

- **Primary (idiopathic) OA** does not yet have an identified cause and is likely to result from a combination of factors related to aging. Other known associations are; genetic predisposition, female gender and repeated/abnormal loads placed on the joint.

- **Secondary OA** can occur as a result of other pathologic processes effecting the joint, such as trauma or infection. Less frequently, conditions such as crystal arthropathy, metabolic, developmental, neurologic, hematologic and inflammatory conditions may also result in secondary degeneration.

## PATHOGENESIS

## Normal Cartilage

The articulating surfaces of bones within synovial joints are covered in smooth **hyaline cartilage**, which reduces friction and provides shock absorbance. Whilst the depth of cartilage.

Healthy hyaline cartilage is predominantly composed of water (>70%), with proteoglycans and collagen forming 25% of the structure and chondrocytes, as the only cellular component, comprising the remainder (**Fig. 1.1**). Due to its low metabolic requirements, there is no direct blood supply to the cartilage, with nutrition and perfusion occurring via diffusion from subchondral bone and the synovial fluid.

Type II collagen provides mechanical support for the joint surface, which must resist both horizontal shearing and axial loading forces. This collagen network (**Fig. 1.1**) must also anchor sufficiently to the underlying bone. Therefore the arrangement of collagen fibers changes from the superficial level, where the fibers are oriented horizontally, to the deeper levels, where they become oblique; finally, they are vertical at the cartilage-bone interface (the 'tidemark'), where the cartilage is calcified and anchored to the bone with hydroxyapatite. Superficially, there is a proportionally large water content, which decreases in deeper layers and is maintained by the hydrophilic nature of proteoglycans.

### ✅ Key Points

- Healthy cartilage is composed of approximately 70% water.
- Collagen fibers are predominantly type 2 collagen.
- Proteoglycans are noncollagenous proteins that act to retain water.
- Cartilage is anchored to the subchondral bone.

- Chondrocytes maintain the matrix and derive nutrition via the synovial fluid rather than the blood supply.

Following skeletal maturity, cartilage has low metabolic activity; however, there remains a slow rate of turnover, repair mediated by chondrocytes and the activity of matrix metalloproteinases (MMPs). Cartilage repair is mostly locally controlled, but there is more distant hormonal, cytokine, and growth factor mediation of chondrocytes including interleukins (ILs), tumor necrosis factors (TNFs), fibroblast growth factor (FGF), parathyroid hormone (PTH), and insulin-like growth factor (IGF).

Smooth joint gliding is achieved via a combination of contact ('boundary') and noncontact ('hydrodynamic') **lubrication**. Surface deformation reduces contact points between surfaces so as to increase contact area (spreading force during loading); the extrusion of a fluid film separates articulating surfaces from contact during unloaded movement (e.g., leg swing). A combination of static fluid interference and dynamic deformation of collagen with associated release of fluid occurs to minimise surface friction.

## Degeneration

Tightly bound and arranged collagen fibers, anchored to bone, with water retention and lubrication are key to the maintenance of an effective joint surface. Impairment of any of these features leads to a cascade of changes that increase friction, decrease shock absorption, and wear resistance. This leads to degradation of structure and function.

As the disease progresses, there is a net loss of cartilage however, some areas may see an increased cartilage presence as greater water content in the pathologic collagen network causes swelling and reduced structural properties. With loss of structural integrity, resistance to trauma is reduced; moreover, given the poor blood supply, lacerations above the tidemark line do not heal, and the proliferating chondrocytes do not adequately heal the resulting gaps. Synovial fluid fills the gaps, prevents contact between surfaces and reduces opposition. Injuries that extend deep to the tidemark and into subchondral bone cause damage to capillary beds and instigate a hematoma-driven inflammatory pathway. This causes the formation of fibrocartilage (type I collagen), which is less effective at lubrication and mechanical resistance.

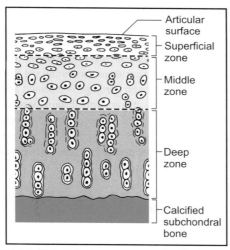

Fig. 1.1 Histological appearance of articular cartilage. The superficial zone is comprised of tangential collagen fibres and flattened chondrocytes. The middle zone contains proteoglycans and absorbs compressive forces. The deep zone contains radially orientated fibres that resist shear and compression. The chondrocytes are arranged in columns.

In normal aging there is a natural decline in number of chondrocytes and synthesis that **does not** result in OA. OA is an abnormal degenerative process. With age, the cartilage becomes stiffer but does not include the same fibrillation and structural collapse or the enzymatic lysis of cartilage proteins.

| Table 1.1 | Histologic changes in cartilage resulting from osteoarthritis |
|-----------|--------------------------------------------------------------|
| **Component** | **Changes** |
| Collagen | Initial increase in synthesis but disorganisation in orientation and size with weaker links. Late loss of collagen content. |
| Proteoglycans | Reduction due to enzymatic activity and loss into the synovium. |
| Water content | Increase initially due to penetration of the collagen network but not retained by strong hydrophilic links with proteoglycans. |
| Chondrocytes | Initial increase in number and synthetic activity. Late formation of clusters, production of matrix enzymes/cytokines, and finally apoptosis. |
| Matrix enzymes | Marked increase in activity, cleaving proteoglycans and collagen. |
| Cytokines | Produced from chondrocytes, which drive the activity of matrix metalloproteinases. |
| Subchondral bone | Cyst formation due to the penetration of synovial fluid. Inflammatory response causing sclerosis and osteophytosis. |

OA is thought to arise from an initiating insult that leads to progressive degeneration of cartilage in primary OA or an insult from a secondary cause (e.g., trauma). There is likely to be a dynamic balance between the magnitude of damage to the extracellular cartilage versus the synthetic capacity of the cartilage (which is driven by the availability of growth factors/cytokines and inhibited by matrix enzymes/hydrostatic fluid interference) (**Table 1.1**). There are also genetic risk factors for the development of OA.

The degeneration begins with **fibrillation** and loss in the superficial zone (reducing resistance to shear stress) followed by the exposure of subchondral bone (fissuring) and penetration of synovial fluid into the bone, resulting in **subchondral cysts** and a mild inflammatory response (**Fig. 1.2**). The subchondral bone responds by strengthening (**sclerosis**). At the joint margins, periosteal cells multiply and differentiate into chondrocytes, which ossify as they progressively protrude, filling gaps under the capsule and become **osteophytes**.

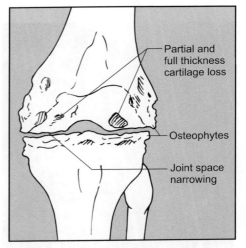

Fig. 1.2 Changes seen in OA.

Labels: Partial and full thickness cartilage loss; Osteophytes; Joint space narrowing

## FEATURES OF OSTEOARTHRITIS

### Clinical

The most commonly affected joints are the knees, hips, feet and hands; however, this is subject to variation geographically. For example, hip OA is common in the United Kingdom but very rare in India. Most patients complain of pain and stiffness in a single joint. The pain is poorly localised throughout the joint and related to activity; that is, stiffness is often worse after activity and immobility. The stiffness classically short lived (<30 minutes) in duration and can be loosened up by motion of the joint. Mechanical symptoms, such as locking or giving way, can indicate loose intra-articular fragments or muscle weakness.

Examination specific to each joint can be found in the relevant chapters of this book, but many features are common to all joints. Joint swelling can occur due to a combination of abnormal bone morphology, joint effusion and synovial hypertrophy. Joint tenderness may be present if a particularly florid secondary synovitis is present; however, this is uncommon. Pain and thickening of the joint capsule cause a reduction in the range of motion, which is worsened by inactivity of the joint due to pain and weakness and can be quantified using a goniometer. Late disease may progress to problems in alignment, such as the varus deformity commonly seen in knee OA.

## Radiologic Features

X-rays are the primary modality of investigation. The appearances (**Fig. 1.3**) include the following:

- Loss of joint space (especially on weight-bearing radiographs)

- Osteophyte formation

- Subchondral sclerosis

- Subchondral cysts

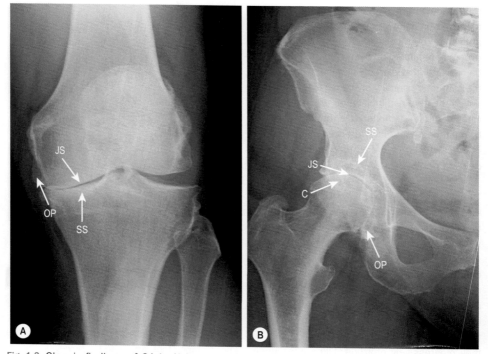

Fig. 1.3 Classic findings of OA in A) knee and B) hip (JS–loss of joint space; SS–subchondral sclerosis; C–cystic change; OP–osteophytes).

- Avascular necrosis (stages of collapse)

- Ankylosis (rare; seen in end-stage disease)

## PRINCIPLES OF MANAGEMENT

### Nonoperative

In all instances, a trial of nonoperative management shoulder be initially considered. The aims are to reduce joint reaction forces while maintaining range of motion and improving joint control. This includes

- Patient education and support

- Pharmacologic treatment with analgesia (including nonsteroidal anti-inflammatory drugs (NSAIDs))

- Physiotherapy to improve muscle balance, joint support, strengthening, and range of motion

- Weight loss for lower-limb OA

- Walking aids

### Operative

If nonoperative care is unsuccessful, surgery may be considered. The aims of surgery are to either improve joint loading by removing damaged structures and/or replace worn articular surfaces.

- *Total joint arthroplasty/replacement.* The damaged cartilage surface and supporting metaphyseal bone are removed and replaced (e.g. total hip replacement).

- *Hemiarthroplasty.* One side of the joint is replaced; it then articulates with the remaining native cartilage (e.g. shoulder hemiarthroplasty).

- *Partial joint arthroplasty.* Part of a joint is replaced with artificial bearing surfaces (e.g. unicompartmental knee replacement).

- *Resurfacing arthroplasty.* The cartilage of the joint is removed, along with minimal subchondral bone (e.g. femoral head resurfacing).

- *Excisional arthroplasty.* Removal of a part or all of the joint (e.g. trapeziectomy).

- *Interposition arthroplasty.* Tissue is placed and usually sutured in between joint surfaces to reduce bone contact and maintain space between the joints (e.g. elbow interposition arthroplasty).

- *Osteotomy.* Bones are realigned to realign the mechanical axis away from the area of disease (e.g. high tibial osteotomy).

- *Microfracture.* Small, contained 'microtrauma' to exposed subchondral bone is implemented so as to stimulate the formation of fibrocartilage to replace hyaline cartilage (e.g. microfracture of the knee).

- *Fusion (arthrodesis).* Involves removal of remaining articular cartilage and opposition of exposed ends to fuse joints together (e.g. ankle fusion).

## OSTEONECROSIS

### Background

Osteonecrosis (ON), often called avascular necrosis (AVN), is the progressive death of bone tissue in the absence of infection. It usually occurs at weight-bearing joints. Osteochondritis dissecans (OCD) specifically describes bone loss around a joint surface. The majority of bone is extracellular; thus ON begins with the death of bone cells followed by the loss of extracellular maintenance and then structural failure, most commonly involving the subchondral bone. Approximately 3000 cases per year are estimated to occur in the United Kingdom. Although there are many risks for the development of AVN, the cause remains unclear in many (40%) cases (**Table 1.2**)

## Table 1.2  Risk factors for the development of avascular necrosis/osteonecrosis

- Trauma
- Embolic/microembolic (e.g., hypercoagulable state)
- Hyperbaric (Caisson disease)
- Alcohol
- Steroids
- Bone marrow disorder (hemochromatosis)
- Endocrinological (diabetes/Cushing disease)
- Hyperlipidemia
- Hematological (sickle cell, malignancy)
- Inflammatory (systemic vasculitis, sepsis, inflammatory bowel disease)
- Marrow infiltration (Gaucher disease)
- Transplant

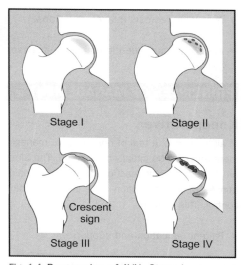

Fig. 1.4 Progression of AVN. Stage I - Ischaemia (normal x-rays). Stage II - Resorption (no collapse). Stage III - Collapse. Stage IV - Arthrosis on both sides of the joint.

## Pathophysiology

The extracellular matrix cannot remodel in response to repetitive microtrauma arising from daily activity. The disease progresses through several stages (**Fig. 1.4**). The surrounding zone becomes hyperemic, and cells die. New vessel formation occurs from the margins, creeping along the trabeculae (cancellous bone) and through the old Haversian canals (cortical bone). The final common pathologic pathway is engorgement of the microvascular circulation, coagulation and finally interosseous hypertension, resulting in cell ischemia and death. This is followed by the resorbing and remodeling of old bone into weak woven bone, which calcifies as hyperdense zones on X-ray from 6 months onward if no collapse has occurred. Remodeling of cortical Haversian canals takes longer and remains structurally weak for up to 18 months. Should remodeling not occur before structural collapse, advanced arthritic deformity and cartilage loss occur.

This race between the reestablishment of perfusion and cellular activity versus repeated subchondral decline of integrity results in collapse of the joint surface and is irrecoverable by the time that subchondral lucency (the 'crescent sign') becomes visible on X-rays (**Fig. 1.5**). The final pathway results in degeneration and collapse of the joint. Early changes are visible on magnetic resonance imaging (MRI) but not plain X-rays (**Fig. 1.6**)

## Presentation

AVN can present throughout the skeleton (**Table 1.3**). The symptoms and signs are discussed in greater details in the individual chapters of this book. In general, pain occurs initially during activity and later at rest. It is common for there to be an initial period of pain which maybe due to the acute inflammation. Over time this subsides and is replaced with the typical pain and stiffness of arthritis.

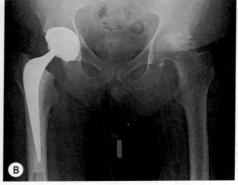

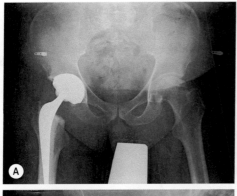

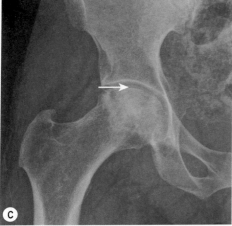

Fig. 1.5 AVN of the left hip. A) Early disease. B) Progression to femoral head collapse. C) Radiological crescent sign. A thin black line is noted in the superior subchondral area.

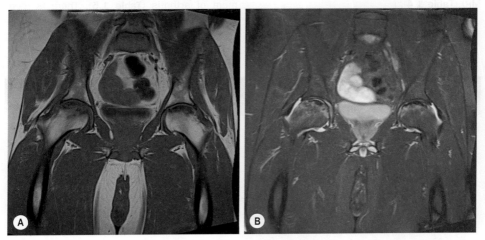

Fig. 1.6 MRI findings in AVN. A) T1 weighted image demonstrating low signal in the superior femoral head bilaterally. B) T2 weighted image showing high signal (inflammation) in the subchondral area below the low signal in the superior head.

**Table 1.3   Locations and eponymous names of types of avascular necrosis**

| Site | Eponymous Name |
|------|----------------|
| Femoral head | Legg–Calvé–Perthes disease (skeletally immature) Chandler disease (adults) |
| Medial femoral condyle | — |
| Lunate | Keinböck disease |
| Scaphoid | Preiser disease |
| Capitellum | Panner disease |
| Metatarsal head | Freiberg disease |
| Navicular | Köhler disease |
| Calcaneus | Sever disease |
| Distal pole of patella | Singding–Larsen–Johansson disease |
| Tibial tuberosity | Osgood–Schlatter disease |
| Spine | Scheuermann disease |

## Investigation

Care should be taken to identify and manage any untreated causal factors. X-rays can be normal in early disease. If there is a high index of suspicion, MRI should be obtained (100% sensitivity and 98% specificity). The Ficat classification was originally based on X-ray findings but has been modified (by Steinberg) to include MRI (**Table 1.4**).

## Treatment

The first stage of treatment should include investigation and optimisation of the underlying cause (such as statins for hyperlipidemia, alcohol cessation, diabetes control, anticoagulants).

Surgery is considered when there is progression (more often in adult patients) and development of arthritis (**Table 1.5**). There is more potential for remodeling in children and intervention is rarely required.

**Table 1.4   Modified Ficat (Steinberg) classification of osteonecrosis**

| Stage | X-ray appearance | MRI |
|-------|------------------|-----|
| 0 | Normal | Normal |
| I | Normal | Oedema |
| II | Cystic changes | Defined subchondral cysts |
| III | Crescent sign | Crescentic fluid collection |
| IV, Mild | Flattening of chondral surface | Cortical collapse and chondral destruction |
| V, Moderate | Joint space narrowing | Loss of cartilage |
| VI, Severe | Advanced degeneration | Exposed subchondral bone with gross deformity |

## Table 1.5    Management of avascular necrosis/osteonecrosis

Active alteration of disease progression (precollapse)

- Bisphosphate therapy
- Core decompression
- Trapdoor/light bulb excision of necrotic tissue
- Protected weight-bearing
- Vascularised bone graft

Symptomatic relief (postcollapse)

- Analgesia
- Physiotherapy (to optimise residual range of motion)
- Realignment osteotomy
- Arthroplasty

## INFLAMMATORY ARTHRITIS

## Introduction

Inflammatory arthritis comprises a range of conditions in which immune-mediated synovial inflammation occurs. In contrast to osteoarthritis, these conditions tend to affect younger adults of working age bringing significant limitation to quality of life and employment.

These conditions can be categorised according to their clinical, biochemical, and genetic features (**Table 1.6**).

In recent decades, modern biologic pharmacologic therapies have drastically reduced the need for surgical intervention, which had previously been inevitable.

## RHEUMATOID ARTHRITIS

## Background

Rheumatoid arthritis (RA) is the most common and often most debilitating of the inflammatory arthropathies. Females are three times as likely to be affected, typically presenting in the fourth decade of life, with relatively strong genetic links having been identified (HLA-DR4, HLA-DRB1). The trigger is not known, but macrophage and T cell activity is increased in the synovium, with enhanced fibroblast activity and mast cell activation. These produce a range of inflammatory mediators (IL-1, 2, 4, 6, 8, TNF-α, interferon), resulting in the formation of abnormal lymphoid tissue and widespread inflammation of synovial tissue (**Fig. 1.7**). The synovium becomes hypertrophic and hypervascular, with pannus formation as well as the infiltration of macrophages, lymphocytes and plasma cells (**Fig. 1.8**). This drives ulceration of hyaline cartilage and activation of osteoclasts, causing reduced bone mineral density, which is seen radiologically as periarticular osteoporosis. Treatment is multifaceted and co-ordinated by rheumatologists as part of a multidisciplinary approach (**Table 1.7**)

## Symptoms and Signs

The classic inflammatory arthritic symptoms of stiffness and pain are found in multiple small joints bilaterally, which persist for more than 1 hour after rest (sleeping, sitting, etc.). A variety of patterns can be described, ranging from transient or 'palindromic', remitting (present for several years and then ceasing), to slowly or rapidly progressive. Deformity arises as a result of intraarticular damage, tendon sheath inflammation, attrition rupture of ligaments and compression of nerves from s ynovial hypertrophy. Disuse and inflammation drive osteopenia and muscle wasting, giving rise to capsular fibrosis. Systemic extraarticular features of RA usually result from

**Table 1.6   Inflammatory arthritis**

| Condition | Epidemiology | Commonly affected joints | Genetic association[a] |
|---|---|---|---|
| Rheumatoid arthritis | 0.5%–1% Worldwide F > M 30–50 | Hands, wrists, elbows, feet, ankles | HLA-DR4 and HLA-DRB1 |
| Crystal arthropathy | 4% M: F 10: 1 | Toes, interphalangeal joints (gout), knee, wrist (pseudogout) | HPRT1 (Lesch–Nyhan syndrome) |
| Ankylosing arthritis | 0.5%–1% M: 1 2.5: 1 | Spine, sacroiliac joints | HLA-B27 |
| Reactive arthritis | | Lower limb joints | HLA-B27 |
| Enteropathic arthritis | | Lower limb joints, spine | HLA-B27 |
| Psoriatic arthritis | 0.1%–0.2% (6%–40% of patients with psoriasis) M = F 30–40 years | Distal interphalangeal joints ('pencil-in-cup' erosions); 'ray' involvement (multiple joints in same phalanx); associated with skin plaques | HLA-B27 and HLA-DR7 |
| Juvenile arthritis | M > F (oligoarticular) M < F (polyarticular) M = F (systemic) | Large joints (oligoarticular), small joints (polyarticular) | HLA-B27 (oligoarticular), HLA-DR4 and HLA-DR5 (polyarticular), HLA-DR8 (poly- and pauciarticular), HLA-DW4 (polyarticular) |

[a]The major histocompatibility complex (MHC) comprises a group of genes found on chromosome 6 that code for cell-surface proteins. These MHC classes can help to differentiate among inflammatory arthropathies.

vasculitis (**Table 1.8**). They are more common with rheumatoid factor (RF)–positive disease and form part of the diagnostic process. Diagnosis is made based on the combination of symptoms (**Fig. 1.9**), signs, laboratory investigations, and X-ray findings (**Table 1.9**).

## Imaging

Plain X-rays are used for both diagnosis and the quantification of deformity. They can also guide the planning of surgical interventions. The classic X-ray appearances of rheumatoid arthritis (**Fig. 1.9**):

- Loss of joint space

- Periarticular erosions

- Soft tissue swelling

In some cases, particularly in the era of modern biologic treatments, many of the classic radiologic features may not be present. In some cases, patterns of radiologic disease more in keeping with OA can be observed. In these patients, the history and laboratory investigations will be helpful in diagnosis.

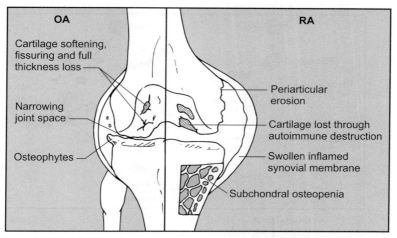

OA

Cartilage softening, fissuring and full thickness loss

Narrowing joint space

Osteophytes

RA

Periarticular erosion

Cartilage lost through autoimmune destruction

Swollen inflamed synovial membrane

Subchondral osteopenia

Fig. 1.7 Comparison of changes in rheumatoid arthritis versus osteoarthritis.

## SPONDYLOARTHROPATHY

## Introduction

Seronegative spondyloarthritis, or spondyloarthropathy comprises a family of autoimmune diseases that target ligamentous and tendinous insertions (entheses) rather than the entire joint; they are summarised in **Table 1.10**. The term *spondyloarthropathy* (meaning 'spine joint problem') is perhaps a misnomer, as it is used to refer to a range of autoimmune syndromes associated with rheumatoid arthritis that do not necessarily always affect the spine. However, when present, these syndromes can result in uveitis, sacroiliitis, inflammatory back pain and skin rash. They have variable associations with the HLA-B27 MHC genotype.

## Ankylosing Spondylitis

**Ankylosing spondylitis (AS)** is the most common spondyloarthropathy; it is characterised by sacroiliitis and enthesitis (inflammation of tendinous and ligamentous insertions) of the spine, resulting in intervertebral fusion (ankylosis). There are three types of pathologic changes to the entheses: inflammation, erosions and syndesmophytes mediated by TNF, cathepsin/MMP1 and Bone Morphogenetic Proteins (BMPs). As has a strong

genetic association (HLA-B27) and typically effects younger males with characteristic sacroiliitis. Mean delay to diagnosis is 5 to 7 years due to the symptomatic overlap with mechanical back pain. Symptoms of back pain, improved by exercise but not relieved by rest, and inflammatory stiffness raise suspicion of AS. Some 75% of patients with AS respond well to NSAIDs. as opposed to 15% with mechanical back pain. Diagnosis requires evidence of sacroiliitis on X-ray or MRI and clinical features such as more than 3 months of pain/stiffness and limited relief with rest. The mainstay of treatment is with NSAIDs and anti-TNF in patients with progressive disease. In patients with a fused spine, traumatic fractures have a greater severity owing to the lack of flexibility and increased length of lever arms. Clinicians should have a very low threshold for computed tomography (CT) evaluation.

Ankylosing spondylitis should be distinguished from **diffuse idiopathic skeletal hyperostosis (DISH)**, which is a much more common nonrheumatologic condition (6%–12%) in which nonmarginal syndesmophytes (osteophytes beginning 2–3 mm from the vertebral baseplate) fuse four consecutive vertebrae (over three intervertebral discs). It predominantly

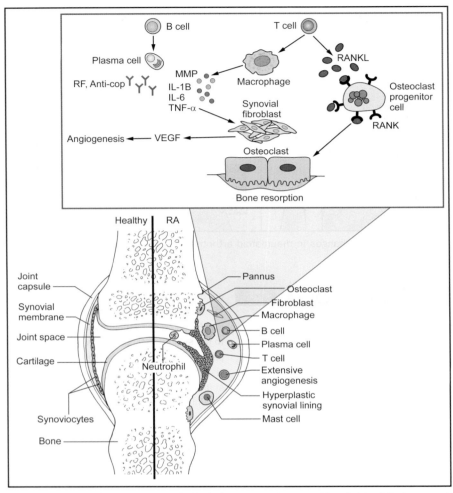

Fig. 1.8 Molecular pathways and histological changes in rheumatoid arthritis. *RF*, rheumatoid factor; *VEGF*, vascular endothelial growth factor; *IL*, interleukin; *RANK*, receptor activator of nuclear factor kappa beta; *RANKL*, receptor activator of nuclear factor kappa beta ligand; *RA*, rheumatoid arthritis; *TNFalpha*, tumour necrosis factor alpha.

occurs in those above 50 years of age and is associated with diabetes; the intervertebral disc space is maintained and importantly spares the facet and sacroiliac joints.

## Psoriatic Arthritis

Psoriatic arthritis (PsA), an inflammatory arthritis, is associated with psoriasis (which may be asymptomatic–e.g., scalp psoriasis). Although it is pathogenetically different from rheumatoid arthritis, rheumatoid factor may be present in up to 13% of patients with psoriatic arthritis, and PsA produces similar synovial histologic features.

Typically, the distribution of inflammation is in the distal interphalangeal joints; however, it can also follow a 'ray' type distribution affecting multiple joints in individual digits, called dactylitis, and occasionally affecting the spine (15%).

**Table 1.7  Therapeutic strategies for inflammatory arthritis**

| Treatment type | Description | Examples |
|---|---|---|
| Nonpharmacologic treatments | Physical and manual interventions to improve joint mechanics/function and to relieve symptoms | • Physical therapy<br>• Massage<br>• Occupational therapy<br>• Smoking cessation<br>• Weight loss |
| Symptomatic relief | Drugs that improve symptoms but do not necessarily alter disease progression | • Nonsteroidal anti-inflammatory drugs<br>• Oral steroids<br>• Corticosteroid injection |
| Oral small molecules | So called because they enter cells owing to their molecular size (<900 Da [Daltons]); many of these are used in more traditional therapies | • Sulfasalazine<br>• Methotrexate<br>• Cyclosporine |
| Biological agents | Large-molecule 'targeted' therapies engineered to modulate biologic processes | • TNF-alpha receptor blockers (e.g., etanercept)<br>• Monoclonal antibiody to TNF-alpha (e.g., infliximab)<br>• Interleukin inhibitor (e.g., anakira)<br>• JAK (Janus kinase) inhibitor (e.g., tofacitinib) |

Clinically the patient will likely have a history of psoriasis (however, in 10%–15%, arthritis presents first). Whilst the joints involved may vary, 80% to 90% will have nail pitting and onycholysis. There are no specific blood markers for PsA, but the presence of psoriasis, nail changes, raised C-reactive Protein (CRP)/Erythrocyte Sendimentation Rate (ESR), and absence of RA criteria (anti-cyclic citrullinated peptide [CCP] and RF) is sufficient for diagnosis.

Radiographically, joints may be fused in a typical 'pencil-in-cup' fashion, have periosteal reaction, and show enthesitis (inflammation at tendon insertions). Progression is typically less aggressive than that of RA, although approximately half of patients will have five or more joints involved by 10 years, and 5% develop rapidly progressing arthritis mutilans.

## Reactive Arthritis

Reactive Arthritis (ReA), involving acute joint inflammation, can be attributed to a recent (or impending) infection, usually of the gastrointestinal tract (*Salmonella enteriditis, Campylobacter jejuni, Clostridium difficile*) or urinary tract (*Chlamydia trachomatis, Neisseria gonorrhoea*). Overall, ReA is relatively rare (0.02%); however, it is a relatively common complication of urinary tract infection (2%–4%) or gastroenteritis (≤15%). It has a weak association with HLA-B27, and is thought to occur when systemically circulating bacteria prompt a T cell response, causing the attack of self-antigens in the synovium, urinary endothelium and cojunctivae.

**Reitier Syndrome** is a particular form of reactive arthritis consisting of joint pain, conjunctivitis/uveitis and urethritis.

**Table 1.8    Extraarticular manifestations of rheumatoid arthritis**

**Tissue Type**

| | |
|---|---|
| Respiratory | Pleural plaques (50%) |
| | Effusion |
| | Interstitial lung disease and fibrosis |
| | Cavitation |
| | Pneumoconiosis (Caplan disease) |
| Cardiac/vascular | Pericarditis (50%) |
| | Atherosclerosis (including cerebrovascular) |
| | Myocardial infarction |
| | Myocarditis |
| | Endocarditis |
| | Valvular dysfunction |
| | Vasculitis |
| | Raynaud syndrome |
| Soft tissue | Rheumatoid nodules (20%) |
| | Splinter hemorrhages |
| | Leg ulcers |
| | Bursitis (e.g., olecranon) |
| | Trigger finger |
| Nervous | Sensorimotor peripheral neuropathy |
| | Mononeuritis multiplex |
| | Compression neuropathy (carpal tunnel syndrome) |
| | Glove-and-stocking sensory loss |
| Renal | Mesangial glomerulonephritis |
| | Amyloidosis |
| | Nephrotic syndrome |
| Hematologic | Anemia |
| | Neutropenia |
| | Thrombocytopenia |
| | Thrombocytosis |
| | Eosinophilia |
| | Malignancy |
| | Lymphadenopathy |
| | Felty syndrome |
| Ocular | Keratoconjunctivitis (10%) |
| | Episcleritis |
| | Scleritis ± ulceration |
| Gastrointestinal | Mesenteric vasculitis and infarction |
| Other | Xerostomia (dry mouth) |
| | Sjögren syndrome |

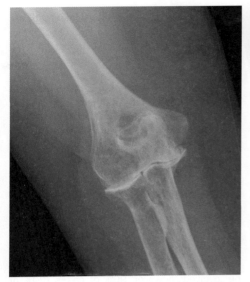

Fig. 1.9 X-ray findings of rheumatoid arthritis: loss of joint space, periarticular osteopaenia, periarticular erosions.

Nonspecific blood markers (ESR and CRP) may be raised, and joint aspiration to exclude other causes of inflammation (e.g., sepsis, crystal arthropathy) will show no specific white cells. Histologically progressive arthritis or pannus formation is very rare; symptoms are usually self-limited to several days/weeks, and intervention following treatment of the initial infection is seldom required.

## Enteropathic Arthritis

Similar to psoriatic arthritis, patients with autoimmune inflammatory bowel disease (Crohn's disease and ulcerative colitis) can have immune complex deposition in the synovial joint lining, typically in peripheral joints of the lower limb. This condition can affect the entire spine as well. Approximately 20% of patients who have

| Table 1.9 American College of Rheumatology classification of rheumatoid arthritis | |
|---|---|
| **Criteria** | **Score** |
| **Joint involvement** | |
| 1 large joint | 0 |
| 2–10 large joints | 1 |
| 1–3 small joints | 2 |
| 4–10 small joints | 3 |
| >10 joints (at least 1 small joint) | 5 |
| **Serology** | |
| –ve RF and –ve ACPA | 0 |
| low + ve RF or low + ve ACPA | 2 |
| high + ve RF or high + ve ACPA | 3 |
| **Acute-phase reactants** | |
| normal CRP and normal ESR | 0 |
| abnormal CRP or abnormal ESR | 1 |
| **Duration of symptoms[a]** | |
| <6 weeks | 0 |
| ≥6 weeks | 1 |

[a]A score of 6 or more is diagnostic.

Source: Jonathan Kay, Katherine S. Upchurch, ACR/ EULAR 2010 rheumatoid arthritis classification criteria, *Rheumatology*, 2012;51(6):vi5–vi9.

*ACPA*, anticitrullinated protein antibody; *CRP*, c-reactive protein; *ESR*, erythrocyte sedimentation rate; *RF*, rheumatoid factor

| Table 1.10 Seronegative spondyloarthropathies | |
|---|---|
| **Spondyloarthropathy** | **Characteristics** |
| Ankylosing spondylitis (AS) | Strong genetic association; back pain and stiffness with sacroiliitis on X-ray |
| Psoriatic arthritis (PsA) | Psoriasis present, distal interphalangeal/finger arthritis |
| Reactive arthritis (ReA) | Recent urinary or gastrointestinal infection; involvement of joints, eyes and urinary tract |
| Enteropathic arthritis (EnA) | Known inflammatory bowel disease; intermittent joint pain affecting the lower limbs joints and spine |

irritable bowel disease (IBD) develop entero-pathic arthritis (EnA), which has no predisposition for gender and is associated with smoking. Only 20% of patients with EnA have the HLA-B27 gene; in those who do, the inflammation can be more pronounced, with spinal involvement and persistent bowel symptoms despite adequate IBD disease management.

No specific test for EnA exists, although the diagnosis may be made in the presence of intermitted joint inflammation on a history of IBD, in particular with sacroiliitis and raised inflammatory markers.

## Juvenile Idiopathic Arthritis

Juvenile Idiopathic Arthritis (JIA) is a persistent inflammatory condition of joints in children under 16 years of age. The pathophysiology is similar to that of RA; however, RF is absent, and the joint erosions/deformities are less severe. Small joints of the hands are affected and, less frequently, knees and ankles.

An initial flu-like illness may occur, with persistent pain/swelling of joints and classic morning stiffness over 30 minutes. Three distinct patterns of JIA are described:

- **Oligoarticular** (50%) in up to four joints; it is asymmetric, affecting larger joints (knees ankles, elbows).

- **Polyarticular** (40%) in five or more smaller joints (hands, neck, temporomandibular joint); half progress into adulthood, causing significant disability.

- **Systemic** (10%) an intermittent condition with high fever, rash, and the inflammation of multiple joints. More severe extraarticular features are also seen (hepatosplenomegaly, tenosynovitis, hepatitis, lymphadenopathy). This condition, also described as adolescent-onset Still disease, can have a very rapid onset and is associated with mortality rates of 5% to 20%.

Any form of JIA can have extraarticular features, with uveitis being the most common and cardiomyopathy having the greatest impact on long-term function.

Joint disease can be treated with NSAIDS and intraarticular steroids, methotrexate and/or biologic agents. Unlike RA, which naturally 'burns out,' JIA can enter remission in 7% within 1.5 years to almost 50% by 10 years following the initial diagnosis.

## Relapsing Polychondritis

Relapsing Polychondritis (RP) is a rare HLA-DR4-linked autoimmune inflammatory condition with an affinity for proteoglycan-rich tissues such as cartilage. Any tissue containing cartilage can be involved; however, 90% of cases (20% at presentation) develop pathognomonic intermitted auricular inflammation, with repetitive flares culminating in the so-called "cauliflower ear". Synovial joint inflammation and costochondritis are second most common, with over 80% of individuals developing sporadic pain. Histology shows plasma cells, interleukins and autoantibodies targeted against type II, IX and XI collagen alongside cartilage matrix protein matrilin-1. The associated polyarthritis is non-erosive. Blood markers are nonspecific, and clinical diagnosis is made using the Michet criteria (scored on the inflammation of cartilage of the ears, nose, larynx, eyes and joints along with ear dysfunction). Patients with type II collagen antibodies can have titers used to monitor disease progress, but these are present in less than 50% of cases. Owing to the rarity of the disease, there is no high-quality evidence for treatment. A combination of NSAIDs, colchicine, immunosuppressants, and TNF inhibitors can be employed.

### Crystal Arthropathy

The joint inflammation of crystal arthropathy occurs as a result of the deposition of sodium urate (gout) or calcium pyrophosphate (pseudogout) crystals in joints.

Gout is a disorder of hyperuricaemia culminating in the deposition of monosodium urate monohydrate crystals predominately in joint fluid, causing flares of acute joint inflammation and pain. Deposition also occurs in other tissues throughout the body as 'gouty tophi' in kidneys, bone, bursae and cutaneous/auricular tissue. The pathogenesis involves a number of factors culminating an imbalance of uric acid breakdown and hyperuricemia as a common final feature. Uric acid is formed by the metabolism of purine; uricemia results from an imbalance of excessive synthesis (increased purine synthesis or turnover) versus excretion via intestine and kidneys (**Fig. 1.10**).

Diagnostically, elevated serum urate levels can be used; however, this measure is unreliable, particularly in acute flares, where it may be normal or reduced. Serum urea and creatinine may also be raised.

Joint aspiration and inspection using a compensated polarised light microscope is the most effective diagnostic tool, which can serve to demonstrate **negatively birefringent, needle-shaped monosodium urate crystals**.

Treatment strategies involve cessation of all nonessential contributing medication (e.g., diuretics) and the minimisation or treatment of comorbidities (hypertension, obesity, diabetes, etc.). Treatment with NSAIDs for acute flares is effective; however, repeated doses, particularly in the elderly, can lead to the progression of disease by impairing renal function. Prophylactic pharmacologic management is indicated for patients with two or more attacks per year, tophi, renal failure or urolithiasis. Short courses of colchicine can be prescribed for those who do not tolerate NSAIDs. Allopurinol or febuxostat (xanthine oxidase inhibitors) can be used beyond a month after an attack to reduce serum urate.

**Calcium pyrophosphate deposition (CPPD),** or **pseudogout**, is the deposition of calcium pyrophosphate in cartilage, which may be seen as **positively birefringent rhomboid pyrophosphate crystals** on microscopy. The shedding of these crystals into the synovial space induces an inflammatory response causing joint pain and pyrexia. No serum biomarker has been identified; a raised white blood cell count may be detected.

**Chondrocalcinosis** describes calcium deposition seen on X-rays and is pathognomonic particularly with calcification of the menisci. Joint aspiration may show rhomboid, weakly positive birefringent crystals on polarised light microscopy.

## TENDINOPATHY

## Background

Tendons are fibrous structures arising directly from muscle and inserting into the apophyses of bone; they act to transmit the contractile

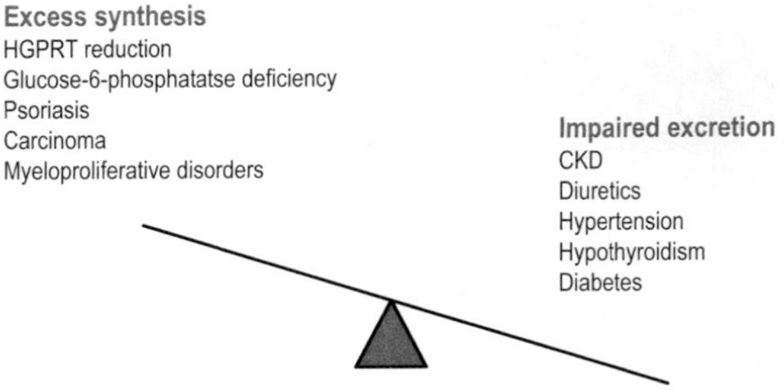

Excess synthesis
HGPRT reduction
Glucose-6-phosphatatse deficiency
Psoriasis
Carcinoma
Myeloproliferative disorders

Impaired excretion
CKD
Diuretics
Hypertension
Hypothyroidism
Diabetes

Fig. 1.10 Causes of hyperuricaemia. *HGPRT,* hypoxanthine-guanine phosphoribosyltransferase; *CKD,* chronic kidney disease.

force of muscles into bone movement at joints—that is, they connect muscle to bone. They are similar in structure to ligaments, which connect bone to bone. However, tendons undergo more cyclic loading and thus have a more organised histologic appearance and lower elasticity. The composition of tendons is predominantly extracellular, with dense and regularly arranged **type 1 collagen** in parallel to the axis of motion, with individual fibrils held together with proteoglycans and a small amount of elastin to aid with recoil. **Tenocytes** are a type of fibroblast; they are the native cells found within the tendon substance, residing in gaps between fibroblasts. They are very mechanically sensitive and are responsible for the synthesis of procollagens in response to mechanical load.

No nerve cells exist within the deep tendon substance, but they are present in the para-tenon and the musculotendinous junction, where they also provide proprioceptive feedback. The blood supply to tendons is relatively low, given tendons' low cell count and metabolic rate. For most tendons, blood is supplied via longitudinal vessels arising from the apophyses and myoten-dinous junctions. Some tendons (such as finger flexors) have synovial sheaths to promote gliding, which isolates them from surrounding blood vessels. These sheathed tendons derive their blood supply from the nearby specific vessels (vincula) and synovial diffusion rather than from intrinsic vessels.

Tendons concentrate the large forces gener-ated by muscles onto relatively small foot-prints, at which point they need to transmit force to stiff mineralised bone. This insertional tissue (enthesis) consists of four distinct zones (**Fig. 1.11**):

1. Tendon—collagenous tendon tissue

2. Uncalcified fibrocartilage with larger, less parallel collagen bundles

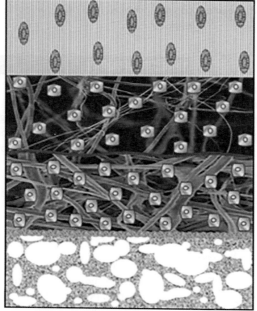

*Tendon*

Aligned collagen fibrils

*Uncalcified fibrocartilage*

Larger, less parallel collagen bundles

*Calcified fibrocartilage*

Mineralised tissue

*Bone*

Interdigitation at interface

Fig. 1.11 Tendon insertion on bone.

3. Calcified fibrocartilage

4. Bone

The stiffness gradually increases from zones 1 to 4, distributing the stress and minimizing focal areas that would be liable to rupture.

Owing to the arrangement of type 1 collagen, tendons have considerable stiffness in traction (i.e., they are resistant to lengthening), with an increase in length of less than 5% under maximal load. However, muscle reflexes also work to relax and shield tendons from exerting loads more than one-third of the ultimate tendon failure strength.

Tendons reach maximal collagen density (and thus strength) in the third decade of life, after which they tend to degrade. Other factors associated with a more rapid deterioration in strength include obesity, hypertension, steroid use, hyperlipidemia, and the individual patient's activity profile. A tendon's loading behavior can be visualised in a stress–strain curve, where stress can be considered as the force applied (i.e., tension) and strain as the relative change in length (**Fig. 1.12**).

Tendons, like most musculoskeletal tissue, exhibit **viscoelastic behavior,** which is a complex interaction of forces within the tissue resulting in a mixture of fluid and solid properties (**Table 1.11**).

## Response to Abnormal Loading

As tendons undergo cyclic loading, they are subject to macro- and microtrauma and have intrinsic/extrinsic mechanisms for repair. This typically occurs over three phases:

1. **Inflammatory (days 1–7).** A cascade of local inflammatory mediators is recruited, polymorphs remove debris and fibroblasts begin to migrate.

2. **Proliferation (days 5–21).** Local fibroblasts migrate, and there is an increased synthesis

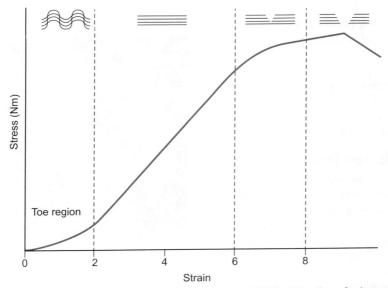

Fig. 1.12 Stress–strain relationship of tendons. There is initial straightening of crimped fibres in a nonlinear 'toe-region'. This is followed by a linear elastic relation, followed by microscopic failure of some fibres and then total failure of the tendon.

**Table 1.11   Viscoelastic properties of tendons**

| Property | Definition | Relevance to tendons |
| --- | --- | --- |
| Creep | Increasing deformation of a material under constant load | When placed under prolonged tension, tendons will lengthen slowly. |
| Stress relaxation | Reduction of internal forces following deformation | Stretching a tendon for a long time and then removing the force will leave the tendon elongated. |
| Hysteresis | Difference in response to force during loading and unloading | Repetitive loading and unloading of a tendon will give different responses (due to internal 'friction'). This property reduces after several repetitions (e.g., 'cycling' a cruciate ligament graft during reconstruction). |
| Rate-dependent behavior | Response of a material to a force as dependent on the rate of force applied | Rapid loading of tendons (and ligaments) results in increased stiffness, whereas slower loading will facilitate more lengthening for the same force. |

of procollagen. Furthermore, angiogenesis occurs alongside the extrinsic recruitment of fibroblasts, resulting in the rapid laying down of relatively weak type III collagen. It is during this phase that the tendons are weakest.

3. **Remodeling (weeks 2–6).** Weak type 3 collagen is remodeled into stiffer, parallel type 1 collagen.

4. **Maturation.** Finally, over the subsequent months to years, the collagen matures, cross links, and aligns along the axis of mechanical load.

## Chronic Tendinopathy

Chronic tendinopathy, occasionally referred to as overuse tendinopathy, is a pathologic failure of tendon healing following injury and is characterised by localised pain and weakness (**Fig. 1.13**). It is a degeneration in the absence of true inflammation. As a pathologic process, tendinopathies are poorly understood, but persistent degeneration and apoptosis despite a lack of ongoing stimulus for inflammation are histopathologic hallmarks. Previously chronic

tendinopathy was thought to be related to inadequate rest; however, more a complex inflammatory malfunction is known to be a core feature. Degeneration persists within the tendon substance, with tenocyte cell death and failure

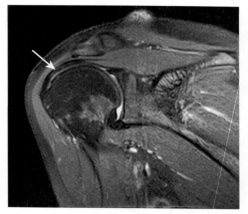

Fig. 1.13 MRI of shoulder with supraspinatus tendinopathy. High signal (white band), but no tear, is evident in the supraspinatus in the T2 weighted coronal image. Normal tendon should appear homogeneously black (low signal).

to convert type III collagen to type I; thus the tendon remains structurally weak. This process gives rise to pain, and the tendon may eventually progress to full failure and tearing.

## Calcific Tendinopathy

In some cases, calcium deposits can be found in chronically tendinopathic tissues typically in the supraspinatus tendons of women 40 to 60 years of age. Metabolic disorders such as diabetes and thyroid disease are often implicated. The exact mechanism is unknown, however, metaplasia of tenocytes into chondrocytes and subsequent ossification have been observed. Although it is most commonly observed in the shoulder, calcific tendinopathy can be found in tendons throughout the body.

## Principles of Management

Tendinopathy, as opposed to acute tendinitis, is refractory to simple NSAIDs and corticosteroid injections. Treatment of this multifactorial condition relies on several modalities:

- **Rest** aims to allow dysfunctional inflammation to cease by removing the ongoing mechanical loading that has led to failure.

- **Eccentric and isometric exercises** may provide mechanical cues to aid the conversion of type II to type I collagen along with realignment of fibers in a parallel manner during healing. The aim is to load the tendon at a level below that which caused the initial damage.

- **Transdermal glyceryl trinitrate** can aid local blood flow and collagen synthesis.

- **Platelet-rich plasma,** autologous blood injections and ultrasonic therapy have failed to demonstrate consistent evidence for their use in tendinopathy.

- **Surgery** may be offered in specific cases where there treatment with other modalities has failed. Surgical management includes decompression, debridement and the stimulation of a healing response.

## INVESTIGATION TECHNIQUES IN ORTHOPAEDICS

History and examination are the cornerstones of clinical practice. Once several differential diagnoses have been identified, investigation is used to confirm or refute the diagnostic hypothesis. Investigations are also used to determine the severity of the disease process and to guide treatment. Investigations should be well targeted to answer specific diagnostic and treatment questions. If they are used in a nondiscriminatory manner, excess cost will be incurred, along with the introduction of diagnostic uncertainty. This section outlines commonly available investigations available to orthopedic surgeons.

## Imaging

Imaging is one of the most important modalities of investigation available. Bones and soft tissues can be visualised by the detection of X-rays (e.g. radiographs and CT), radiofrequency waves (e.g. MRI), sound waves (ultrasound scanning) and other ionizing radiation (e.g. isotopic bone scans).

## X-rays

X-ray technology has been in use for over a century, having been discovered by Wilhelm Röntgen in November 1895; since then, predictions regarding the natural history of injuries and disease have been inferred from the visualisation of bone and soft tissue. X-rays are absorbed by dense tissues, particularly mineralised bone. As an imaging modality, X-ray films (or plain radiographs) can be obtained quickly, are low in cost and are relatively easy to interpret. Typically orthogonal views (at 90-degree angles to one another) are obtained (e.g., anteroposterior and lateral). However, oblique views can also be sought, most frequently in the hands and feet. X-rays can also be obtained in the operating theater, during procedures, to check on bone position and implant positioning. In this case, the machine is usually operated by the surgeons themselves, after receiving additional training in radiation safety.

- Plain radiographs are created by X-rays passing from a source, through the body. Those that are not absorbed by bone or soft tissue strike photographic film that is then developed. More recently, the X-rays are detected by a digital receiver plate and stored directly in a computer system (**Fig. 1.14A**).

- Fluoroscopy is a method of generating an amplified live X-ray image onto a screen by converting X-rays to photons, which are ultimately projected by a video camera (**Fig. 1.14B**). Thus the fluoroscope is also known as an image intensifier. It allows the use of relatively low doses of X-rays, which can then be further reduced by closing the aperture to focus on a smaller area.

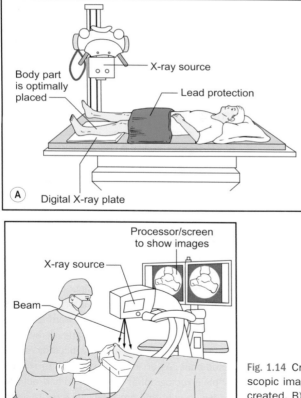

Fig. 1.14 Creation of radiographs and fluoroscopic images. A) Plain radiograph being created. B) 'Mini C-arm' fluoroscopy being used during a procedure by a surgeon. A highly focused beam results in less scatter and low radiation exposure to the patient and other team members.

## Computed Tomography

Developed by Sir Godfrey Hounsfield in 1967, CT enables a series of multidirectional X-rays to be computationally combined. This overcomes the two-dimensional limitation of plain radiography and can provide measured information on density (expressed in Hounsfield units). The X-ray source is collimated (narrow and parallel) and projects X-rays through the patient to a detection plate, which moves through a series of directions to obtain cross-sectional images at predetermined intervals (**Fig. 1.15**).

Modern CT scanners have a series of tubes and corresponding detectors, which means that multiple slices can be obtained simultaneously (commonly 128, but 256- and 320-slice systems exist) while the patient moves through the imaging segment, making scans quicker and subject to less motion artifact.

CT has a very high resolution for dense tissue (such as bone); it can delineate between small fragments, and its views can be reconstructed into three-dimensional surface images. Soft tissue (such as cartilage or blood vessels) is less effectively differentiated; this can in part be overcome by the use of contrast (administered intravenously, intraarticularly, intrathecally and so on).

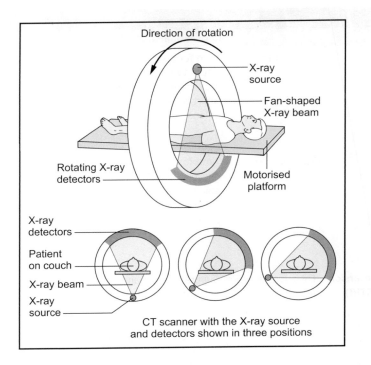

Fig. 1.15 CT scanner: The patient lies in the centre of the scanner. An X-ray source is directly across from a detector. This source and detector spin as the patient is passed through. Plain X-rays are obtained from multiple angles and are then computationally combined to produce an 'axial slice'. These slices can then be reformatted in multiple planes and rendered into 3 dimensional models.

# Magnetic Resonance Imaging

MRI uses a large magnet that lines up hydrogen atoms (protons in water molecules in the body) parallel to the magnetic axis. It is therefore useful to image tissues with higher water content, such as ligaments, tendons, and other soft tissue. It is important in the local staging of tumors and in surgical planning. After the hydrogen atoms line up with the magnetic field, radiofrequency (RF) pulses are released from several angles, which causes the atoms to 'wobble' and synchronise their spin. Protons in different tissues take different times to return to their parallel state (T1) or desynchronise their spin (T2). These perturbations are detected and then processed by computers. Different imaging sequences can be used in the course of examining different anatomic structures and pathology (**Table 1.12**). Depending on the tissue and sequence, tissue is visualised as either white (having a high signal) or dark (having a low signal) (**Table 1.13**).

# Ultrasound Scanning

Ultrasound scanning (US) is a safe, inexpensive, noninvasive imaging technology–has been used since 1940. It was first applied clinically by Glasgow obstetricians in 1958. Ultrasound scanning emits sound waves of 1 to 18 MHz (above the audible range of humans) using a linear array of piezoelectric transducers; then the same transducers serve to detect the reflected sound waves. Tissues that reflect more sound waves appear brighter. The Doppler effect

| Table 1.12 | Magnetic resonance sequences | | |
|---|---|---|---|
| **Sequence** | | **Description** | **Clinical Use** |
| **Spin echo** | T1 weighted | Time for protons to return to parallel state with the magnetic axis. Short time between RF pulses. | **Clear definition of anatomy,** particularly those areas that are separated by fat. Fat appears bright; fluid and other tissues are relatively dark. |
| | T2 weighted | Time for desynchronisation of spinning Longer time between RF pulses | **Clear definition of pathology** as fluid and fat appears bright, demonstrating edema. Fluid is bright and fat less so. The remaining bone/muscle/cartilage is relatively dark. |
| **Short-tau inversion recovery (STIR)** | Fat suppression sequence | Suppresses fat and helps delineated edema from tissues that have high proportions of fat. Fluid appears bright in contrast to the remaining dark tissues. | |
| **Metal artifact reduction sequence (MARS)** | Reduces signal from metal | Used for imaging around metal implants. | |

**Table 1.13   Tissue appearances on magnetic resonance imaging: increased signal is represented visually by tissue being 'whiter' and decreased signal by tissue being 'darker'**

| Tissue | T1 | T2 | STIR |
|---|---|---|---|
| Cortical bone/ligament/tendon | ↓ | ↓ | ↓ |
| Muscle/spinal cord/cancellous bone | - | - | - |
| Fluid/cartilage/synovium/intravertebral disc | ↓ | ↑ | ↑ |
| Fat | ↑ | ↑ | ↓ |

is a physical phenomenon where the frequency of a wave changes when it bounces off a moving object. Doppler sequences demonstrating flow can be obtained (e.g., in blood vessels).

US can image bone surface, muscle, soft tissue and fluid-filled spaces very well, and it provides a dynamic demonstration of pathology (e.g., in a rotator cuff) (**Fig. 1.16**).

US is user-dependent, requiring skill and training to obtain diagnostic images and make

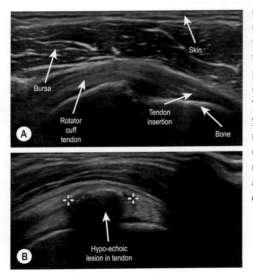

Fig. 1.16 Ultrasound image of shoulder. A) Longitudinal image at rotator cuff insertion. B) Longitudinal image demonstrating hypo-echoic lesion consistent with calcific deposit.

accurate interpretations. Scanning is usually effective only for superficial structures, and artifact is often limited by acoustically dense bone. US can also be limited by body habitus in patients with more adipose tissue.

## Bone Densitometry

Bone mineral density (BMD) can be estimated subjectively on plain X-rays or by following a history of low-energy fracture. For a diagnosis of osteoporosis, however, BMD can be measured quantitatively by CT, ultrasound scanning, or most commonly dual-energy X-ray absorptiometry (DEXA) (**Fig. 1.17**). This device emits two X-rays of different intensities, and the relative absorbance is used to infer density at that point. Typically two anatomic sites are measured: the lumbar spine and proximal femur. A **T score** compares the patient's results with a young population of the same gender and ethnicity and diagnoses osteoporosis and/or osteopenia. A **Z score** compares the patient's results with those of a population of the same age and gender to gives insight into secondary causes for low BMD.

● Osteoporosis is defined by a T score less than 2.5 standard deviations below the matched average.

● Osteopenia is defined as a T score between 1 and 2.5 standard deviations below the matched average.

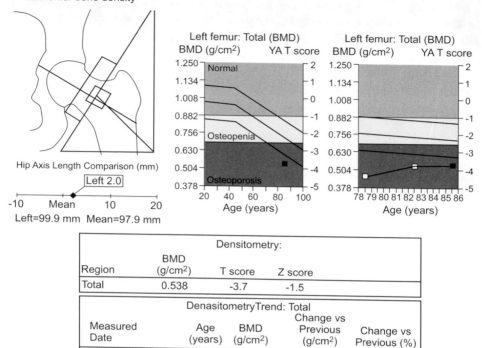

Left femur bone density

Left femur: Total (BMD)

Hip Axis Length Comparison (mm)

Left 2.0

-10    Mean    10    20

Left=99.9 mm  Mean=97.9 mm

| Densitometry: | | | |
|---|---|---|---|
| Region | BMD (g/cm²) | T score | Z score |
| Total | 0.538 | -3.7 | -1.5 |

| Denasitometry Trend: Total | | | | |
|---|---|---|---|---|
| Measured Date | Age (years) | BMD (g/cm²) | Change vs Previous (g/cm²) | Change vs Previous (%) |
| 23/03/2021 | 85.6 | 0.538 | 0.004 | 0.7 |

Fig. 1.17 Typical DEXA Results. Femoral neck analysis. The bone density (BMD) is plotted against age (left hand graph) demonstrating the T score to be -3.7 and therefore in the osteoporotic region NHANES (National Health and Nutrition Examination Survey) – comparative dataset used to calculate T score and Z score.

## Radionuclear Studies

Although plain radiographs and CT scans measure the absorption of X-ray beams as they pass through the body, radionuclear studies place radioactive materials into the body and measure their distribution using external sensors to pick up the radiation (e.g., gamma camera scintigraphy). The radioactive isotopes are attached to carriers that cause them to be taken up by the tissues of interest (**Table 1.14**). The most commonly used scan in orthopaedics is a technetium-99m bone scan. It is attached to methylene diphosphonate (MDP). This chemical tag assists in adsorption onto the bone mineral matrix. As a result, the scan highlights skeletal uptake and activity. It can show areas

of increased bone turnover, particularly related to neoplastic disease (**Fig. 1.18**).

## Nerve Conduction Studies

Nerve conduction studies (NCSs) are a noninvasive way of gaining information about sensory, motor or mixed peripheral nerves. Although direct nerve stimulation can be performed intra-operatively, most are undertaken using transcutaneous stimulators and recording electrodes. Broadly, NCSs give information on **amplitude** ('quantity' of conduction related to the number of neurons carrying signal) and **latency/ velocity** (quality of conduction related to myelination). In general, upper limbs conduct faster than lower limbs, more proximal nerves conduct faster and lower temperatures reduce velocity.

**Table 1.14 Radioisotopes used in orthopaedic imaging**

| Radioactive tracer | Scan type | Tissue affinity | Clinical utility |
| --- | --- | --- | --- |
| Technetium-99m | Bone scan | Osteoblasts | Occult fracture, osteomyelitis, metastatic disease |
| Gallium-67 | Bone scan | Inflammatory proteins | Osteomyelitis, rheumatoid arthritis |
| Indium-111 (attached to autologous leukocytes) | White cell scan | Inflammatory sites | Localising low-grade infection (e.g., low-grade prosthetic infection) |
| Positron emitting isotopes (e.g., carbon 11, fluorine-18) | Position emission tomography (PET) | Various, depending on the chemical tagged | Limited in orthopaedics at present. Occasionally used in Musculoskeletal (MSK) oncology or infectious diseases. |

## Motor nerves

Motor function is studied via a cutaneous stimulator placed over the nerve proximal to the suspected compression. The distal muscular response is measured with a recording electrode placed over a muscle (e.g. the abductor pollicis brevis). A 'supramaximal' stimulating potential is used in order to ensure that all the axons evoke a potential. The time to detect a muscle response is dependent upon nerve conduction, synaptic transmission in the muscle and eventually myocyte contraction. Therefore the nerve conduction velocity is additionally measured via two stimulating electrodes a known distance from each other. The time to respond from the distal electrode is subtracted from that of the proximal electrode and represented in millimeters per second to give a velocity of conduction between the two electrodes (**Fig. 1.19A**).

## Sensory Nerves

These nerves can be stimulated in an anterograde or retrograde fashion, with amplitude and latency directly measured and velocity calculated from time and measured distance (**Fig. 1.19B**).

## Proximal Compression

Proximal nerves are difficult to measure directly owing to their deep anatomical locations. The induction of an action potential in a nerve distally also transmits proximally along the nerve and causes synaptic changes at the spinal root ganglions, before sending a signal back along the nerve to the recording electrodes. This occurs after the main action potentional, and it is demonstrated as an 'F response' (**Fig. 1.19C**). The absence or increased latency of this response can imply a proximal lesion (for example, in the brachial plexus or at the nerve root). However, as nerves arise from several roots of the spine/plexus, the F response can be less reliable and can indeed be absent in normal individuals over 60 years of age.

**Electromyography (EMG)** is used to measure muscle recruitment from a specific motor unit. A surface or needle electrode is placed into a muscle and measures the baseline activity (e.g., fibrillations). The muscle is then voluntarily contracted, and the motor unit action potential is measured to give information on the quantity of motor unit recruitment from a nerve. This can be useful in the examination of more

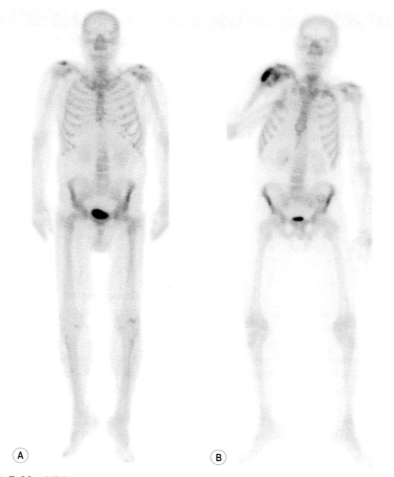

Fig. 1.18 Te99m-MDP bone scan. A) Normal findings, with tracer collecting in bladder. B) Abnormal uptake in right proximal humerus in association with a metastatic lesion.

proximal motor function (i.e., around the shoulder).

## PRINCIPLES OF ARTHROPLASTY

### Introduction

The term *arthroplasty* (from the Greek meaning 'joint moulding') refers to the surgical manipulation of joints in order to restore normal kinematic motion and typically involves the use of implants to replace degenerate joint surfaces.

Arthroplasty has evolved to maximise range of motion and function while also minimizing complications such as loosening, wear, and dislocation. Meticulous attention to sterility and tissue handling is required to avoid infection, which can be a devastating complication.

### Types of Arthroplasty

There are various arthroplasty techniques. Selection of the appropriate one is based on the severity of disease, the affected joint, and the patient's age and functional demands (**Fig. 1.20**).

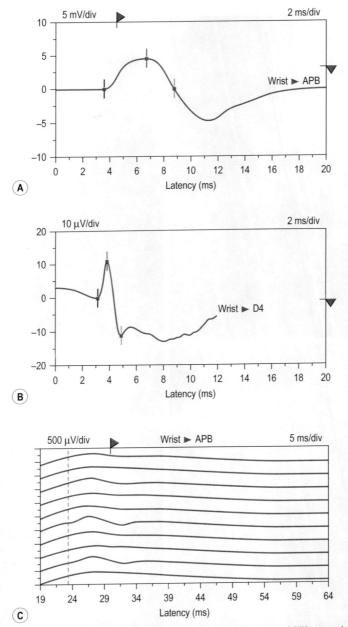

Fig. 1.19 Nerve conduction studies. A) Motor. B) Sensory. C) F waves. Milliseconds (ms), abductor pollicis brevis (APB), D4 (represents ring finger sensory electrode).

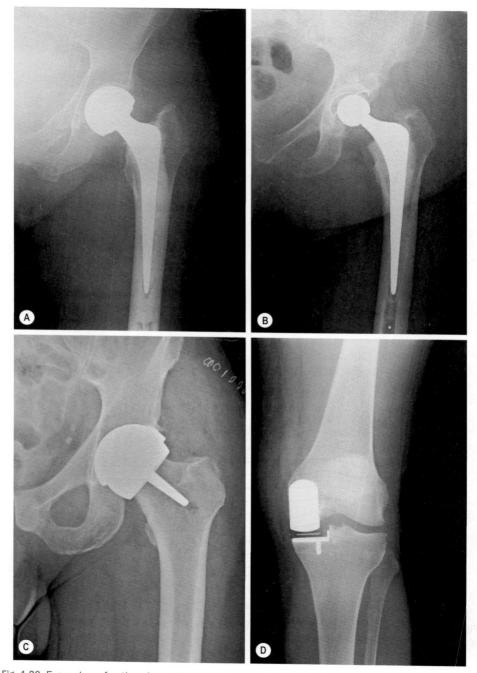

Fig. 1.20 Examples of arthroplasty. A) Hemiarthroplasty. B) Total joint replacement. C) Resurfacing. D) Partial joint.

**Interposition arthroplasty** is the simplest form of arthroplasty wherein soft tissue or an implant is placed as a spacer between two joint surfaces in order to reduce surface contact without resecting the chondral surfaces. Soft tissue interposition is still used in a few techniques, such as ligament reconstruction and tendon interposition (LRTI) following trapeziectomy.

**Excisional arthroplasty** completely removes part of a joint to reduce reaction forces between pathologic cartilaginous surfaces. It is still used in the wrist (trapeziectomy). It may also be used as a salvage procedure when a previous implant has failed (Girdlestone procedure). Following the procedure, the joint capsule fills with hematoma, and the subsequent inflammation causes fibrosis of the bone ends, which is painless. This occurs at the cost of impaired biomechanics and function.

**Cheilectomy** is the excision of impinging osteophytic areas of bone, which cause impingement and irritation. The most common example of this is removal of the dorsal osteophyte seen in hallux rigidus.

**Hemiarthroplasty** replaces one side of a joint by removal of the cartilage and the supporting bone. The most common example of this is hip hemiarthroplasty for an intracapsular fracture involving the neck of the femur. It is also used in the shoulder. More recently, distal humeral hemiarthroplasty has been described in the management of unreconstructable distal humeral fractures.

**Resurfacing arthroplasty** removes and replaces cartilage and a small amount of subchondral bone while retaining most of the supporting bone. Such procedures have been used in the shoulder and hip. From a technical standpoint, total knee replacement is actually a resurfacing arthroplasty. These procedures maintain 'bone stock' for future revisions; therefore they tend to be indicated in younger patients. As the underlying bone is kept, there is limited scope for the correction of any deformity.

**Total arthroplasty** addresses both sides of a joint by excising cartilage and more of the underlying bone. This resection enables the correction of periarticular deformities and flexible reconstruction to improve or restore joint kinematics. Total joint arthroplasty (such as total hip or knee replacement) aims to place the joint in an accepted neutral alignment, thus correcting any 'pathologic' joint alignments (e.g., varus knee).

**Unicompartmental arthroplasty** can be performed in joints with multiple articulations in which one of the articulating areas is arthritic but the remainder are preserved. Both surfaces of the compartment are replaced, as in unicompartmental knee replacement; however, the rest of the joint compartments must be symptomless, and limited correction can be achieved.

## Alternative Techniques Without Arthroplasty

**Fusion (arthrodesis)** is not an arthroplasty but rather an important form of joint alteration in which surgical debridement of the joint surface and stabilisation result in fusion of the articulation. This is commonly performed in small joints of the hand, wrists, ankle and feet and is effective at removing arthritic pain, but at the cost of joint motion.

**Osteotomy** does not alter joint surfaces but realigns forces transmitted through the joint (e.g. high tibial osteotomy). This can reduce symptoms and alter the progression of degenerative joint disease.

## MATERIALS AND BEARING SURFACES

## Materials

A number of biocompatible materials have proven useful over the last century and have been employed in various forms in orthopaedic surgery (**Table 1.15**).

Knowledge of a material's physical and biological characteristics is fundamental to its

**Table 1.15   Common materials employed in orthopaedics**

| Material | Use | Strengths | Limitations |
|---|---|---|---|
| **Polymers** • Ultra-high-molecular-weight polyethylene ± high crosslinking via radiation (XLPE) | • Prosthetic bearing surface | • Cheap • Improved wear properties when highly crosslinked | • Soft • Particulate wear • Relatively short follow-up for XLPE (highly cross-linked polyethylene) |
| • Polymethyl methacrylate | • Bone 'cement' | • Similar stiffness to bone • Can contain antibiotics | • Challenging to remove |
| **Ceramics** • Zirconium | • Prosthetic bearing surface (withdrawn) | • Scratch resistance • Scratches are trough only • Low wear rates • Low friction | • Brittle • Difficult to revise • Expensive • Squeak • Edge loading |
| • Aluminum oxide (Alumina) | • Prosthetic bearing surface | | |
| **Metals Alloys** • Cobalt chrome | • Prosthetic components • Prosthetic bearing surface | • Cheap • Long-term data | • Scratches cause peaks and troughs, leading to wear • Metallosis • Stiffness mismatch with bone |
| • Stainless steel (iron alloy with a minimum of 10.5% chromium and 0%–1.2% carbon) | • Plates, screws, wires • Prosthetic components • Prosthetic bearing surface | | |
| • Titanium alloys | • Plates, screws | • Closer stiffness to bone • Resistance to corrosion | • Softer • Limited fatigue resistance |
| **Silicone** • Silicone elastomer | • Interposition arthroplasty | • Cheap • Flexible | • Soft • Unpredictable wear profile |

application in orthopaedics. In cases such as joint arthroplasty is essential that such a material be biologically inert so that it will not produce a host reaction, however other materials are designed to evoke a biological response (e.g. ligament reconstruction or osseointegration). Articulating surfaces should also be hard-wearing and resistant to corrosion and should tolerate normal physiologic stresses and strains over time, thus resisting fatigue. Implants are termed load-bearing when they are expected to fully assume normal physiologic loading. Load-sharing implants tend to be used more commonly in trauma applications as temporary devices while bones heal. In arthroplasty, devices need to be fully load-bearing.

Materials change in length in response to the application of force. The change is termed elastic if the material can return to its previous state when the force is removed. Beyond elastic deformation, plastic deformation occurs, in which the change in length is irrecovarable. Each material will exhibit a point of force/stress at which it will break. Stress–strain curves are commonly used to represent how materials respond to load (**Fig. 1.21**). Different materials respond to stress in different patterns of elastic and plastic deformation along with their breaking points (**Fig. 1.22**).

- Stress is the applied force divided by the area through which it is acting.

- Strain is the proportional change in length that occurs due to the applied stress.

## Tribology

Tribology is the study of how different bearing surfaces interact with each other through friction and wear. Each combination of surfaces has benefits and drawbacks; therefore no single one of these surfaces is uniformly used.

For total joint arthroplasty, four bearing options are commonplace:

- Metal-on-polyethylene (MoP)

- Metal-on-metal (MoM)

- Ceramic-on-polyethylene (CoP)

- Ceramic-on-ceramic (CoC)

Most current large joint replacements (knee, shoulder, and elbow) are predominantly metal-on-plastic. In younger patients, metal–ceramic bearings may have reduced overall long-term wear. Ceramic can, however, exhibit brittle features and is more prone to fracture. MoM has been found to have unacceptably high wear patterns in many implants. Metal wear results in metal-ion release, which in turn can be associated with the formation of aseptic lymphocyte-dominant vasculitis-associated lesions (ALVAL) and pseudotumors. Patients with MoM articulations require specific counseling about the associated risks and benefits, along with ion monitoring according to national guidelines.

## Lubrication and Wear

All joints become lubricated in order to minimise friction between articulating surfaces. This can be provided by fluid–film lubrication (in which surfaces have a contained layer of fluid between surfaces through which load is transmitted) or boundary lubrication (where the fluid layer is too thin to bear load but interferes with surface adhesion). Most arthroplasties rely on boundary lubrication owing to the small size of the components and the nature of their material properties.

## Wear

Wear can be defined as the progressive loss of material due to mechanical means. There are several types of mechanisms and two patterns. Mechanisms of wear can be

- **Two-body abrasive:** two rough surfaces rubbing to create debris

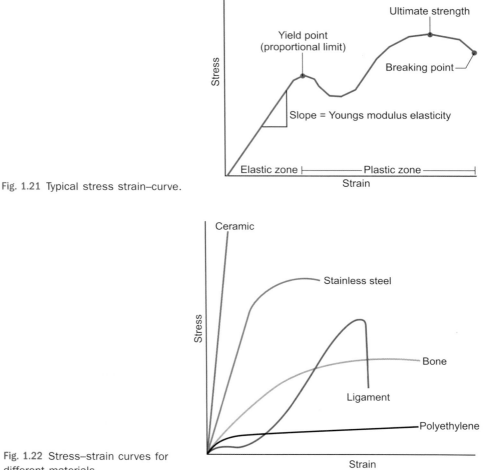

Fig. 1.21 Typical stress strain–curve.

Fig. 1.22 Stress–strain curves for different materials.

- **Third-body abrasive:** an additional particle at the interface of two surfaces creating further debris

- **Adhesive:** temporary molecular adhesion between surfaces in contact, which then detaches particles

- **Delamination:** fatigue failure of a material below the contact surface following repetitive stress and structural failure of the material

Wear can be described in two ways:

- **Volumetric wear** is the volume (cubic millimeters per year) of material detached from the softer surface. This is a product of force and sliding distance and is inverse to the material's hardness. Large bearing surfaces are therefore more liable to volumetric wear.

- **Linear wear** is a loss in height (millimeters per year) of a surface caused by a harder material 'burrowing' into it.

As part of the wearing process, debris is created. In the case of polyethylene-containing replacements, causing a cell-mediated inflammatory response from macrophages and osteoclasts (as polyethylene debris is similar size to bacteria). These cells not only phagocytose the wear debris but also release inflammatory mediators that cause bone lysis. In a similar manner, metal debris from MoM bearings releases cobalt and chromium locally and systemically, causing a physiologic response ('metallosis'). Metal debris is much smaller and penetrates cells creating large areas of metallic debris and immune response locally (osteolysis and pseudotumors) along with reported cases of systemic effects (e.g., neuropsychological changes and cardiomyopathy).

## Implant Fixation

Implants need to be securely fixed to the neighboring bone. The two main methods of fixation are cemented and uncemented.

- Uncemented implants are impacted directly against bone and rely on the biologic ingrowth of bone to maintain mechanical coupling. To accomplish this, the surface of the implant is manufactured to be rough (e.g., sandblasted), porous (e.g., trabecular metal) or coated with an osteoinductive material (e.g., hydroxyapatite).

- Cemented implants use a polymer cement between the bone and implant. It acts more like a grout than a glue. The cement interacts at the implant–cement and cement–bone interfaces, transmitting load from implant to bone.

## Bone Cement

Bone cement is polymethylmethacrylate (PMMA). It is a polymer with good biocompatibility (**Fig. 1.23**). It has similar biologic properties to bone and therefore efficiently transmits stresses and strains from the implant to the skeleton.

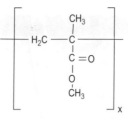

Fig. 1.23 Chemical structure of methylmethacrylate (MMA) subunit.

Bone cement has to be mixed during surgery. It is supplied as both a powder and a liquid (**Table 1.16**). The liquid contains the monomer methylmethacrylate (MMA) and is mixed with the polymer found in the powder. After a period of waiting (usually a couple of minutes), it reaches its working phase and is ready to be inserted. For medullary fixation, it is applied in a retrograde manner with a 'gun' having a long nozzle (**Fig. 1.24**). The handle is squeezed as the nozzle is withdawn, filling the canal. The cement is pressurised so that it will adequately fill the grooves in cancellous bone. The implant is then inserted. For the resurfacing of implants, it is usually applied to the cut bone surface and also to the back of the implant. As the polymerisation reaction occurs, heat is generated. This can cause thermal necrosis in adjacent tissue, so it is important to optimize blood flow and irrigation.

Bone cement can degrade and wear over time, leading to implant loosening (aseptic loosening). Loosening can occur at the implant–cement interface. It can also occur at the cement–bone interface, where changes in bone can lead to debonding.

## Revision Arthroplasty

There are many reasons why a joint arthroplasty may need to be revised. These include infection (e.g., periprosthetic joint infection (PJI)), dislocation, loosening, implant failure or periprosthetic fracture. Revision for pain alone, where there is no identified cause for the symptoms, is associated with a lower chance of success.

**Table 1.16  Components of bone cement**

| | Chemical | Role |
|---|---|---|
| **Powder** | Polymethyl methacrylate | Polymer–used to act as a surface for the initiation of polymerisation |
| | Antibiotic | Antimicrobial (reduces deep periprosthetic infection) |
| | Zirconium dioxide/barium sulfate/ | Radioopacity |
| **Liquid** | Methyl methacrylate | Monomer |
| | Dye (chlorophyll) | Coloration (green) |
| | N,N-dimethyl-p-toluidine | Initiator |
| | Benzyl peroxide | Accelerator |
| | Hydroquinone | Stabiliser |

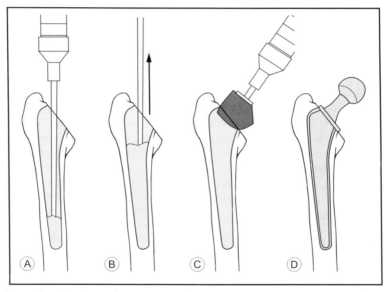

Fig. 1.24 Cementing the femoral component of a total hip replacement: A and B) The canal is filled with cement in a retrograde fashion. C) A stopper is placed to occlude the top of the canal, and further cement is squeezed in to pressurise the cement. D) The final implant is placed.

Revision can broadly be categorised into implant retention, single-stage revision, and multistage revision. Prior to surgery, the diagnosis is confirmed by history taking, clinical and radiologic examination, serum blood markers (ESR, CRP) or more specific investigations (e.g., joint aspiration and microbiologic culture) (Fig. 1.25). Newer techniques are becoming available, measuring levels of synovial fluid alpha-defensin and using next-generation genetic sequencing techniques to identify lower levels of bacteria.

| Major criteria (at least one of the following) | Decision |
|---|---|
| Two positive cultures of the same organism | Infected |
| Sinus tract with evidence of communication to the joint or visualisation of the prosthesis | |

| | | Minor criteria | Score | Decision |
|---|---|---|---|---|
| Preoperative diagnosis | Serum | Elevated CRP _or_ D-dimer | 2 | ≥ 6 infected |
| | | Elevated ESR | 1 | |
| | Synovial | Elevated synovial WBC count _or_ LE | 3 | 2–5 possibly infected |
| | | Positive alpha-defensin | 3 | |
| | | Elevated synovial PMN (%) | 2 | 0–1 not infected |
| | | Elevated synovial CRP | 1 | |

| | Inconclusive preop score _or_ dry tap | Score | Decision |
|---|---|---|---|
| Intraoperative diagnosis | Preoperative score | - | ≥ 6 infected |
| | Positive histology | 3 | 4–5 inconclusive |
| | Positive purulence | 3 | |
| | Single positive culture | 2 | ≤ 3 not infected |

Fig. 1.25 Defining periprosthetic joint infection (PJI). C-reactive protein (CRP), WBC (White blood cell), leukocyte esterase (LE), polymorphonuclear (PMN). Source: The 2018 Definition of Periprosthetic Hip and Knee Infection: An Evidence-Based and Validated Criteria, Parvizi, Javad et al. _The Journal of Arthroplasty_, 2018;33(5):1309–1314.e2.

The surgical options for arthroplasty revision are as follows:

- **Implant retention** may be attempted if aseptic or acute infection the (immediately postoperative or late hematogenous). This involves a debridement and implant-retention (DAIR) procedure along with exchange of some components (i.e., bearing surfaces). Surgery may be followed by a period of antibiotic therapy tailored to the sensitivities of any cultured microbes.

- **Single-stage revision** is the removal of all implants and meticulous debridement of all surrounding superficial soft tissue that has been in contact with the infected cavity before the insertion of new implants. This can be performed in a fit patient with an infection that is known and sensitive to antibiotic therapy.

- **Two-stage revision** removes infected implants and debrides infected soft tissues at the first stage. There is an interim period (e.g., 6–12 weeks) between debridement and definitive reconstruction during which antibiotics are administered locally (typically via a cement spacer) and systemically. Second-stage reconstruction is then undertaken. This is still considered the gold standard treatment, especially in cases with unidentified or more resistant organisms.

Occasionally, following multiple revision attempts, the only option left may to, excise, fuse (arthrodese) the joint or undertake an amputation. Decisions regarding the management of failed arthroplasty and PJI are best taken in a multidisciplinary team environment, including microbiology support.

## PRINCIPLES OF ARTHROSCOPY

### Background

Arthroscopy is used for both diagnostic and therapeutic purposes. Although there were sporadic reports of arthroscopic examination in the early twentieth century, it started to become more popular in the 1960s, following research by the Japanese surgeon Masaki Watanabe. Techniques were further refined during the 1970s and 1980s with the introduction of fibre-optic technology.

Arthroscopy is now commonly used to examine and treat conditions in the knee, shoulder, hip, elbow, wrist and ankle. The introduction of arthroscopic instruments, shavers and radiofrequency ablation devices has opened up the field of arthroscopy to a wide range of therapeutic interventions to debride and reconstruct damaged soft tissue, cartilage and tendons.

### Key equipment

- Arthroscopy stack (**Fig. 1.26**)

  - Monitor

  - Camera unit

  - Light source

  - Data input/recording unit

  - Fluid management unit

  - Shaver console and handpiece

  - Radiofrequency ablation unit and handpiece

- Other

  - Camera head

  - Cannulas

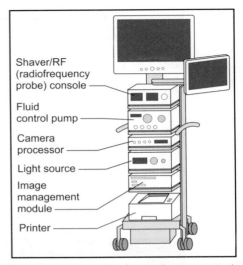

Shaver/RF (radiofrequency probe) console

Fluid control pump

Camera processor

Light source

Image management module

Printer

Fig. 1.26 Components of an arthroscopy stack.

- Tubing for fluid management

- Specialist drapes

- Arthroscopic instruments

- Suture anchors

- Traction device (for joints such as hip/ankle)

### Patient Positioning

Correct patient positioning is of vital importance to successful arthroscopy. For knee arthroscopy, patients are commonly positioned so that the knee can be flexed. A bolster or holding device may be used to provide a fulcrum so that the medial compartment may be opened to provide better access and visualisation. The leg is then manipulated into a 'figure of eight' position to open the lateral compartment.

For shoulder arthroscopy, patients may be placed in either the beach chair or lateral position. Both positions have advantages and disadvantages; the choice is usually determined by whatever the surgeon has been most exposed to during training.

Ankle and wrist arthroscopy both require traction, which can be manual or implemented via a specialised distraction device.

## Procedure

The general principle of arthroscopy relies on the creation of small surgical incisions that act as 'portals' and are placed in safe zones. A cannula is inserted into the joint (**Fig. 1.27**).

The cannula is connected to the fluid management system. Sterile normal 0.9% saline is instilled into the joint. This may be under gravity flow. In situations where more control of bleeding and swelling is needed due to extravasation, a dedicated fluid management unit may be used to control pressure. Outflow cannulas can be used if continuous fluid flow is required for irrigation and are useful for clearing the joint of debris.

A second portal is usually introduced to allow insertion of a probe, arthroscopic instruments, shavers, or radiofrequency (RF) ablation probes.

A hypodermic needle can be used to assess the placement and trajectory of the resulting portal.

A range of arthroscopic procedures may be undertaken. These fall into three categories:

- **Diagnostic arthroscopy** to evaluate the chondral surfaces, assess for loose bodies, and detect damage to soft tissue such as menisci, ligaments and tendons

- **Removal of loose bodies** such as residual osteochondritis dissecans lesions or osteochondral fractures

- **Reconstruction** of damaged anatomic structures such as menisci, ligaments and tendons

The knee and shoulder are the joints where most arthroscopic procedures are performed.

*Knee*

- **Meniscectomy** or repair

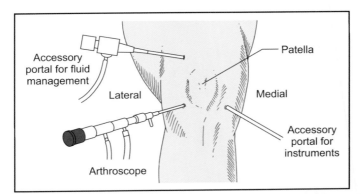

Fig. 1.27 Knee arthroscopy. The arthroscope is connected to a light source via a fibre-optic cable. It is also connected to a camera which transmits images to a screen. Fluid inflow is connected to this cannula to inflate the joint. Instruments are passed through an accessory portal. Occasionally, a further portal is placed to allow for more accurate fluid management and irrigation.

- **Ligament reconstruction** (or repair) can be used to reconstruct the ACL (anterior cruciate ligament), PCL (posterior cruciate ligament) and MPFL (medial patellofemoral ligament) ligaments

- **Chondral procedures,** including repair, microfracture or debridement

*Shoulder*

- **Arthroscopic subacromial decompression** excision of subacromial bursae with RF ablation and shaving of the undersurface of the acromion

- **Arthroscopic stabilisation** repair of detached glenoid labrum

- **Arthroscopic acromioclavicular joint excision** of a degenerative AC joint with shaving from below through the subacromial space

- **Arthroscopic rotator cuff repair** of acute or degenerative rotator cuff tears, usually using anchors that are preloaded with sutures

*Other Joints*

- **Elbow**–used to remove loose bodies. Can also be used to debride and perform arthrolysis in osteoarthritis and posttraumatic stiffness.

- **Ankle**–for debridement of chondral lesions.

- **Hip**–for debridement of chondral lesions along with management of femoroacetabular impingement and labral pathology.

# INTRODUCTION

The hip is a ball and socket synovial joint between the pelvis and femur (**Fig. 2.1**). The acetabulum is formed by the fusion of the triradiate cartilage between the three ossification centres of the pelvis: ilium, ischium and pubis. It is further deepened by the labrum and surrounded by a strong capsule with three ligamentous condensations (iliofemoral, ischiofemoral and pubofemoral ligaments) (**Fig. 2.1**). The iliofemoral ligament in particular is one of the strongest ligaments in the body and is tight in hip extension to reduce energy expenditure during stance. The acetabulum is anteverted 15° and covers the femoral head at an angle of 45°. An important landmark in elective practice is the transverse acetabular ligament, which represents the inferior portion of the acetabular labrum. It has a constant alignment in nondysplastic hips and can provide a useful guide to acetabular implant orientation (**Table 2.1**).

The femoral head is predominantly covered with a cartilage cap to permit a large range of movement. The hip capsule attaches anteriorly along the intertrochanteric crest and posteriorly part way up the femoral neck. The blood supply to the femoral head penetrates through the capsular attachment, which is important in hip pathology such as femoral neck fracture or avascular necrosis. In the adult the blood supply is predominantly through the medial femoral circumflex artery, which reaches the capsule through the quadratus muscle and must be protected during joint preserving surgery through a posterior approach. The normal femoral neck is anteverted 15° with a neck-shaft angle of 125°. The greater and lesser trochanters are bony protuberances from the proximal femur that permit numerous muscle attachments around the proximal femur, predominantly from muscles originating around the pelvis.

# ADULT MANIFESTATIONS OF HIP DYSPLASIA

## Clinical Summary

Developmental dysplasia of the hip in childhood (Chapter 10) can result in long-term acetabular and/or femoral anatomical abnormalities. The presence of dysplastic features on imaging is associated with a four-fold increase in the development of osteoarthritis. Dysplasia can affect both the acetabulum and femur.

A reduced joint contact area is responsible for point loading and reduced lubrication. This culminates in loading and accelerated chondral and labral damage. Patients commonly present with onset of symptoms in their third to fifth decade of life.

## Symptoms

Symptoms arise from progressive degeneration and tearing of the anterosuperior labrum followed by chondral surface and eventually degenerative joint disease. There may be an associated femoroacetabular impingement (FAI) due to reduced femoral offset and abnormal femoral version (**Table 2.2**).

● Fatigue weakness and trochanteric pain

● Hip pain when sitting (common in FAI due to impingement)

● Progression from intermittent pain to a constant dull ache

● Clicking or locking during activity

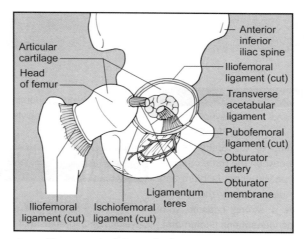

Fig. 2.1 Hip joint anatomy. The capsule follows the intertrochanteric crest anteriorly and incorporates the iliofemoral ligament. Posteriorly the capsule attaches part way up the femoral neck and incorporates the ischiofemoral ligament. This is important in hip preservation surgery as the retinacular vessels penetrate the femoral head through the capsular attachment. The transverse acetabular ligament is a constant anatomical structure that can aide implant alignment during arthroplasty.

| Table 2.1 | Radiological Evaluation of Hip Dysplasia | |
|---|---|---|
| **Measure** | **What is Evaluated** | **How It's Measured** |
| Acetabular Index | Femoral head coverage | Line through the tear drops (Hilgenreiner's line) transecting a line from teardrop to superolateral rim of acetabulum. Normal <35° |
| Centre-Edge Angle | Femoral head coverage and subluxation | Vertical line from centre of head to superior apex of femoral head and oblique line from centre of head. Normal >25°, borderline 20–25°, abnormal <25° |
| Crossover Sign | Retroversion | The anterior wall should be medial to the posterior wall. A retroverted acetabulum will result in crossing of the walls and a prominent ischial spine. |
| Posterior Wall Sign | Anteversion | The posterior wall of the acetabulum should be medial to the centre of the femoral head. If it lies laterally, this is indicative of an anteverted acetabulum. |
| α-Angle | Femoral offset | Line along centre of femoral neck to centre of head transecting line from superior head-neck junction to centre of head. A value >60° signifies "cam impingement" |

**Table 2.2   Differentiating Hip Dysplasia and Femoroacetabular Impingement**

| Hip Dysplasia | Femoroacetabular Impingement |
|---|---|
| • Wide range of motion | • Limited range of motion (especially internal rotation) |
| • Shallow, vertical acetabulum | • Normal or over-coverage |
| • Uncovered femoral head | • Cam or Pincer lesion on X-ray |
| • Hypertropic labrum | • Pistol grip femurs |

When later degenerative changes occur, symptoms are more typical of hip osteoarthritis (OA), namely groin, buttock or thigh stiffness/pain related to activity levels. The differential diagnoses of extraarticular hip pathologies should be considered, particularly in the presence of normal imaging.

## Clinical Examination

● Inspection – Antalgic, stiff or Trendelenburg gait (due to reduced femoral offset and abductor failure)

● Palpation – Femoral triangle pain

● Movement – Limited range of motion, crepitis, excessive internal rotation (femoral anteversion), and pain on hip flexion and internal rotation, signifying femoro-acetabular impingement

## Imaging

The aims of imaging in adult hip problems are to:

1. Establish the presence of dysplasia (acetabulum and femur)

2. Gauge severity of dysplasia

3. Identify focal pathology (e.g., FAI, labral or chondral damage)

4. Evaluate presence/absence of irreversible chondral degeneration

5. Plan for surgery

## Plain X-rays

The typical presentation of a dysplastic hip is a shallow acetabulum. Plain X-rays are usually adequate to evaluate adult manifestations of developmental dysplasia of the hip (DDH) (**Table 2.1** and **Fig. 2.2**). The later findings are similar to OA changes: joint space narrowing, osteophytosis and subchondral sclerosis.

Patients with missed DDH, may present in young adulthood with hip pain and leg shortening. Plain X-rays can demonstrate low and high chronic hip dislocation (**Fig. 2.3**).

## Computed Tomography

Computed tomography (CT) can be helpful for more detailed appreciation of coverage and version of the hip joint. It is not routinely required unless there is uncertainty regarding the anatomy and version of the acetabulum and femur.

## Magnetic Resonance Imaging

Magnetic resonance imaging (MRI) is usually undertaken as an arthrogram with intraarticular contrast to determine if any of the following are present:

● Labral pathology

● Impingement (bone oedema, chondral changes)

● Chondral lesions

● Joint erosions

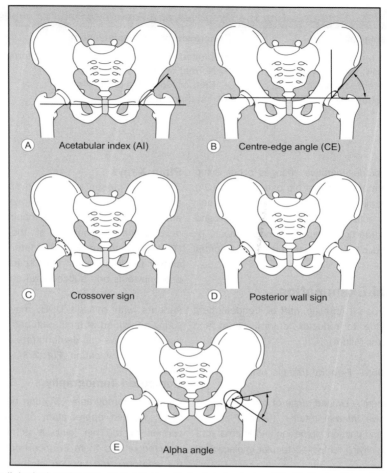

Fig. 2.2 Radiological evaluation of dysplasia. A) Acetabular Index (AI), B) Centre-Edge Angle (CE), C) Crossover Sign, D) Posterior wall sign, E) Alpha angle.

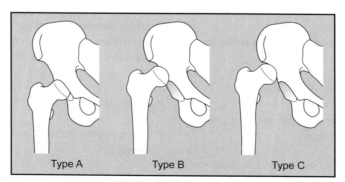

Fig. 2.3 Hartofilakidis classification of late consequences of DDH. A) Dysplasia, B) Low dislocation, C) High Dislocation.

## Hip Arthroscopy

Hip arthroscopy is an effective way of evaluating joint surface damage if there is an indication for a targeted therapeutic procedure, especially in borderline cases (CE angle 20–25°):

- Labral tear/detachment

- Focal chondral defect (for debridement or microfracture)

## Treatment

### Nonoperative

There is limited scope for nonoperative management in dysplastic hips due to the pathoanatomy and abnormal mechanics. Weight modification and gait training may give some symptomatic relief.

### Operative

*Hip Arthroscopy* – Hip arthroscopy can be used to treat a focal lesion such as a labral detachment or partial chondral damage. It is usually only be successful in those with a borderline centre-edge angle.

*Periacetabular Osteotomy* – A periacetabular osteotomy (PAO) aims to increase cover of the femoral head with articular cartilage, improving the contact area in the weight-bearing zone. A range of periacetabular osteotomies have been described; however, the Ganz PAO (while technically challenging) is the predominant procedure for acetabular realignment (**Fig. 2.4**). This is successful in symptom relief in 85% of cases; however, if full-thickness chondral damage exists, then the failure rate is 80%.

*Femoral Osteotomy* – Varus osteotomy can both increase offset and reduce the femoral head back into the joint (**Fig. 2.5**). Additional excessive femoral anteversion or retroversion can be neutralised with derotation during this procedure.

*Arthroplasty* – The younger age of presentation brings additional challenges of functional expectations, return to work and implant longevity

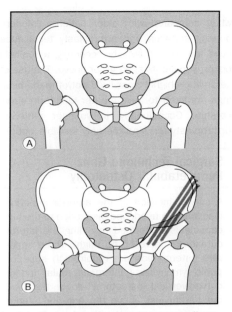

Fig. 2.4 Ganz osteotomy. A) Osteotomy lines, B) Rotation to provide additional femoral head coverage.

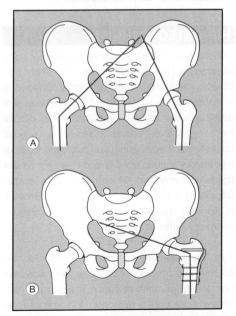

Fig. 2.5 Femoral osteotomy. A) Demonstrating valgus left hip. B) Varus osteotomy to increase head coverage in acetabulum.

when compared with older patients. Modern bearing surfaces and arthroplasty techniques have led to arthroplasty becoming a realistic option in patients aged 40 or above. The use of ceramic on highly cross-liked polyethylene bearings are likely to have greater long-term survivorship. Occasionally, in younger patients, arthroplasty remains the only feasible option.

## Surgical Technique Ganz Periacetabular Osteotomy

A curved incision of the anterior superior iliac spine is used, and dissection to the hip capsule is performed (avoiding the lateral cutaneous nerve of the thigh). Three separate osteotomies are required: i) superior pubic symphysis, ii) inferoacetabular and iii) curved-vertical osteotomy down the iliac crest from just above the anterior inferior iliac spine to connect with cut (ii). The acetabulum is then mobilised to cover the femoral head using fluoroscopic imaging and held with threaded wires (**Fig. 2.4**).

## HIP OSTEOARTHRITIS

The hip joint is the second most common joint affected by OA, after the knee. It is likely that genetic risk factors contribute to an underlying vulnerability to joint damage. This combines with developmental risk factors such as hip dysplasia, Legg–Calvé–Perthes disease or slipped upper-femoral epiphysis as an adolescent. Other risk factors include obesity and lower limb malalignment. Secondary OA can also be seen after trauma to the acetabulum or proximal femur. It is also the final pathway observed in avascular necrosis of the hip.

The pathological processes observed are common to other OA conditions, with subchondral and synovial inflammation, articular cartilage loss and osteophyte formation. In some forms of hip OA, osteophytes form on the floor of the acetabulum, leading to hypertrophic OA.

## Symptoms

- Pain is noted anteriorly in the groin. Where pain is mostly posterior pelvic, other pathology such as low back pain and sacroiliac joint disease should be considered.

- Stiffness, particularly for extended periods on waking

- Reduced walking distance

- Requirement for a walking aid, such as walking stick

## Clinical Examination

- Look

  - Gait: Patient is observed to have either an antalgic or Trendelenburg gait

  - Leg length: Should be initially assessed while standing to judge the degree of pelvic tilt Further examination of leg lengths is undertaken with the patient lying on the examination couch. The apparent and true leg lengths should be appraised. Apparent leg length deformity occurs through the effect of flexion and adduction contractures on pelvic tilt, and this the apparent length. True leg length deformity arises from shortening due to pathology in the femoral head and acetabulum.

- Feel

  - The greater trochanter should be palpated to exclude a differential diagnosis of lateral hip pain (trochanteric bursitis).

- Move

  - Flexion, extension, abduction and adduction should be examined individually and compared with the contralateral side.

Extension is examined in the supine position by flexing the patient's contralateral hip fully. If the leg being examined remains on the bed, extension has occurred at the hip joint to account for the pelvis tilting while flexing the other side. This manoeuvre is called the Thomas test.

## Investigation

Plain radiographs of the pelvis are most useful in determining if there is loss of joint space, osteophyte formation, subchondral cysts and sclerosis.

- Plain radiographs are also vital for preoperative planning through templating. This allows the surgeon to determine the anticipated component sizes. This improves situational awareness during surgery.

- In cases where diagnosis is unclear, through the presence of symptoms such as coexisting back pain, injection testing can be performed. Local anaesthetic and corticosteroid are injected into the hip joint under fluoroscopic or ultrasound control. A positive response will result in a temporary improvement in symptoms.

- In cases where other pathology such as labral injury and FAI is considered, magnetic resonance arthrography is useful.

## Treatment

- *Nonoperative management* – Education and advice on activity modification and weight loss. A walking stick may also be advised for use in the contralateral hand.

- *Operative management* – There is little place for nonarthroplasty surgical interventions because of the success of hip replacement surgery. In a total hip replacement (THR) both the femoral head and acetabulum are replaced. There are a variety of approaches,

bearing surfaces and implant fixation techniques.

## AVASCULAR NECROSIS OF THE HIP

## Clinical Summary

Avascular necrosis (AVN) of the hip is infarction of the bone following loss of blood supply to the femoral head. It is sometimes called osteonecrosis. It covers a spectrum of severity from minor interruption with subsequent revascularisation to collapse of the subchondral bone and severe arthritis of the hip joint (**Fig. 2.6**). The blood supply of the head arises mainly from the medial femoral circumflex artery, with lesser contribution from the lateral circumflex artery. These vessels run with the hip capsule and ascend the neck to the head. There are smaller supplies from within the bone and the artery of the ligamentum teres.

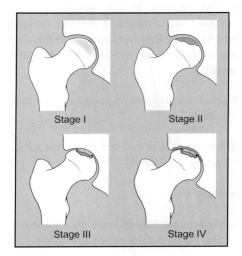

Fig. 2.6 Stages of avascular necrosis of the hip – Stage 1 with symptoms but no obvious changes on imaging. Stage 2 with normal femoral head shape but early imaging changes to suggest osteonecrosis. Stage 3 with subchondral collapse and/or flattening of the femoral head. Stage 4 with secondary arthritis affecting acetabulum.

AVN of the hip tends to present earlier in life than OA and often involves both hips within 2 years of each other, especially if atraumatic. It is more commonly seen in men and at a younger age, typically around 35 years old, compared with 65 years old in females.

AVN usually follows a pattern of infarction then collapse, which is followed by overt. The process occurs over a period of approximately 2 years. It is the third most common reason for hip replacement in those under 50 years of age.

Bone infarction arises from an insult to the microcirculation within the bone. Without a blood supply the bone gradually undergoes necrosis. In favourable conditions, such as a small area of necrotic bone, maintenance of subchondral support and no further insult to the microcirculation, the bone will revascularise. The necrotic bone is gradually replaced and support to the cartilage restored. In more severe cases the necrotic bone collapses in the weight-bearing area of the femoral head, causing deformation and collapse of the femoral head and subsequent OA.

Several risk factors have been identified, including:

- Previous AVN of the contralateral hip particularly within 2 years

- Male sex

- Previous trauma either directly to hip joint or altering mechanics of pelvis/limb

- Genetic factors – family history

- Smoking

- Alcohol abuse

- Obesity

- Coagulopathies and haemaglobinopathies (e.g., sickle cell disease)

- Steroids and immunosuppressants

- Occupational exposure to high pressure (such as divers, eponymously known as Caisson disease)

- Previous radiotherapy to the pelvis/upper leg

- Cancer patients due to hypercoagulability: steroids, radiotherapy and chemotherapy treatment

## Symptoms
- Pain

  - Persistent anterior hip and groin pain, often of insidious onset

  - Aggravated by movement especially uphill or stairs

- Stiffness especially with later stages of collapse/arthritis

- Reduced walking distance

## Clinical Examination
The findings are similar to OA of the hip; however, pain may be more severe than in primary OA and out of proportion to the X-rays, which may appear normal. Examination should always include the lumbar spine, contralateral hip and ipsilateral knee. Around 3% of patients may have multiple site involvement so be prepared to examine other symptomatic joints.

## Investigation
- Plain X-rays of the pelvis can detect subchondral collapse of the femoral head (including the crescent sign) and secondary arthritis of the hip joint. In early cases there may not be any changes seen on X-ray.

- MRI is useful when there is persistent pain but changes on X-ray. Approximately 15%–20% of early AVN is detectable on MRI but not X-ray.

- At present there are no blood tests or other serological investigations for AVN.

# Treatment

## Nonoperative

Nonoperative treatment may be considered for early stages of hip AVN before subchondral collapse. Identification of the underlying cause and changing medical treatment (such as stopping steroids or immunosuppressants when possible) can prevent further necrosis. Additional nonoperative measures have limited evidence to support their efficacy but include activity modification with or without partial or non-weight-bearing through the affected side and bisphosphonates or prostacyclin analogues. Bisphosphonates and prostacyclin analogues have been trialled with variable results, with some weak evidence they may reduce pain and time to revascularisation. However, their efficacy and cost benefit are not well established at present.

## Surgical Management

Surgical treatment is divided into joint preservation and joint replacement. Joint preservation procedures are reserved for precollapse AVN.

Once the subchondral bone has collapsed, arthroplasty is the only viable alternative.

## Joint Preservation

Core decompression involves drilling into and removing or decompressing the necrotic bone within the femoral head (**Fig. 2.7**). This may be augmented with porous metal rods or one of several forms of bone grafting such as injectable synthetic bone graft (calcium sulphate or phosphate), allograft or autograft including vascularised or nonvascularised fibular graft. The evidence for these procedures is weak, but core decompression may offer symptomatic relief and delay arthroplasty in younger patients without subchondral collapse.

## Joint Replacing

Once the subchondral bone has collapsed the recommended treatment for ongoing symptoms is joint replacement. There are several issues to consider in a patient with AVN.

- Age – Younger patients with higher premorbid activity levels and expectations. Implant choice for proven longevity and ease of revision. Uncemented acetabular implants are generally favoured as these have improved longevity in terms of bone fixation compared with cemented implants and allow for the use of ceramic-on-ceramic bearings.

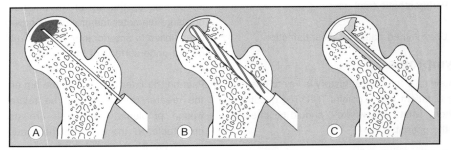

Fig. 2.7 Core decompression of the femoral head. A) Femoral head with area of AVN without collapse of the overlying cartilage. B) Drill used to 'decompress' the necrotic bone. C) The subsequent drill tract filled with either metal augment or bone graft, synthetic, allograft or fibular autograft.

- Comorbidity – Patients with hip AVN may have significant other comorbidities that contributed to the process. For example, patients on steroids or chemotherapy are at significantly higher risk of wound complications and deep infection, alcoholics are at higher risk of dislocation and patients with clotting disorders have a higher risk of bleeding or thrombosis. These patients require a robust shared decision making consent process and preoperative optimisation.

## THE PAINFUL TOTAL HIP REPLACEMENT

### Clinical Summary

THR is one of the most successful surgical operations undertaken. It is rare for patients to experience significant pain or complications. When a patient experiences pain and/or dysfunction following THR there can be several reasons:

- Periprosthetic joint infection

- Soft tissue irritation (i.e. iliopsoas impingement)

- Aseptic loosening

- Component malalignment

- Periprosthetic fracture

- Unexplained pain and dissatisfaction

### Symptoms

Obtaining a full clinical history is key to assessing a patient with a painful THR. The questions 'when? what? and where?' should be directed to the patient:

*When was the hip implanted? When did it start to become painful?*

A recently performed hip replacement that has been painful since day 1 suggests a problem arising from the procedure. There may have an intraoperative complication, or the components could be misaligned. Alternatively, there may be an early infection arising from contamination during or just after surgery. Later onset symptoms may indicate late infection and/or loosening.

*What brings the pain on, and what does it feel like?*

Pain and snapping in the groin that occurs during movement should prompt thoughts of iliopsoas impingement or the iliotibial band snapping over the greater trochanter due to an increased offset.

Pain that worsens with weight bearing is concerning for instability and loosening. Early on, this could be loosening of an uncemented component. Later, in both cemented and uncemented implants, septic and aseptic loosening must be considered.

*Where is the pain?*

- Hip joint pain is normally felt in the groin, but radiation to the thigh or knee is common. A failing acetabular component will usually cause groin pain, whereas a failing stem more often presents with thigh pain.

- Snapping in the groin can indicate impingement of the iliopsoas tendon. Most likely it is catching on the rim of the acetabulum, but large diameter femoral heads have also been linked to anterior impingement rubbing on the undersurface of the tendon.

- Pain on the lateral aspect of the hip around the greater trochanter can be related to wound problems, but these are usually detectable to the eye. Another cause is increased offset.

- Trochanteric pain results from excessive offset putting the fascia lata under tension. This then snaps over and back on the trochanter with movement.

## Investigation

In the clinic or the emergency department plain radiographs, bloods and a set of observations will be the main tools available and can provide a large part of the diagnosis.

- Clinical Examination – May reveal wound issues such as a sinus

- X-rays – Used to examine component orientation, loosening and fracture (**Fig. 2.8**)

- CT Scan – May be useful to look for subtle fractures around the acetabulum or femur

- MRI – May be useful, particularly if there is a metal-on-metal articulation and risk of pseudotumour formation and acute lymphocyte dominant vasculitis-associated lesion (ALVAL)

- Blood tests (white cell count and C-reactive protein) – Used to examine the pattern of systemic inflammation

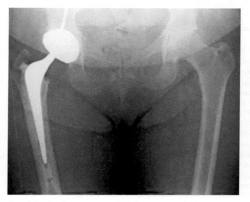

Fig. 2.8 An intraoperative fracture of the greater trochanter. This patient may have pain from the time of operation that fails to settle in the expected time frame. Pain on abduction may also be present or a positive Trendelenberg's test if the fragment displaces further. In this case, the fracture was noticed and held down with a fibrewire repair.

- Aspiration – Should be undertaken using aseptic technique. This procedure is usually image-guided using ultrasound or fluoroscopy in a clean environment. Samples are sent for microbiological examination (Gram stain and subsequent culture and sensitivity). Cultures should be for an extended period. Care should be taken to ensure the laboratory receives the samples in a timely manner. Failure to identify the infective organism at this stage can cause significant problems with subsequent treatment and require a staged technique. Antibiotics should be avoided until a sample for microbiological sample has been obtained. If a patient has signs of sepsis and urgent treatment is required, aspiration under aseptic conditions, along with blood cultures, should be performed immediately prior to starting antibiotics.

- Other "near-patient" tests – There is increasing potential for tests that can be undertaken at the bedside, such as synovial analysis for α-defensin, using a lateral-flow device.

## Treatment

The treatment of a painful hip replacement is based on the specific diagnosis.

### Periprosthetic Joint Infection

In 2021, the European Bone and Joint Infection Society published a consensus paper on the investigation and diagnosis of periprosthetic joint infection. Based on the investigations detailed, it is possible to place a patient into one of three categories: infection unlikely, infection likely and infection confirmed (**Fig. 2.9**).

Treatment of an infection can be described in four broad categories:

- **Suppression** is reserved for patients in whom surgery is no longer an option. Long-term antibiotics are taken to keep the infection quiescent, accepting that it will never clear.

| | Infection unlikely (all findings negative) | Infection likely (two positive findings)[a] | Infection confirmed (any positive finding) |
|---|---|---|---|
| **Clinical and blood workup** | | | |
| Clinical features | Clear alternative reason for implant dysfunction (e.g., fracture, implant breakage, malposition, tumour) | 1) Radiological signs of loosening within the first five years after implantation 2) Previous wound healing problems 3) History of recent fever or bacteraemia 4) Purulence around the prosthesis[b] | Sinus tract with evidence of communication to the joint or visualisation of the prosthesis |
| C-reactive protein | | >10 mg/l (1 mg/dl)[c] | |
| **Synovial fluid cytological analysis[d]** | | | |
| Leukocyte count[c] (cells/µl) | ≤1,500 | >1,500 | >3,000 |
| PMN (%)[c] | ≤65% | >65% | >80% |
| **Synovial fluid biomarkers** | | | |
| Alpha-defensin[e] | | | Positive immunoassay or lateral-flow assay[e] |
| **Microbiology[f]** | | | |
| Aspiration fluid | | Positive culture | |
| Intraoperative (fluid and tissue) | All cultures negative | Single positive culture[g] | ≥ two positive samples with the same microorganism |
| Sonication[h] (CFU/ml) | No growth | >1 CFU/ml of any organism[g] | >50 CFU/ml of any organism |
| **Histology[c,i]** | | | |
| High-power field (400x magnification) | Negative | Presence of ≥ five neutrophils in a single high power fields | Presence of ≥ five neutrophils in ≥ five |
| | | | Presence of visible microorganisms |
| **Others** | | | |
| Nuclear imaging | Negative three-phase isotope bone scan[c] | Positive WBC scintigraphy[j] | |

**Summary key**

a. Infection is only likely if there is a positive clinical feature or raised serum C-reactive protein (CRP), together with another positive test (synovial fluid, microbiology, histology or nuclear imaging).

b. Except in adverse local tissue reaction (ALTR) and crystal arthropathy cases.

c. Should be interpreted with caution when other possible causes of inflammation are present: gout or other crystal arthropathy, metallosis, active inflammatory joint disease (e.g. rheumatoid arthritis), periprosthetic fracture, or the early postoperative period.

d. These values are valid for hips and knee periprosthetic joint infection (PJI). Parameters are only valid when clear fluid is obtained and no lavage has been performed. Volume for the analysis should be >250 µL, ideally 1 ml, collected in an EDTA containing tube and analyzed in <1h, preferentially using automated techniques. For viscous samples, pre-treatment with hyaluronidase improves the accuracy of optical or automated techniques. In case of bloody samples, the adjusted synovial WBC= synovial WBC observed − [WBC blood / RBC blood x RBC synovial fluid] should be used.

e. Not valid in cases of ALTR, haematomas, or acute inflammatory arthritis or gout.

f. If antibiotic treatment has been given (not simple prophylaxis), the results of microbiological analysis may be compromised. In these cases, molecular techniques may have a place. Results of culture may be obtained from preoperative synovial aspiration, preoperative synovial biopsies or (preferred) from intraoperative tissue samples.

g. Interpretation of single positive culture (or <50 UFC/ml in sonication fluid) must be cautious and taken together with other evidence. If a preoperative aspiration identified the same microorganism, they should be considered as two positive confirmatory samples. Uncommon contaminants or virulent organisms (e.g. Staphylococcus aureus or gram negative rods) are more likely to represent infection than common contaminants (such as coagulase-negative staphylococci, micrococci, or Cutibacterium acnes).

h. If centrifugation is applied, then the suggested cut-off is 200 CFU/ml to confirm infection. If other variations to the protocol are used, the published cut-offs for each protocol must be applied.

i. Histological analysis may be from preoperative biopsy, intraoperative tissue samples with either paraffin, or frozen section preparation.

j. WBC scintigraphy is regarded as positive if the uptake is increased at the 20-hour scan, compared to the earlier scans (especially when combined with complementary bone marrow scan).

**Fig. 2.9** European Bone and Joint Infection Society Summary Diagram for diagnosis of periprosthetic joint infection. McNally M, Sousa R, Wouthuyzen-Bakker M, Chen AF, Soriano A, Vogely HC, Clauss M, Higuera CA, Trebše R. The EBJIS definition of periprosthetic joint infection. *Bone Joint J.* 2021 Jan;103-B(1):18–25.

- **Debridement and implant retention** consists of washout and debridement along with exchange of any modular components. A femoral head or the liner of an uncemented acetabulum can be exchanged, but well-fixed implants are retained. Biofilm should ideally not have had the chance to form so this is only appropriate early on in acute infection.

- **Revision** is used in situations where biofilms have had the time to form. Nothing will clear the infection without removal of foreign material along with aggressive debridement and washout. Revision procedures can be single-stage or two–stage. In a single-stage revision, a prosthesis is reimplanted after a thorough washout and debridement and removal of all the previous cement and components. This is only possible if the responsible organism has been identified from aspirates preoperatively. If the pathogen is known, the correct antibiotics can administered to prevent any bacteria left behind infecting the new metalwork. Antibiotics will be given for a prolonged course, usually starting with intravenous followed by oral if possible. High-risk, aggressive bacteria and immunosuppressed or diabetic patients should be considered for two-stage revision. At the first operation, complete implant and cement removal, debridement and washout are performed. A cement spacer is then inserted. Spacers are loaded with antibiotics, and the patient undergoes a prolonged course of antimicrobials (**Fig. 2.10**) When the infection has settled clinically, blood markers are normal and the antibiotic course complete, new implants can be inserted. Multidisciplinary teams are best placed for the management of these cases and clinical networks with centralisation of services are developing to concentrate expertise.

- **Amputation** may be rarely required when reconstructive options are no longer possible or the patient wishes a definitive surgery

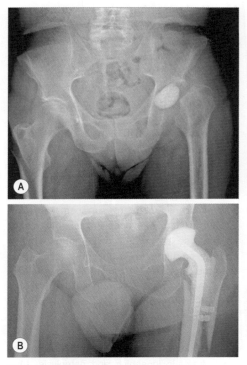

Fig. 2.10 Spacers for staged revision arthroplasty of the hip. A) Nonarticulating cement spacer on the left for an infected hemiarthroplasty. B) An articulating spacer that can allow the patient to manage mobilising in the house and transfers.

with predictable results. This is particularly important when someone has had multiple operations to attempt to clear infection, usually over a number of years. An amputation can remove all infection and allow someone to get their life back.

Fluid and tissue samples must be sent to the laboratory at each procedure. Multiple samples, generally five to seven, allow the best chance of isolating a bacteria or fungus. Samples at various stages can also pick up any changing resistance patterns. A multidisciplinary team approach with microbiologists and infectious diseases is crucial to successful management.

## Aseptic Loosening

This is a diagnosis of exclusion. Patients present with start-up pain, which is pain when standing from a seated position when force is greatest across the hip. The pain will often worsen gradually, with the frequency and intensity of discomfort increasing and function decreasing.

Wear particles from bearing surfaces, especially from polyethylene, are the main cause of the osteolysis seen as part of this phenomenon. Wear is a feature of expendable surfaces moving against one another, but it can also occur at nonbearing surfaces (**Table 2.3** and **Fig. 2.11**). Advances in technology such as the use of ceramic-on-ceramic bearings and the production of highly crosslinked polyethylene aim to reduce normal particulate wear and decrease loosening. It is up to the surgeon to implant components correctly to avoid other causes.

Submicron particles of polyethylene produce the most dramatic loosening and osteolysis. Macrophages phagocytose these particles and then activate osteoblasts. The osteoblasts, in turn, produce RANK (receptor activator of nuclear factor kappa-beta) ligand which binds with its receptor on the osteoclast to start the resorption of bone. The mineral, inorganic phase of bone is dissolved by acid produced by carbonic anhydrase while the protein, organic phase of bone is enzymatically degraded.

When managing a patient with suspected osteolysis, infection must be excluded as it can coexist with or be a cause of loosening. History, examination and basic tests and investigations will give the most information. For anyone with early failure, aspiration is mandatory. Where suspicion remains high, further investigations mentioned previously may be required. Repeat aspiration can be considered with extended cultures or cultures for fungi, and nuclear medicine tests can also help in ambiguous cases.

In a long-surviving prosthetic hip, wear and loosening are to be expected. If the history, exam, bloods and X-ray do not suggest infection, then most surgeons would be happy to

| Table 2.3 Types of Wear in Arthroplasty | |
|---|---|
| Two body wear | Wear between two articulating surfaces – intentional or not. |
| Adhesive wear | Two body wear due to one surface pulling material off another. Occurs when the bond between the surfaces is stronger than the bonds in the material undergoing wear. |
| Abrasive wear | Two body wear due to a rough, hard surface gouging a softer surface. A scratched metal femoral head ploughing furrows in a polyethylene liner is one example. |
| Third body wear | Wear due to an interposed piece of material such as cement between two articulating surfaces. |
| Backside wear | Wear between a liner and its shell – two surfaces that should not form an articulation. |
| Trunionosis | Wear between the morse taper of the stem and the femoral head. Again, this should not be a mobile articulation. |
| Volumetric wear | Volume of particles removed – $mm^3$/year – higher with larger femoral heads. |
| Linear wear | Depth of the erosion into the bearing surface in mm/year. Increased by small femoral heads |

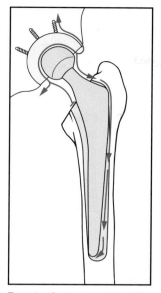

Fig. 2.11 Transit of wear particles throughout articulation and interfaces. After early loosening, fluid and particles can access further distally, in turn causing wider spread loosening.

proceed with single-stage revision albeit often after a negative aspirate. At the time of revision tissue samples are sent to microbiology just in case of low-grade infection.

A rare cause of aseptic bone resorption, particularly in the older population, is malignancy (primary, metastatic or haematological).

## Component Malorientation

A malpositioned acetabulum can protrude and can irritate the nearby soft tissues. This can be due to excessive retroversion leading to a prominent anterior edge, whereas anteversion uncovers the posterior rim. Failure to deepen the acetabulum can leave the entire implant proud. This is usually the result of failing to ream out the central osteophyte. Malpositioning is more commonly associated with instability and dislocation. In rarer cases the iliopsoas tendon catches over the anterior acetabular rim. A snapping sensation may be reported. Axial slices on CT scan will allow assessment of version, and coronal slices will show if the socket has been placed on the true floor and how open or closed it is. Treatment involves activity avoidance and/or steroid injection, fascia lata release or revision of implants.

## PERIPROSTHETIC HIP FRACTURE

The management of periprosthetic fractures is challenging and usually undertaken by specialists. Familiarity with the Vancouver classification system is important to guide treatment (**Table 2.4** and **Fig. 2.12**) but has limitations when applied to cemented implants.

Intraoperative periprosthetic fractures are caused by patient, implant and surgical factors. Late fractures can be a result of implant design

### Table 2.4 Extraarticular Hip Pathology

Muscular injury – Gluteus maximus, iliopsoas, hamstrings, etc.

Greater trochanter pain syndrome – Umbrella term for bursitis and tendinopathies

Impingement – Bony (greater trochanter/acetabular) or soft tissue (rectus femoris, psoas tendon, etc.)

Neuralgia/nerve entrapment – Sciatic (e.g., piriformis syndrome), cluneal and lateral femoral cutaneous nerves (meralgia paraesthetica)

Snapping hip – Internal (psoas tendon) and external (iliotibial band, gluteus maximus)

Groin pathology – Ilioinguinal hernia, Gilmore groin

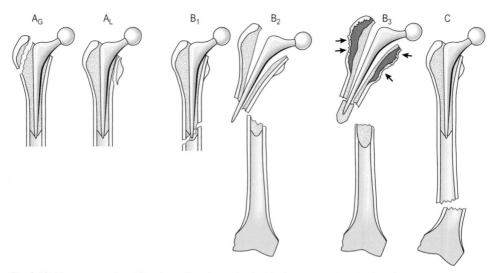

Fig. 2.12 Vancouver classification of periprosthetic hip fractures (Ag - isolated greater trochanter, Al, isolated lesser trochanter, B1 around tip with stable cement mantle and implant, B2 around stem tip with loose implant/mantle, C distal to tip).

features leading to stress risers, osteoporosis and loosening of the implant.

Each implant system has its own characteristics with which the surgeon must be familiar. Intraoperative periprosthetic features are more likely to occur when implanting uncemented prostheses.

## Treatment

The key treatment decision in managing a periprosthetic hip fracture is implant stability, which can be difficult to assess (particularly in a cemented femoral situation), and sometimes it is an intraoperative decision. Clues to a loose stem may be thigh pain or loss of function prior to fracture indicating that the stem was failing, evidence of subsidence when comparing pre- and postfracture radiographs, osteolysis of the surrounding bone, comminution of the fracture or the cement mantle and, in the case of uncemented implants, early fracture before the bone has bonded to the stem.

With the availability of locking plates, fixation of more fractures has become possible.

Cement–in–cement revisions can be performed rather than removing all the cement, which prevents the inevitable bone loss associated with cement extraction (**Fig. 2.13**). Other fractures with proximal bone loss may require bypassing with a long uncemented stem (**Fig. 2.14**).

Fracture with loose implants, cement and poor bone are best dealt with using a proximal femoral replacement, which requires no bony healing, and the patient can weight bear immediately, both of which are key surgical aims when treating elderly patients, who are most likely to have these injuries.

## HIP EXAMINATION

The hip is a deep joint, and pain in this area can be referred from a variety of sources. A thorough history regarding the nature and location of pain is required prior to examination to distinguish hip symptoms from knee, lower back, groin, intraabdominal and neurological or vascular origins. It is important to distinguish between intraarticular and extraarticular causes

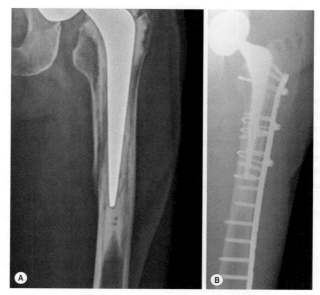

Fig. 2.13 Combined open reductional and internal fixation (ORIF) with cement-in-cement revision. A) A spiral periprosthetic fracture around a polished tapered, cemented implant. The cement mantle is disrupted, and the implant loose, but there is good bone stock – this is a Vancouver B2 fracture. B) The treatment of this fracture was with a cement-in-cement revision following ORIF with cables and a periprosthetic locking plate.

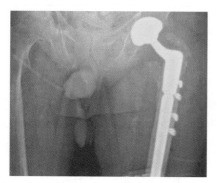

Fig. 2.14 Reconstruction with long uncemented revision implant. The conical shape of the distal stem provides fix within the diaphysis, distal to the fracture, and the bony fragments are then cabled onto the implant and will bond to the hydroxyapatite coating as they heal. The proximal body comes in various sizes to restore offset and leg length. It is bolted to the distal stem and can be rotated prior to final tightening to allowing adjustments of anteversion.

of hip pain (**Table 2.4**). A screening examination of the spine should also be undertaken to assess whether any pain or dysfunction is arising from this area.

## Look

- The patient should be undressed to underwear from the waist down. Prior to focussing on the hip, a brief screen of the lower back and knee should be undertaken by assessing forward and lateral flexion of the spine and range of motion of the knee.

- Beginning with the patient standing, look for scars (**Fig. 2.15**), muscle wasting (particularly of gluteus maximus and the quadriceps) and relative leg length (pelvic tilt). Of note, any scars as a result of surgery in childhood may become less obvious or change shape or location by the time skeletal maturity is reached.

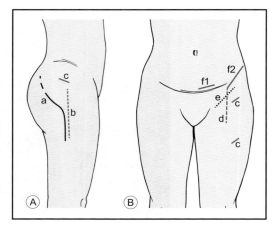

Fig. 2.15 Hip scars. A) Lateral view B) Anterior view. Scar locations: a) Posterior approach to hip (dotted line posterior approach to acetabulum). b) Lateral/anterolateral approach. c) Hip arthroscopy portals. d) Anterior approach to hip. e) Anterior approach (bikini line inscision). f1 & 2) Periacetabular approaches – f1 medial window (intrapelvic) approach and f2 lateral window.

- The gait is observed for speed and symmetry. Antalgic or Trendelenburg gaits are the commonly observed findings.

- Leg length discrepancy is assessed supine and can identify where shortening is a result of spinal or other pathology leading to pelvic

tilt (**Fig. 2.16**). A screening measurement for global leg length from the anterior superior iliac spine to the medial malleolus is performed, and if equal, then no further measurements are usually required. If a discrepancy is measured, then femoral lengths are measured from the greater trochanter to the medial

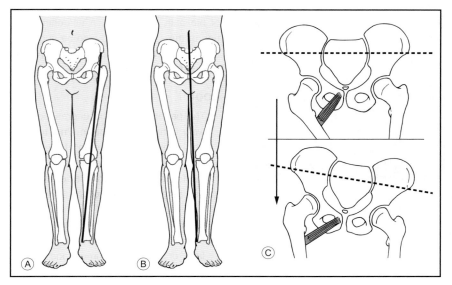

Fig. 2.16 Apparent versus real leg length. A) Real leg length is measured from the ASIS to the medial malleolus B) Apparent leg is measured from the umbilicus to the medial malleolus. It is affected by real shortening of the leg, along with other issues resulting in pelvic tilt (spinal pathology or hip adductor contracture), C) Adductor contracture leading to pelvic tilt.

femoral condyle and tibial length from the tibial tuberosity to the medial malleolus.

## Feel

The hip joint itself is too deep to assess for effusion or heat, but localised tenderness around the hip region can indicate important pathology. Palpate the following areas:

- Superior pubic ramus – Feel along its length by finding the pubic symphysis then palpating along its border laterally.

- Hip joint/femoral triangle – Located just inferior to the midinguinal point (halfway between the pubic symphysis and the anterior superior ischial spine); firm pressure over an irritable hip will be uncomfortable.

- Greater trochanter – The most prominent bony prominence on the lateral proximal thigh, 10–15 cm interior to the iliac crest.

## Move

Hip movements can be examined supine. Patients should perform active movements, and further passive motion should be noted in degrees for flexion/extension, internal/external rotation and abduction/adduction (**Fig. 2.17**).

## Additional Tests

- **Thomas test** – Due to a compensatory flexion of the pelvis, a fixed flexion deformity of the hip can be difficult to visualise. The Thomas test (**Fig. 2.18**) flexes the contralateral hip to flex the pelvis (confirmed by placement of a hand at the lower back and feeling the lumbar spine pressing down). If a flexion contracture is present, extension is not possible, and the affected hip lifts from the couch.

- **Trendelenburg test** – This test assesses hip abductor muscle (gluteus medius and minimus) integrity, which can fail as a result of anterolateral approaches to the hip, following anterior hip dislocations or neuropathy of the superior gluteal nerve (e.g., L5 radiculopathy). During single leg stance (e.g., swing phase of gait), the abductors of the limb in contact with the ground act to prevent gravity tilting the pelvis (**Fig. 2.19**). Therefore, this test involves the examiner placing their hands on a bony pelvic landmark (typically the anterior superior iliac spines) and asking the patient to bend the knee and lift one foot off the ground to test the contralateral hip abductors. A positive test is a downward tilt in the pelvis within 30 seconds of the test beginning.

- **Impingement test** – Femoroacetabular impingement can be examined by application of the FADIR position (**Fig. 2.20**). The hip is passively placed into flexion, adduction and internal rotation. Reproduction of pain may represent impingement pathology, such as a labral or cam lesion. It is not specific, so it may be positive in other hip conditions such as OA.

## Neurovascular Examination

To complete the examination the distal neurovascular status should be assessed with a screening test of the major myotomes and dermotomes (**Table 2.5**). This is accompanied by palpation of the peripheral pulses.

## Surgical Procedure: Total Hip Replacement

### Before the Operation

A patient should have previously undergone a thorough assessment to determine that a hip replacement is the most appropriate treatment. Discussion of the risks, benefits and alternatives should take place prior to the day of surgery to allow time for adequate shared decision making (**Table 2.6**).

**Templating** – Templating provides the surgeon with an anticipated stem and acetabular size, femoral neck offset, head

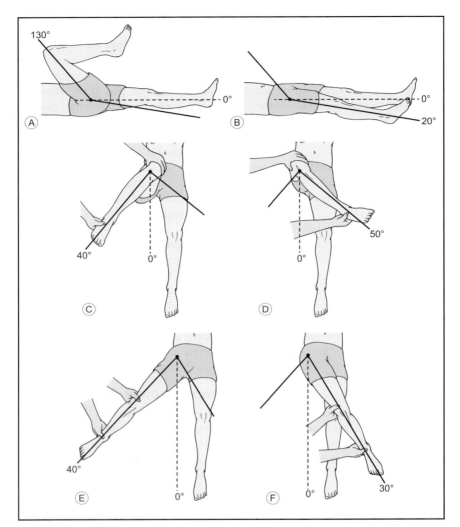

Fig. 2.17 Examination of hip movements. A) Flexion. B) Extension. C) Internal rotation. D) External rotation. E) Abduction. F) Adduction.

size and length (**Figs. 2.21**, **2.22**). It can be performed with traditional acetate overlays or with more modern software packages. It is important to set the scale correctly. The height of the neck cut should also be planned. Effective templating ensures accurate implant placement, soft tissue tension and leg length equality. Head and socket size and material are selected to maximise stability while minimising wear (**Fig. 2.23**). This results in optimal function and reduced complications such as dislocation.

**Surgical Briefing and Checklist** – Check that the entire armamentarium is available and whether any surgical or anaesthetic issues are expected for each case. The World Health Organization checklist should be used before the first incision is made

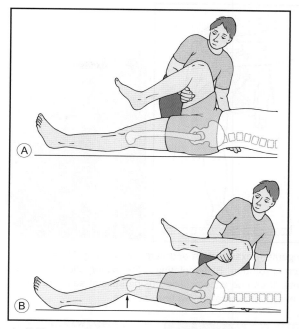

Fig. 2.18 Thomas test. A) The examiner places one hand underneath the patient's back while flexing the contralateral hip to that being examined. B) If there is a flexion contracture, Thomas test is noted to be positive if the contralateral knee lifts off the examination couch. The examiner's hand detects loss of lumber lordosis and appropriate pelvic tilt by the placement of their hand behind the patient's back.

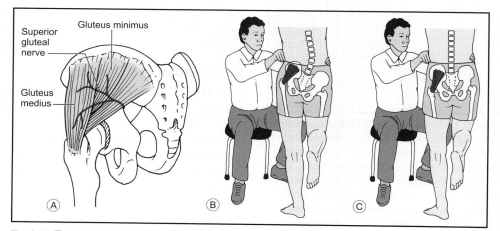

Fig. 2.19 Trendelenburg test. A) Abductors of the hip. B) Negative and C) Positive Trendelenburg sign of the left hip.

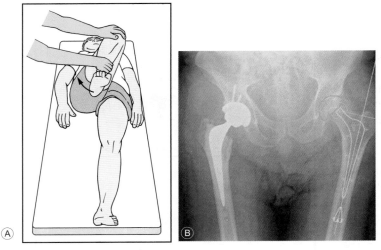

Fig. 2.20 Hip impingement examination and surgical planning A) FADIR position: flexion, adduction and internal rotation. B) Templating – Templating allows estimation of bony cuts and anticipated implants. It can be accomplished using special software packages within a PACS (Picture Archiving and Communication System) system.

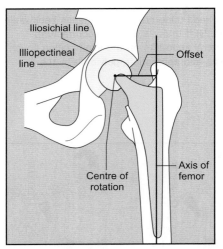

Fig. 2.21 Important anatomical considerations during THR. Offset: the perpendicular distance from the anatomical axis of the femur to the centre of rotation of the femoral head.
Centre of rotation: the point about which the hip rotates – restoring this is a key goal.
Iliosichial line: represents the posterior column of the hemipelvis. The acetabulum should normally lie lateral to this.
Illiopectineal line: represents the anterior column of the acetabulum.

(https://www.who.int/teams/integrated-health-services/patient-safety/research/safe-surgery/tool-and-resources).

## Operative Positioning

The patient is usually turned on their side into the lateral decubitus position (**Fig. 2.24**) and held with supports. The pelvic tilt should be assessed and placed in a neutral position. The anterior supports are placed on the anterior superior iliac spines while the posterior one supports the sacrum.

## Preparation and Draping

To avoid contamination it is important to pay attention to the following:

- Avoid gown contamination against the table when prepping or holding the leg; place an approach drape over the lower leg and table end.

- Externally rotate the leg and lock the knee in extension. This prevents the knee from buckling and the leg collapsing down and becoming contaminated.

## Table 2.5 Relevant Nerves to Hip Examination

| Nerve | Sensory Component | Motor Component |
|---|---|---|
| Femoral Nerve | Anteromedial thigh | Knee extension (anterior compartment of thigh) |
| Saphenous Nerve (branch of femoral) | Anteromedial lower leg | No motor innervation |
| Sciatic Nerve | Anterolateral and posterior lower leg (peroneal, sural and tibial branches) | Knee flexion. All ankle, foot and toe movements |
| Obturator Nerve | Proximal medial thigh | Hip adduction |
| Lateral Cutaneous Nerve of the Thigh | Lateral thigh | No motor innervation |

## Table 2.6 Complications to Discuss During the Consent Process

**General**

Bleeding and blood transfusion

Infection

Damage to nerves, blood vessels, tendons/muscles

Blood clot in leg or lung

Heart attack, stroke, pneumonia, organ failure

COVID–19

Death

**Specific for the operation**

Dislocation

Leg length difference

Fracture during or after operation

Need for revision

**Specific to the patient**

Increased risk of infection with diabetes, immunosuppression, smoking

Increased risk of dislocation with neurological dysfunction

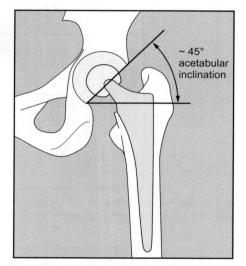

Fig. 2.22 Acetabular inclination. This is measured in the coronal plane and the angle between the horizontal (pelvic axis) and the surface of the acetabulum.

- After prepping the foot, that swab is immediately handed off. Alternatively, the foot may be left unprepared but wrapped in a fluid-impervious drape or stocking.

- The last place to be prepped is the groin. This swab should be immediately discarded.

## Approach

The posterior approach is most commonly used. The incision should be approximately split in the middle by the greater trochanter and curve slightly posterior at the proximal end (**Fig. 2.25**). For obese patients, a larger

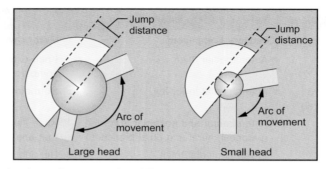

Fig. 2.23 Head size, jump distance and stability. A larger head has a larger arc of movement before the neck impinges on the edge of the socket. When this happens, the radius of the head being larger, it must jump a larger distance before it will dislocate. There is a larger articulating area so volumetric wear increases. A smaller head has a smaller arc of movement before it impinges, and a smaller radius means less distance for it to escape the socket.

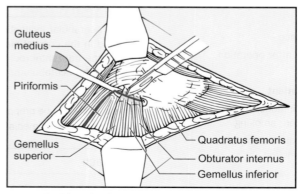

Fig. 2.24 Lateral positioning for hip replacement. It is essential to ensure the pelvis is perpendicular to the operating table. This is achieved with the use of well placed supports.

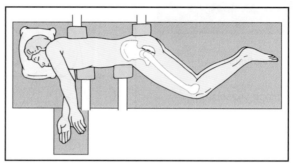

Fig. 2.25 Posterior approach. After the fascia lata is divided, the posterior aspect of the hip joint is revealed. A finger protects the nerve while a cut is made along the superior border of piriformis and then continued distally along the femur, detaching the tendon and the short lateral rotators. Following this, the capsule is divided and reflected.

wound is essential. Struggling with access and a steeper angle of approach for instruments is avoided by planning a longer wound from the start.

The fascia lata is incised in line with the skin wound. Proximally, fibres of the gluteus maximus are split using the index fingers of both hands. Residual trochanteric bursa is removed.

The patient's leg is internally rotated by the assistant, and the piriformis is identified at the back of the hip. It has a rope-like feel. The sciatic nerve is felt and protected with a finger. Incise along the cranial border of piriformis, above the finger placed on the nerve and head up to the greater trochanter (**Fig. 2.25**). The incision is then turned sharply 90° to transect the piriformis close to bone and run along the femur caudally. Do not enter the quadratus femoris if possible. It can be undermined and usually contains vessels that will bleed if cut. This can be done in one layer straight down to bone or in two layers, muscles first then capsule.

The next step is to cut the neck (the location depends on the system used). Mark the cut with diathermy. With the thigh parallel to the floor and the tibia vertical, make the cut. The saw should be at full speed before gently touching down on the bone. Stabilise the saw with the other hand resting on the patient. Start medially to avoid the oscillating blade contacting the greater trochanter. It is often necessary to complete the cut at its lateral aspect using an osteotome striking down into the neck proximal to distal.

## Acetabular Preparation

Remnants of the ligament teres and fat fill the floor of the acetabulum and can be cleared using a gouge, scraping from the centre to the transverse acetabular ligament. Central osteophytes are also removed with an osteotome.

With the true floor now visible, reaming can begin. Start small and work up sequentially until the reamer takes up the entire acetabulum and all the cartilage is removed. All but the first reamer should be reaming concentrically.

The first reamer, with a small diameter, can be used to ensure the remaining medial osteophyte is cleared. The reamers should match the desired position for the final cup. Version is normally taken from the transverse acetabular rim, setting the reamers parallel to the ligament. The inclination is altered by raising the operator's end of the reamer to achieve a more open position and lowering it to obtain a closed position. A good target is 45°.

When cement is used for the acetabulum, a mantle of 2 mm on either side of the socket requires the final reamer to be 4 mm larger than the cup to be inserted. Uncemented implants are usually reamed line-to-line or slightly under-reamed.

The cup should be seated as instructed by the manufacturers (**Fig. 2.26**). Screws are an option in uncemented cups if there is a concern about bone quality or integration. Some surgeons use them routinely to provide additional fix prior to integration; others almost never use them.

## Femur

Femoral preparation will vary depending on whether the implant is cemented or uncemented. A view of the calcar, the apex of the neck, is important for establishing version. Rasps and broaches are used to prepare the canal for the femoral implant.

Trial implants are placed, and then an assessment of position and stability is undertaken.

- Leg Length – Check leg lengths by comparing the distal femora with the preincision lengths. The relative positions of the knees can be assessed.

- Stability – Externally rotate in extension and internally rotate in flexion. The hip should not sublux or dislocate. No impingement should occur between the greater trochanter and the poster wall of the socket.

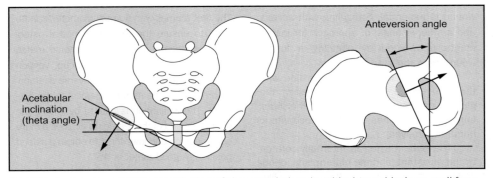

Fig. 2.26 Acetabular position. Positioning of the acetabulum is critical to achieving a well-functioning total hip replacement.

- Offset – Using the swab, apply traction in the line of the neck while supporting the leg with the other hand in neutral abduction. A few millimetres is good; none means the offset is excessive, and a centimetre or more indicates too little offset. Offset can often be varied using modular options of the head or stem.

### Implantation

The acetabulum is implanted first. Cement may be used for both implants, one implant, or none. Different cement brands will set at different rates, which is affected by ambient temperature and storage. Familiarity is required with locally used cement and setting characteristics. Cement is applied to the acetabulum during its working phase, and the cup is placed, paying attention to its inclination and version (**Fig. 2.26**).

Pulsatile saline lavage is used to thoroughly clean the canal, and then the canal is dried with a swab.

Cement is inserted into the femur with a retrograde technique using a gun. Pressurisation is achieved with a rubber collar and requires the nozzle to be shortened (**Fig. 2.27**).

Stem insertion starts on the posterior aspect of this centreline for a centre–centre tip with no cement defects. Sinking the stem should be done smoothly and in stages. The version should match that at trial or the planned change from trialling.

While the cement sets, any movement can torque the stem and create a wider cement void then the stem can fill. If this goes unnoticed, the stem can toggle within the cement mantle causing wear at the cement–implant interface leading to early failure.

A trial reduction is undertaken to confirm the head sizing. Following this the definitive head can be placed and the joint reduced.

### Soft Tissue Repair and Wound Closure

The posterior soft tissue can then be repaired. A heavy nonabsorbable suture is ideal, with the soft tissue repaired to the greater trochanter (**Fig. 2.28**). A running stitch with an absorbable no. 1 suture is performed along the remaining short lateral rotators.

The wound is repaired in layers to reduce dead space and the potential for accumulation of fluid. The skin is ideally repaired with a continuous subcuticular absorbable suture. The addition of wound glue supports this repair and provides a barrier to ingress of contamination.

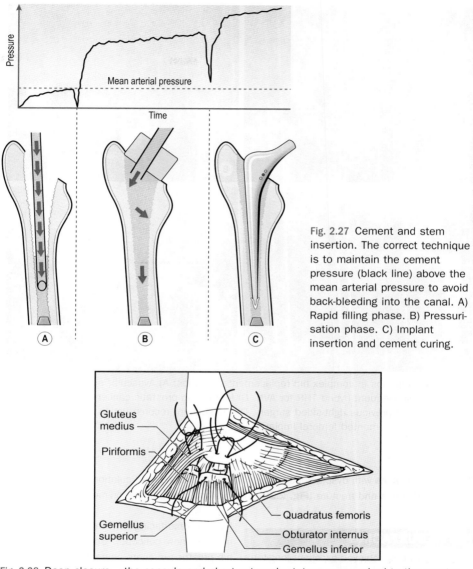

Fig. 2.27 Cement and stem insertion. The correct technique is to maintain the cement pressure (black line) above the mean arterial pressure to avoid back-bleeding into the canal. A) Rapid filling phase. B) Pressurisation phase. C) Implant insertion and cement curing.

Fig. 2.28 Deep closure – the capsule and short external rotators are repaired to the greater trochanter. This step may reduce the dislocation risk and increases the barriers between the external environment and joint.

The surgeon should assist with the subsequent transfer of the patient from the operating table to ensure there is no risk of dislocation during the period where there is reduced protective sensation and muscle tone.

## Hip Replacement in Complex Situations

Some require specialist equipment and expertise. The signs of a potentially more demanding operation can be subtle and easily missed.

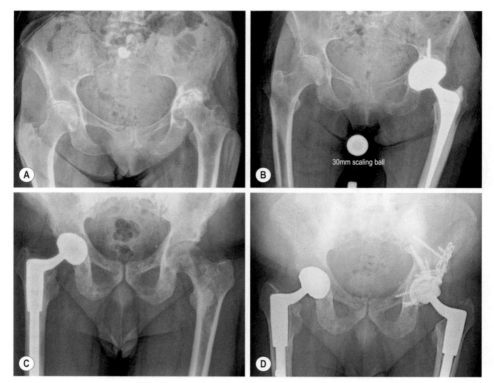

Fig. 2.29 Radiographs in complex hip replacement scenarios: A) Avascular necrosis with head collapse. B) Subsequent hybrid THR for AVN. C) Metastatic prostatic cancer (involving pelvis and femur), with previous right-sided surgery. D) Subsequent reconstruction of acetabulum and long-stem uncemented femoral implant.

These include cases with dysplasia, bone loss, metastatic disease and fracture (**Fig. 2.29**).

## HIP RESURFACING

Although THR has achieved excellent long-term outcomes and patient satisfaction, there has been ongoing research and development to optimise implant design, bone preservation and articulation surface technology (tribology). The modern era of hip resurfacing is an example of how development and implementation of novel orthopaedic implants and techniques can lead to unintended consequences and adverse events. The aim of hip resurfacing is to preserve bone, particularly in younger patients,

and introduce an articulation with superior wear characteristics (metal-on-metal).

Neither resurfacing nor metal-on-metal bearings are new concepts. Some of the earliest hip prostheses share characteristics with their modern counterparts. As far back as 1940 when Ring implanted the first of his eponymous hip replacements, metal-on-metal was chosen. The Ring and McKee–Farrar bearing surfaces were made of Vitalium (a cobalt chrome alloy). Both had good survival rates, especially when considering their novel and pioneering use. Resurfacing was attempted as far back as 1946 when the Judet hemiarthropasty was produced from acrylic. It was later adapted to include a central metal rod to increase the implant strength (**Fig. 2.30**). Acrylic was not ideally suited to life as a bearing surface; nonetheless, some long-surviving examples can be found in the literature. The evolution of Charnley's low-friction arthroplasty and the use of cemented implants with a metal-on-polyethylene bearing (hard-on-soft) marked the started of wide-spread adoption of successful and reproducible arthroplasty techniques.

With the Charnley, a femoral head of 22.225 mm was selected after experimentation with various sizes. This is the metric conversion of the original imperial 7/8 of an inch. This size was a good compromise between volumetric wear (worse with larger bearings) and linear wear (increased by a smaller head which has higher contact forces) and had a lower frictional torque upon the acetabulum. The downside of the small head was the reduced jump distance and susceptibility to dislocation (**Fig. 2.23**). A return to resurfacing and metal bearing surfaces occurred to address these negative features of the total hip replacement.

## Metal-on-Metal Articulation

It was hypothesised that metal-on-metal resurfacing should theoretically allow for anatomical sized heads that reduce dislocation rates and replicate normal hip anatomy (**Fig. 2.31**). It should also have reduced stress shielding. The low-wear characteristics should have avoided the problems of aseptic loosening observed with polyethylene debris. Unfortunately, it was later discovered that metal-on-metal bearings could lead to the release of cobalt and chromium ions during wear. In severe cases, local soft tissue reactions occurred, and these are termed ALVAL (Aseptic lymphocyte-dominant vasculitis-associated lesion), or pseudotumours. These are not malignant but can result in local tissue destruction, pain and loss of function.

In addition, despite being bone preserving for the femur, greater bone removal is required on the acetabular side to accommodate the socket and larger head. Thin metal acetabular components minimise this compared with using cement and polyethylene, which would require excessive bone removal. Attempts to use thinner acetabular shells resulted in unintended shell deformation, point loading and increased wear.

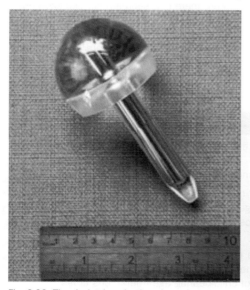

Fig. 2.30 The Judet hemiarthroplasty was an early iteration of hip resurfacing. Note the central, metal stem, indicating that this was a later version of the prosthesis. *Picture courtesy of Andrew C. Macey.*

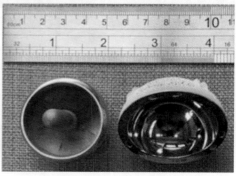

Fig. 2.31 Example of hip resurfacing implants (head on left, socket on right) (Birmingham Hip Resurfacing (Smith & Nephew)). *Picture courtesy of Andrew C. Macey.*

Hip resurfacing may still be a viable option in a small group of patients. Correct patient selection is vital (**Table 2.7**). It is contraindicated in women of child-bearing age due the unknown effects of metal ions on a developing foetus. Lower bone density in older patients and small pelvic geometry in women means the procedure is generally reserved for younger males with a sufficiently large native hip. Smaller head sizes make the implant more susceptible to malposition of the acetabulum, decreasing the load bearing surface, so a minimum of a 48-mm diameter head has also been adopted as part of patient selection.

Implant related complications for hip resurfacing include dislocation, loosening, wear, elevated metal ions, ALVAL/pseudotumour and periprosthetic fracture. The risk of periprosthetic fracture is increased if the implant is malpositioned or the surrounding bone is osteoporotic.

---

## Improving the Outcome from Joint Replacement

### ODEP

This body was set up in the UK to provide a way of assessing the longevity of orthopaedic implants

Manufacturers submit evidence for assessment, and an implant is given a score, e.g., 7B, 13A or 13A*.

The number refers to a benchmark for years of follow-up, with 3, 5, 7, 10, 13 and 15 years being the current benchmarks. These will extend as longer follow-up evidence is available.

The letter given is either A or B and grades the quality of evidence based on the number of contributing centres, total study cohort and the number of surviving patients. A represents implants with higher quality evidence higher quality. Low-volume implants will usually have B ratings.

A* is an indicator of the highest quality of evidence, including from centres outside of the developing centre and a lower revision rate at each benchmark.

### Joint Registries

Joint registries track, at a national level, the operations, complication and revision rates for various joint replacements.

The practice originated in Sweden where there is a separate hip and knee registry. New Zealand had the first English language registry. In the UK, the National Joint Registry (NJR) collects data for England, Wales, Northern Ireland, The Isle of Man and Guernsey. Other large databases include the Norwegian, Danish and American.

| Table 2.7 | Indications and Contraindications for Hip Resurfacing | |
|---|---|---|
| Indications | | • Young, active patient with osteoarthritis<br>• Male<br>• Head diameter of >48 mm |
| Contraindications | Absolute | • Avascular necrosis<br>• Cystic degeneration of the femoral head<br>• Osteoporosis<br>• Fracture |
| | Relative | • Coxa vara (alters biomechanics and predisposes to periprosthetic fracture)<br>• Females of child-bearing age (metal ions cross placenta)<br>• Renal failure (reduced metal ion clearance)<br>• Leg length discrepancy – not correctable with resurfacing |

The Scottish Arthroplasty Project runs in Scotland, but it is not a true registry as it does not collect implant data.

The NJR in the UK produces detailed reports for implant survival which can even be broken down by component combinations, method of fixation and bearing surfaces. Data are also available by age of the patient. A wealth of information is available and allows the surgeon to choose an evidence-based implant.

*Advantages*
- Large body of data – bigger than feasible for prospective trials
- Longitudinal follow-up
- Describes the performance of an implant for an average surgeon – not just the originating centre or high-volume surgeons
- Can pick up early worrying trends

*Disadvantages*
- Costly
- Data quality reliant on high compliance for entry
- Single endpoint of revision
- Variation in definition of revision between registries
- Can be a lag time in data release and then a lag time in reaction

## Follow-up of Patients with Metal-on-Metal Hips

The Medical Healthcare Products Regulatory Agency in the United Kingdom has released guidance on follow-up and investigations for patients with metal-on-metal hip replacements. Follow-up requirements depend on the following:

- Whether it is a resurfacing or a large head THR

- The implant's Orthopaedic Device Evaluation Panel rating

- Head size

- Patient age and sex

## Information: Orthopaedic Device Evaluation Panel (ODEP)

Annual follow-up is advised for most patients and includes blood metal ion levels, radiographs and clinical assessment.

For those with implants having at least an ODEP 10A rating (e.g., a Birmingham hip resurfacing) less frequent follow-up is possible. Any patient with a symptomatic metal-on-metal resurfacing should have serum cobalt and chrome ions measured and a metal artefact reducing sequence MRI of the hip to look for pseudotumours. Any abnormality of bloods, imaging or symptoms is cause to consider revision.

# 3 The Knee

Chloe EH Scott, Tim White, Michael JC Brown

The knee is a complex hinge joint consisting of three functional compartments within the same capsule: the medial, lateral, and patellofemoral compartments. In addition to a range of motion of 140 degrees in the sagittal plane, during flexion there is also anteroposterior (AP) glide and rotation. Rotation occurs around a pivot point in the medial compartment, with AP glide observed most in the lateral compartment: The lateral femoral condyle glides posteriorly across the lateral tibial plateau as the knee flexes. Given the relatively incongruent bony anatomy, several soft tissue structures also control and stabilize motion (**Fig. 3.1**). The medial and lateral menisci are fibrocartilaginous structures that act to increase congruency of the medial and lateral compartments, increase joint surface area, reduce contact stress, accommodate glide/rollback and disperse synovial fluid, which is produced by the lining of the synovial joint. The anterior and posterior cruciate ligaments (ACL and PCL), respectively, limit anterior and posterior translation of the tibia and have key roles in maintaining rotational stability. The collateral ligaments restrain varus/valgus force and have a secondary role in maintaining rotational stability.

50%. There are several additional risk factors, including:

- Genetic predisposition

- Trauma

- Obesity

- Inflammatory joint disease

Pain in knee OA is complex and multifactorial. It is not necessarily proportional to the extent of radiographic change. It is thought to result from the stimulation of subchondral nociceptive pain receptors through a complex interaction of synovial inflammation, venous congestion and increased intraosseous pressure. Pain is also affected by central factors such as comorbidity, response to analgesia and psychosocial influences. A striking feature of OA is that some patients with advanced disease have few symptoms, while others with only minor pathological changes seem to experience debilitating pain and restriction. OA may affect a single compartment of the knee (e.g., the patellofemoral joint [PFJ] or medial compartment), or it may be widespread (or tricompartmental).

## OSTEOARTHRITIS OF THE KNEE

Osteoarthritis (OA) of the knee can be classified according to its aetiology as primary (idiopathic, or nontraumatic) or secondary (e.g., due to trauma or gross mechanical misalignment).

OA has traditionally been viewed as a disease caused by 'overuse' or 'wear and tear' but is arguably better described as 'age-related' as the lifetime risk of symptomatic knee OA is

## Clinical Assessment

### History

Identify the severity and duration of the following symptoms:

- **Pain** is classically mechanical, being worse with weight-bearing activity and better with rest. It is often described as being dull and aching. Pain that wakes a patient at night when moving is particularly intrusive.

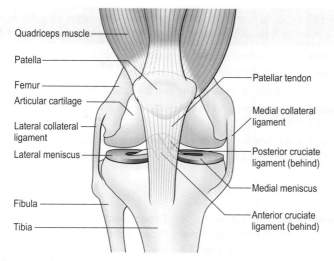

Fig. 3.1 Line diagram of the knee.

- **Stiffness** is usually worse after a period of inactivity and better once the patient has been up and about for some time or when local heat is applied.

- **Swelling** is due to effusion fluid, tissue thickening and osteophytes.

- **Crepitus** is the crunching sensation arising from damaged joints with movement.

- **Catching and subjective instability** are common due to snagging of the damaged joint surfaces and pain inhibition of muscles, and it should be distinguished from locking or true instability [refer to Key Point box page 94].

- **Functional impairment** involves mechanical symptoms that limit activities of daily living, recreation, and occupation.

## Examination

See page 100 [later in this chapter]

## Investigations
### Plain radiographs

Plain radiographs are almost always sufficient for the investigation of OA. **Weight-bearing** AP and lateral views are used initially, complemented by specific compartment or alignment views as required. The radiographic changes of knee OA can be classified (**Table 3.1**) and are easily remembered using the acronym LOSS (**Fig. 3.2**):

- **L**oss of joint space

- **O**steophyte formation

- **S**ubchondral sclerosis

- **S**ubchondral cyst formation

### Special Views

**Merchant's (or skyline) view:** Helpful to visualize the PFJ if there is concern about arthritis and/or patellar maltracking (see **Fig. 3.2C**).

| Table 3.1 | Radiographic classification of knee OA using the Kellgren and Lawrence classification (based on AP weight-bearing x-rays) |
|---|---|
| Grade 0 | No joint space narrowing (JSN) or reactive changes |
| Grade 1 | Possible osteophytic lipping and doubtful JSN |
| Grade 2 | Definite osteophyte formation and possible JSN |
| Grade 3 | Moderate osteophytes and definite JSN and some sclerosis and possible bone end deformity |
| Grade 4 | Large osteophytes and marked JSN and severe sclerosis and definite bone end deformity |

**Long-leg alignment views:** May be useful in context of previous trauma, markedly abnormal alignment or adjacent joint pathology (**Figs 3.3** and **3.4**).

**Rosenberg view:** This is a weight-bearing PA film taken with the knee in 30 to 45 degrees of flexion. It visualizes the lateral compartment where areas of cartilage loss typically engage in flexion and can be missed when radiographs are taken with the knee extended (**Fig. 3.5**).

**AP pelvis radiograph:** The hips should always be assessed clinically when knee pain is being investigated; where there is any irritability or stiffness, radiographs should be obtained.

## Cross-Sectional Imaging

Cross-sectional imaging is rarely required for the assessment of OA, although computed tomography (CT) may be useful when there is significant bone loss to help with surgical planning. Magnetic resonance imaging (MRI) can identify other causes of knee pain, such as osteonecrosis, when initial radiographs fail to provide diagnostic clarity.

## Treatment
### Nonsurgical Treatments
The first line of treatment for OA of the knee is nonsurgical; two-thirds of patients never require knee surgery:

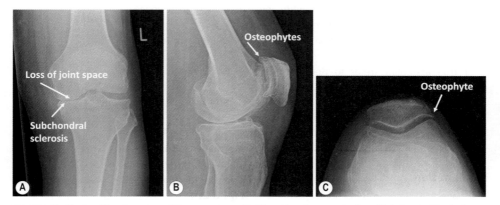

Fig. 3.2 Radiographic changes of knee osteoarthritis. A) anteroposterior; B) lateral; C) skyline.

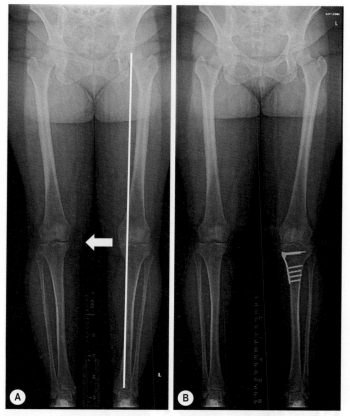

Fig. 3.3 Hip–knee–ankle radiographs before and after high tibial osteotomy (HTO). A) The line of mechanical axis runs from the centre of the femoral head to the centre of the ankle and passes through the medial compartment indicating varus. Surgery aims to move the knee toward the midline. B) Postoperative image after corrective HTO.

- **Exercise** that involves a programme of muscle building and strengthening should be encouraged at all stages of the disease.

- **Weight loss** is important because obesity both causes and exacerbates knee OA. Weight loss (aiming for 10–20% reduction) improves mobility and reduces joint loading and pain; the knee is a force multiplier – that is, weight reduction by 1 kg reduces the forces in the knee by 4 kg.

- **Pain management** consists of advice regarding simple painkillers and progression up the analgesic ladder. First-line analgesia consists

of regular paracetamol with topical anti-inflammatory application. Topical capsaicin treatment is also safe and effective. Oral nonsteroidal anti-inflammatory drugs (NSAIDs) and opiates have the potential for long-term side effects and should therefore be used with caution, particularly in the elderly. Electrotherapy via transcutaneous electrical nerve stimulation (TENS) has been shown to provide an effective form of pain relief.

- **Orthoses** are important because off-loading braces are effective where there is predominantly unicompartmental OA, particularly with a correctable coronal deformity. Walking

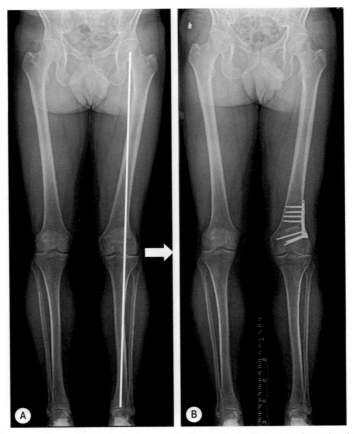

Fig. 3.4 Hip–knee–ankle radiographs before and after DFO. A) The line of mechanical axis passes through the lateral compartment indicating valgus. Surgery aims to move the knee away from the midline. B) Postoperative image after corrective DFO.

aids can maximize function and facilitate exercise.

- **Injections** such as intraarticular corticosteroids can be used for temporary symptom control when other therapies have failed, but the effects can be short lived. The role of platelet-rich plasma (PRP) and other biological therapies is incompletely understood but evolving.

- **Other therapies** such as glucosamine or chondroitin sulphate supplements are not recommended based on current evidence. Similarly, acupuncture is not supported by scientific evidence for OA of the knee.

## Surgical Treatments
### Knee Arthroscopy

Arthroscopic lavage is not an appropriate or effective treatment for OA of the knee. Arthroscopy is reserved for patients who have localised mechanical symptoms, with confirmed discrete pathology (such as an unstable meniscal tear), with minimal background degenerative changes, who have failed a period of conservative treatment. Arthroscopic debridement of degenerate meniscal tears does not provide sustained benefit. Loose body removal is usually effective at relieving mechanical symptoms.

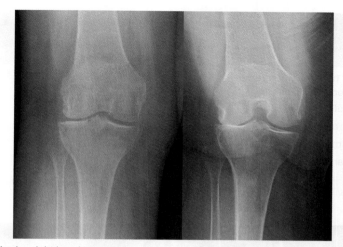

Fig. 3.5 Standard weight-bearing anteroposterior and Rosenberg posteroanterior views of the same knee on the same day.

## Correction of Malalignment

Malalignment may be the cause or the consequence of OA: Patients with primary or post-traumatic malalignment are predisposed to developing OA, and the progress of the OA may be slowed or modified by correction of the alignment. Similarly, joint space loss can result in progressive malalignment, which then exacerbates overloading and pain, the typical varus (bowed-legged) posture in medial compartment knee OA being a very common example. Although for patients with end-stage OA, total knee arthroplasty allows correction of all but the most severe alignment abnormalities, in younger patients, correction of malalignment with bracing or osteotomy can improve symptoms and function and buy time before salvage arthroplasty is considered.

**Bracing,** such as the use of varus or valgus off-loading braces, is effective in restoring alignment and improving symptoms and function, particularly where the malalignment is correctable and the OA affects only the medial or lateral compartment. Bracing can be a helpful indication of likely symptom relief for patients considering osteotomy.

**High tibial osteotomy (HTO)** addresses the most common knee deformity: varus alignment secondary to isolated degenerative change in the medial compartment; it is usually a medial opening wedge (see **Fig. 3.3**). HTO is successful in 80% patients at 10 years, provided patients are selected appropriately (**Table 3.2**). Normal posterior tibial slope in the sagittal plane (~9°) is usually maintained; however, decreasing the posterior slope can be of use in the ACL-deficient knee, and, conversely, increasing the degree of slope can help prevent instability with PCL deficiency.

**Distal femoral osteotomy** is most commonly performed for valgus alignment and lateral compartment OA using a lateral opening wedge (see **Fig. 3.4**). Periarticular osteotomy of the knee can be performed either using measurements taken from full-length preoperative radiographs with intraoperative fluoroscopy or with intraoperative computer navigation software.

## Arthroplasty

When nonoperative or joint-preserving knee surgery fails, knee replacement surgery can be

**Table 3.2   Indications and contraindications for periarticular osteotomy of the knee**

| Indications | Contraindications |
|---|---|
| Young active patients who are not candidates for arthroplasty | Inflammatory arthritis |
| | Obesity |
| Normal vascular supply | Flexion contracture >15° |
| Normal body mass index | Knee flexion <90° |
| Pain interfering with activities of daily living | >20° of correction required |
| Single compartment disease | Patellofemoral arthritis |
| | Significant ligamentous instability |

**Table 3.3   Indications and contraindications for medial unicompartmental knee replacement**

| Indications and contraindications for medial UKR | |
|---|---|
| Indications | Contraindications |
| Symptomatic KL3 OA medial compartment | Inflammatory arthropathy |
| Intact ACL | KL4 patellofemoral OA |
| Intact MCL | Fixed flexion deformity >10° |
| Correctable varus | Flexion <90° |
| FFD <10° | Deficient ACL (mobile bearing UKR) |
| | Absent lateral meniscus |

KL, Kellgren and Lawrence classification; ACL, anterior cruciate ligament; MCL, medial cruciate ligament; FFD, fixed flexion deformity; UKR, unicompartmental knee replacement.

considered. This involves replacing the knee joint, either partially (a unicompartmental knee replacement [UKR]) or completely (a total knee replacement [TKR]).

## KNEE REPLACEMENT

Knee replacement is a highly clinically and cost-effective treatment for end-stage symptomatic degenerative arthritis of the knee. It significantly improves quality of life and indeed can be life-changing. Simple hinges were introduced in the 1950s followed by condylar resurfacing implants in the 1970s, which have subsequently evolved into the modern knee arthroplasty designs we use today. The demand for knee arthroplasty is increasing year on year

with increased life expectancy and increased expectation of quality of life. As mentioned, knee replacement surgery may be partial (UKR) or total (TKR). The relative indications and contraindications for medial UKR and TKR are given in **Tables 3.3** and **3.4**.

**Unicompartmental knee replacement** is an option when only one compartment of the knee is involved (see **Table 3.3**). Approximately 10% of primary knee arthroplasty procedures are currently UKRs, though approximately one-third of patients are potentially suitable. Advantages over TKR include faster rehabilitation; preservation of more normal knee mechanics through ACL retention; shorter length of hospital stay; lower

**Table 3.4    Indications and contraindications for total knee arthroplasty**

| Indications | Contraindications |
| --- | --- |
| Severe symptomatic knee arthritis (KL ≥3) | Knee infection or sepsis from any source |
| Failure of conservative treatment | Medical comorbidity that would make surgery and anaesthesia dangerous |
| Osteonecrosis with subchondral collapse | Significant vascular disease |
| Severe deformity or instability | Soft tissue or skin conditions |
| Failed joint-preserving surgery (HTO, DFO, UKR) | |

KL, Kellgren and Lawrence classification; HTO, high tibial osteotomy; DFO, distal femoral osteotomy; UKR, unicompartmental knee replacement.

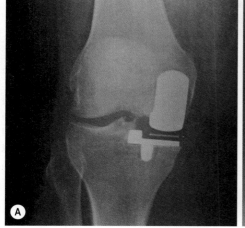 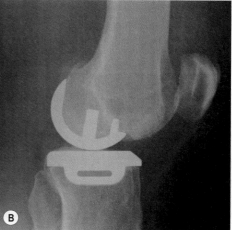

Fig. 3.6  Medial UKR.

blood loss and lower risks of infection, venous thromboembolism, and death. The most common UKR is of the medial compartment (**Fig. 3.6**). More rarely, partial knee replacement of the isolated lateral compartment (**Fig. 3.7**) or the isolated PFJ (**Fig. 3.8**) is performed. All varieties of UKR come with an increased risk of revision surgery by 10 years when compared to TKR, but at 25 years 70% of UKRs are intact and unrevised.

**Total knee replacement** is an effective and reliable treatment for pain when nonoperative or joint preserving techniques have failed (see **Table 3.4**). A persistent 10% to 20% rate of dissatisfaction after TKR continues to drive different philosophies in both implant design and implantation technique.

## Primary TKR Implants

TKR involves resurfacing the tibiofemoral joint of the knee +/- the patella to obtain a pain-free, balanced and stable knee joint. In a standard primary knee replacement, the tibial and femoral components are not linked together, and the stability of the TKR in all planes depends on the native knee ligaments. Femoral components are typically made of cobalt chrome or stainless steel and are highly polished to articulate with a polyethylene insert and the patella; they can be fixed in place with cement or be uncemented with bone on-growth. Tibial baseplates are typically also metallic, most usually titanium, with a short stem or flange to give rotational stability, and again can be cemented or uncemented. Metal tibial

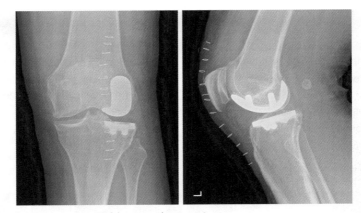

Fig. 3.7 Lateral unicompartmental knee replacement.

components have modular polyethylene inserts that come in 1- to 2-mm thickness increments. Alternatively, tibial components can be non-modular, made entirely of polyethylene, and these must be cemented.

## Cruciate Retention or Sacrifice

Though some rare bicruciate retaining implants are available, TKR typically involves removing the ACL. The PCL can be retained or sacrificed depending on the implant. Cruciate retaining (CR) implants employ a relatively nonconforming polyethylene insert and rely on the integrity of the native PCL to facilitate rollback in flexion (**Fig. 3.9A**). In contrast, posterior stabilized (PS) designs remove the PCL and an additional box of bone on the femoral side and replace it with a cam and post mechanism (see **Fig. 3.9B**). The cam and post interaction guides rollback during knee flexion. Somewhere between these design principles lie more conforming polyethylene inserts, which provide some AP stability due to their deep-dish designs but which do not involve a post.

## Fixed or Mobile Bearing

Where tibial components are modular (a metal tray and a polyethylene insert), these parts can be either fixed together via a click-in mechanism (fixed bearing), or the polyethylene can be designed to rotate on a polished metal tibial base plate surface (mobile bearing). The mobile bearing concept is based on the fact that the native knee rotates during flexion. Motion at this interface does, however, have the potential to generate more polyethylene wear.

## The Ladder of Constraint

The level of constraint refers to how linked the tibial and femoral components of a TKR are in order to achieve a balanced and stable knee joint. Less constrained implants rely on native soft tissue for stability (see **Fig. 3.9A–C**), whereas fully constrained implants include linkage of femoral and tibial components as hinges (see **Fig. 3.9D**), replacing the function of all cruciate and collateral ligaments.

Increasing constraint results in increased stability but comes at a cost: Constraint can conflict with normal knee mechanics, and moreover, increased constraint transmits greater stress to the bone-cement or bone-implant interface, resulting in early loosening. The least level of necessary constraint should therefore be used.

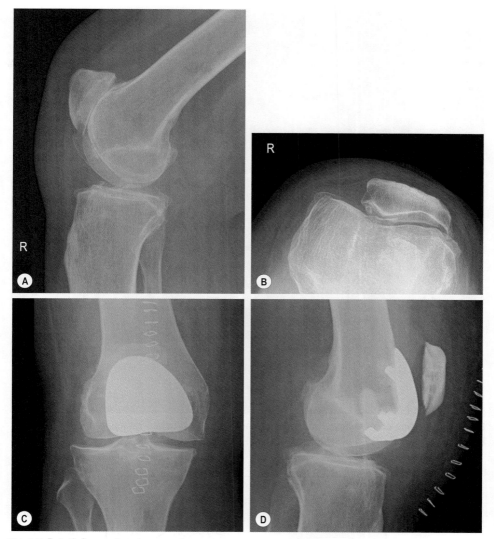

Fig. 3.8 Patellofemoral replacement.

## Alignment

To insert a TKR, sufficient bone must be removed to fit in the implants. The orientation of these bone cuts determines the alignment of both the implant and of the lower limb. These cuts create gaps. The aim is to obtain gaps that are symmetrical and equal in flexion and extension, and throughout a range of motion (**Fig. 3.10**).

The extension gap is governed by

● Distal femoral resection (cut)

● Tibial resection

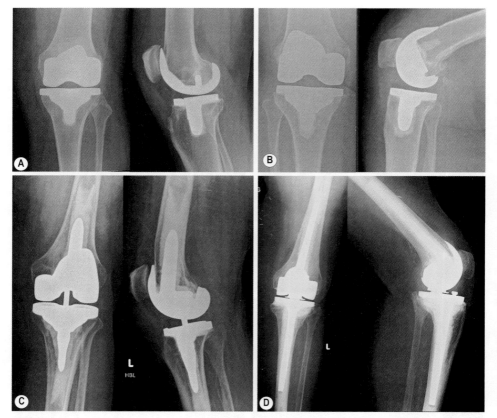

Fig. 3.9 Increasing constraint in total knee replacement. A) Cruciate retaining design. B) Posterior stabilized. C) Constrained condylar. D) Hinge.

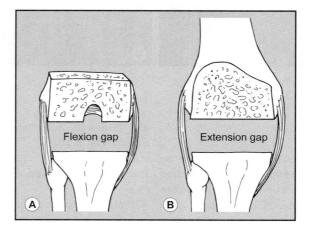

Fig. 3.10 A) Flexion and B) extension gaps.

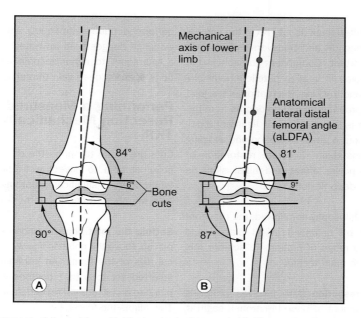

Fig. 3.11 Alignment philosophies. A) Mechanical alignment. B) Kinematic alignment.

The flexion gap is influenced by

- Position of the femoral AP cuts (i.e., amount of posterior condylar resection)

- Rotation of the femoral cuts

- Tibial resection

Different philosophies exist in terms of alignment aims (**Fig. 3.11**):

**Mechanical alignment (MA):** The aim is neutral coronal plane alignment of the limb, with a tibial cut that is perpendicular to the mechanical axis (i.e., parallel to the floor and perpendicular to the tibial anatomical axis). The distal femur is cut in 5 to 7 degrees of valgus (see **Fig. 3.11A**). As the native joint line is most frequently oblique and displays considerable variation, these resections often create an asymmetrical extension gap, and therefore soft tissue releases are required to make this symmetrical and to balance the knee. Asymmetrical flexion gaps can similarly require soft tissue release to obtain symmetrical gaps and a balanced knee.

**Kinematic alignment (KA):** There is marked variation in local native knee anatomy and alignment. The aim of KA is to recreate the 3D anatomy of the knee's prearthritic joint surfaces and match the native flexion–extension axis. In the coronal plane this typically means increased femoral component valgus and tibial component varus resulting in an oblique joint line, though overall mechanical alignment may still be neutral. The posterior tibial slope aims to match native slope as does femoral component rotation, which is referenced from the posterior femoral condyles. This should create symmetrical, rectangular flexion and extension gaps requiring no or minimal soft tissue releases for balance (see **Fig. 3.11B**).

**Restricted KA:** This is KA within a predefined safe zone to avoid extreme outliers that have the potential for early loosening.

Though we often think about TKR in the coronal plane, the sagittal and transverse planes are equally important. Component rotation in the transverse plan is vital to patellofemoral biomechanics and tracking. Recreation of the joint line with appropriate resection depths from the distal femur is key in achieving ligament isometry throughout a range of motion and avoiding midflexion instability. Accurate restoration of posterior condylar offset and tibial slope is required for deep flexion.

Whichever philosophy is followed, the resultant knee must be balanced in all planes and throughout a range of motion. To achieve this there are two main techniques:

**Measured resection** (MR) involves removing the same amount of bone in coronal, sagittal, and transverse planes as is replaced with the implant. This typically involves performing femoral cuts first and can be used to deliver either mechanical or kinematic alignment.

**Gap balancing** (GB) involves cutting the tibia first and using this cut to reference the femoral cuts. This should create rectangular flexion and extension gaps with femoral rotation set according to the tibia, and soft tissue releases should be minimal. GB can be used to deliver mechanical or kinematic alignment.

Achieving kinematic alignment often requires additional technologies such as patient-specific jigs or robotic assistance. Mechanical alignment can be delivered using MR or GB techniques using jigs.

## Surgical Approach

TKR is typically performed via a medial parapatellar or subvastus approach. The lateral parapatellar approach is rarely used for TKR, although some surgeons advocate its use in knees with marked valgus deformity. UKR is performed through less extensive versions of these approaches. Traditionally TKR has been performed under tourniquet, although recent evidence suggests an advantage in not using a tourniquet to minimize pain and complications such as deep vein thrombosis.

## Performing a Measured Resection Mechanically Aligned TKR

Cuts are made to shape the distal femur and proximal tibia to accept well-fitting implants. Where there is significant anatomical variation, cuts will need to be adjusted.

**Setting the joint line.** A femoral entry hole is placed above the notch in line with the anatomical axis of the femur. An intramedullary jig is inserted set to 5 to 7 degrees valgus with a planned distal femoral resection of 8 to 10 mm. This aligns the femoral component perpendicular to the mechanical axis of the lower limb and sets the level of the joint line.

**Sizing and rotation.** Femoral component size is determined according to the AP diameter of the femur. The rotation is referenced as either (a) parallel to the transepicondylar axis, (b) perpendicular to Whiteside line, or (c) at 3 degrees of external rotation to the posterior condylar axis (PCA) (**Fig. 3.12**). Note that in valgus OA, the lateral femoral condyle is often hypoplastic, and referencing rotation from the PCA alone risks an internally rotated femoral component and potentially patella maltracking. A cutting block is used to make the posterior femoral condyle and chamfer cuts. The aim is to maintain posterior condylar offset, minimize anterior femoral offset, avoid notching of the anterior femur and position the trochlea to facilitate patella tracking.

**Tibial cut:** An extramedullary jig is used to measure a cut that is perpendicular to the anatomical axis. Proximally the jig is positioned at the ACL footprint. Distally it is aligned with the centre of the ankle (tibialis anterior tendon at the ankle). Rotation is determined by a line

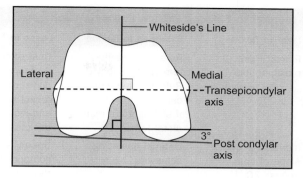

Fig. 3.12 Anatomical references for femoral rotation.

from the medial third of the tibial tuberosity to the PCL insertion. Posterior tibial slope is set according to implant specifications (typically 3°). Enough bone is resected to insert the TKR. If femoral component + tibial baseplate + 9-mm polyethylene = 17 mm, and 8 mm have been taken from the distal femur, then 9 mm must be taken from the proximal tibia. This resection depth is measured from the intact side of the knee, typically the lateral side. Where the medial plateau is used as reference, the resection depth is typically 2 to 4 mm as the proximal tibia is usually varus, and thus the medial plateau is lower than the lateral.

**Osteophytes:** Medial and lateral osteophytes affect coronal balance and must be removed before any soft tissue release. Removing osteophytes is often all that is required for balance. Posterior femoral condyle osteophytes cause fixed flexion and should be removed before distal femoral recuts that raise the joint line are considered for fixed flexion.

**Balancing:** Where flexion and extension gaps are not rectangular and equal, soft tissue balancing is required. **Table 3.5** indicates causes and solutions for common imbalance problems. The tibial surface is common to both flexion and extension gaps, so resecting more tibia will increase both gaps. The femur has different flexion and extension surfaces, so recuts depend upon the specific imbalance encountered.

## Modern Technologies

Optimizing alignment and balance are key areas of research in knee arthroplasty, and modern technologies can aid in delivering accurate patient-specific plans. This includes computer navigation and techniques informed by 3D cross-sectional imaging (CT or MRI) such as patient-specific jigs, customized implants, or robotic-assisted surgery. These techniques can deliver more accurate bone cuts, which may lead to increased longevity. Pressure sensors and robotic assistance also quantify balance throughout a range of motion intraoperatively. The evidence base for these technologies is growing, but benefits in terms of either satisfaction or longevity are currently not proven.

## TKR Complications

TKR has a success rate up to 90% in terms of patient satisfaction. Recovery can be arduous, and significant pain and swelling are expected up to 8 weeks. Most of the benefit is realized by 6 months, but TKRs typically continue to improve up to and sometimes beyond 1 year. Approximately 12% of patients will complain of persisting chronic pain postoperatively despite having no identifiable problem with their implant. Significant complications include:

**Table 3.5   Strategies to balance flexion and extension gaps**

| | Tight in flexion | Balanced in flexion | Loose in flexion |
|---|---|---|---|
| **Tight in extension** | Resect more proximal tibia | Remove posterior femoral osteophytes Release posterior capsule If still tight cut more distal femur | Upsize femoral component and decrease polyethylene thickness or resect more distal femur and increase polyethylene thickness |
| **Balanced in extension** | Increase posterior slope of tibia Recess PCL Downsize femoral component | Optimal balancing achieved | Upsize femoral component or augment the posterior femur or increase polyethylene constraint to CS or PS instead of CR |
| **Loose in extension** | Use a thicker polyethylene AND increase posterior slope of tibia or recess PCL or downsize femoral component | Augment distal femur | Upsize polyethylene or augment the tibial baseplate |

PCL, posterior cruciate ligament; CS, cruciate substituting deep dish; CR, cruciate retaining; PS, posterior stabilised.

- **Mortality** within 90 days occurs in ~1/300 cases and, predictably, this rate increases with age and comorbidity.

- **Infection.** The overall deep periprosthetic infection rate after TKR is ~1%. No single test is diagnostic for this devastating complication, which can present as a profound sepsis, a slightly painful knee, or anything in between. An arthroplasty surgeon must always have a high index of suspicion for infection, and diagnosis is made using a combination of history; examination; blood tests; joint aspirate and radiological investigations, including plain radiographs or nuclear medicine bone scans. Infection is treated with revision surgery and antibiotics, often for prolonged periods, with success dependent on a number of host and organism factors.

- **Stiffness.** The greatest predictor of postoperative knee stiffness is preoperative knee stiffness. Component malpositioning is rarely the cause but is potentially rectifiable with revision surgery. Where components are well positioned, stiffness occurring in the first 3 months of TKR can be treated with manipulation under anaesthesia (MUA). This has a risk of fracture but is usually a successful strategy. Cases of arthrofibrosis can recur.

- **Vascular injury** is thankfully rare, occurring in ~1/10,000 cases, but the sequelae of a missed vascular injury are devasting. Care must be taken intraoperatively to protect neurovascular structures, and the patient's neurovascular status should be reassessed and monitored postoperatively.

- **Intraoperative ligamentous or capsule injury** can occur, requiring conversion to a more constrained implant. Damage to the extensor mechanism can be catastrophic and may require complex reconstruction with allograft or mesh and prolonged splintage in extension for several weeks.

- **Venous thromboembolism.** Symptomatic venous thromboembolism (VTE) occurs in up to 5% of patients, but fatal pulmonary embolism is much rarer (0.05%). VTE prophylaxis protocols vary between centres and individual surgeons. Choosing a regimen involves balancing the risks of VTE with risks of wound leakage and bleeding from other sites.

- **Loosening and wear.** In the medium to longer term, TKRs can wear or loosen, requiring revision surgery. Current evidence demonstrates that, overall, 82% of TKRs last at least 25 years. Risk of revision is age-related, with the lifetime risk of revision being much higher in younger patients: Men under 50 have as high as a one-third lifetime risk of revision.

## Revision Knee Arthroplasty

### Modes of Failure

TKRs can fail in several ways, including infection, aseptic loosening, polyethylene wear, instability and periprosthetic fracture. Revision surgery is more complex than primary surgery, and the outcomes are less certain and dependent upon the mode of failure. TKRs should not be revised for unexplained pain without an identified mode of failure that can be corrected at revision surgery.

### Manging Bone Defects

The mode of failure or the removal of the primary implants may create bone defects in the tibia or the femur. These may be contained (with intact cortical bone surrounding them) or uncontained (where both metaphyseal and cortical bone have been lost). These defects are managed according to their size and location using a range of possible techniques, including cement, bone grafting, metal augments or metaphyseal cones or sleeves (**Fig. 3.13**). Where defects are large,

necessitating extra metalwork such as augments or cones, additional stems are required as well for biomechanical stability. This is dictated by the zone of the defect where the epiphysis is zone 1; the metaphysis, zone 2; and the diaphysis, zone 3; A zone 1 defect will require additional support in zone 1 and possibly zone 2; a zone 2 defect will require additional support in zone 2 and possibly zone 3.

### Managing Constraint

Revision TKR typically involves increasing implant constraint. This may be due to the mode of failure (e.g., revision for instability), bone defects destabilizing ligament attachments or the releases involved in accessing the knee joint and removing the primary components. The ladder of constraint is ascended in a stepwise fashion.

### Soft Tissue Envelope

Failure involving infection or fracture may significantly compromise the soft tissue envelope and may require plastic surgery techniques to obtain soft tissue coverage of revision implants such as a medial gastrocnemius flap.

## ANTERIOR KNEE PAIN (PATELOFEMORAL PAIN)

Anterior knee pain is common and encompasses a range of pathologies, typically presenting with:

- *Pain* felt behind or deep to the patella, often worse after prolonged flexion (e.g., while sitting at a desk) or upon descending stairs or slopes

- *Crepitus* on movement

- *Subjective instability.* It is important to distinguish this from true patella instability (see later). In anterior knee pain, the patient commonly complains of feeling pain and then a sensation of the knee 'giving way',

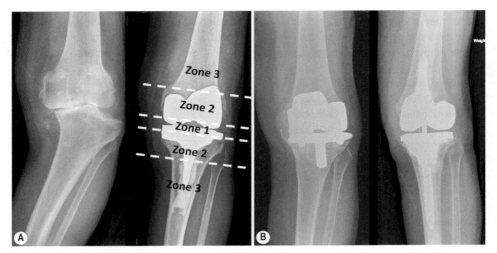

Fig. 3.13 Bone defect management: zone 2 tibial defects managed in a primary total knee replacement with an augment A) and in a revision with a metaphyseal cone B).

resulting from pain inhibition of the quadriceps muscle.

Causes include:

- *Patellofemoral OA.* There is often a history of injury to the PFJ, clear crepitus on examination and narrowing of the joint on the skyline view, with confirmatory MRI changes.

- *Patella overload.* This may result from recurrent instability (see later) or be apparently spontaneous. The term *idiopathic chondromalacia patella* is often used to describe apparent hypersensitivity of the PFJ to pressure and pain in the absence of any identifiable abnormality.

- *Quadriceps or patella tendonitis*, with focal tenderness at the enthesis (tendon insertion)

- *Fat pad impingement* may be seen on MRI and may respond to debridement.

- *Loose bodies* and *anterior meniscal tears* usually result in intermittent, sharp, catching pain.

- *Psychosocial causes* with inappropriate, non-mechanical pain responses

Management is almost always nonoperative with physiotherapy exercises to rehabilitate the quads, vastus medialis obliquus (VMO) and hip girdle muscles. Surgery is likely to be disappointing unless there is a clear biomechanical or radiographic abnormality but occasionally includes:

- Arthroscopic resection of a large plica or inflamed fat pad

- Debridement or radiofrequency ablation of loose chondral flaps on the patella or, rarely, osteochondral grafting of discrete lesions

- Surgery to address underlying patella instability or malalignment where this is demonstrated

- Tibial tuberosity osteotomy – designed to bring the insertion of the patella tendon anteriorly (Maquet) – is somewhat unpredictable.

# PATELLA INSTABILITY

Patients may present with an acute dislocation or subluxation or with recurrent instability and pain. An initial episode of instability may follow a direct blow to the medial aspect of the patella but more usually occurs without contact following external rotation of the trunk on an extended knee. The patella may only partially sublux before knee flexion or a reflex contraction of the quadriceps pulls the patella back into place. Patients with recurrent instability are often young women with hypermobility/generalized ligamentous laxity (GLL).

## Pathoanatomy of PFJ Instability

Stability may be adversely affected by anomalies of the static or dynamic stabilizers of the PFJ or of the patient's rotational profile.

### Static Stabilizers

* *The medial patellofemoral ligament (MPFL)* is a thickening of the knee joint capsule and acts as the principal restraint in the first 20 degrees of knee flexion: the most common position of instability. GLL predisposes to incompetence. Alternatively, the MPFL can be torn or avulsed from the patella, occasionally with a bony fragment. It may become stretched or incompetent with injury. Reconstruction is commonly effective.

* *The trochlear groove*, particularly the lateral wall, acts as the principal static restraint in deeper flexion. Hypoplasia of the lateral femoral condyle may result in a flat, or worse, a convex, trochlea, predisposing to instability. This can be assessed on the lateral knee radiograph by identifying the crossing sign or a supratrochlear spur (**Fig. 3.14**). Trochleoplasty aims to restore normal anatomy, although it is complex and rarely undertaken.

* *Patella alta* can prevent the patella entering the trochlear groove correctly during flexion.

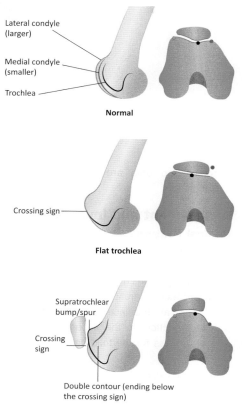

Lateral condyle (larger)

Medial condyle (smaller)

Trochlea

**Normal**

Crossing sign

**Flat trochlea**

Supratrochlear bump/spur

Crossing sign

Double contour (ending below the crossing sign)

**Convex trochlea**

Fig. 3.14 Trochlear dysplasia. On the lateral radiograph, the normal trochlea can be seen deep to the condyles as an extension of the Blumensaat line. The lateral condyle is usually larger and more prominent. Where the trochlea is flat, the trochlea line intersects with the condylar lines: the crossing sign. If the trochlea is convex, the trochlear line becomes the most prominent feature, described as a bump or a spur, and the medial condyle is often small, producing a double contour.

### Dynamic Stabilizers (Fig. 3.15)

* The *Q angle* indicates the degree of lateral pull of the quadriceps, away from the

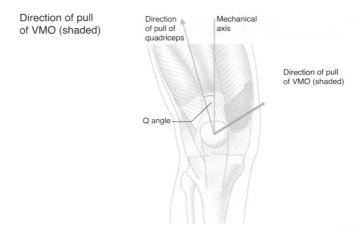

Fig. 3.15 Dynamic patella stabilizers: Q angle and vastus medialis obliquus (VMO).

mechanical axis. A higher Q angle predisposes to instability.

- The *VMO* muscle imparts a medial pull on the patella, resisting lateral instability. Weakness or incomplete rehabilitation of the quads and VMO predisposes to recurrent instability and pain, which is the main target of PFJ physiotherapy.

### Rotational Profile

- The *TT–TG measurement* reflects the location of the tibial tuberosity in relation to the trochlear groove (**Fig. 3.16**). The more laterally placed the tuberosity is in relation to the groove, the greater the lateral pull. A measurement of more than 15 mm predisposes to patellar instability.

- The *miserable malalignment syndrome* comprises three anomalies that predispose to PFJ maltracking: (1) femoral neck anteversion, (2) valgus knee alignment, and (3) external tibial torsion. With the feet parallel, patients with this condition have 'kissing patellae', which can almost touch. This leads to a grossly abnormal Q angle. Double derotational osteotomies of the

femur and tibia are arduous but often successful.

## Assessment and Investigation

### Clinical Features

Acute injury may be accompanied by a haemarthrosis, with tenderness over the MPFL and the lateral condyle (which is often contused during the dislocation). Rarely, the patella may still be dislocated at the acute presentation and require reduction. In the subacute or chronic setting, assess for the following:

- *Increased passive patella translation:* Mentally divide the patella into four vertical quadrants and carefully displace the patella laterally, noting how many quadrants of translation are possible on the injured and uninjured sides (normal is less than two).

- *Patella apprehension:* comprising anxiety and reflex quads contraction which may make this assessment difficult, so be patient.

- *J-shaped tracking:* a 'jump' of the patella into the trochlear groove at the beginning of active flexion, associated with *patella alta*.

- *Increased Q angle* or *miserable malalignment*

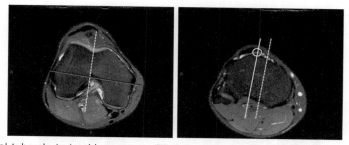

Fig. 3.16 Tibial tubercle to trochlear groove (TT–TG) measurement. The lowest point of the trochlea is identified and Whiteside's line drawn *(white dotted line)* perpendicular to the transepicondylar axis *(orange line)*. This line is copied onto the slice where the tibial tubercle is most prominent *(white circle)*. A parallel line is drawn through the tuberosity at this point *(solid white line)*. The distance between them *(orange arrow)* is the TT–TG measurement.

## Radiographic Features
Radiographs of the knee are used to assess for:

- Loose bodies and fractures (usually seen on the AP view)

- Trochlear dysplasia (assessed on the lateral view)

- Patella alta (also on the lateral image) (see **Fig. 3.17**)

- Patella tilt (assessed on skyline [Merchant] view) (see **Fig. 3.2C**)

- Assessment of overall lower limb alignment using hip–knee–ankle (HKA) films (see **Fig. 3.3**)

## MRI scans are helpful for
- Excluding loose bodies

- Assessing MPFL integrity

- Assessing the rotational profile – that is, measuring the TT–TG distance (see **Fig. 3.16**)

# Management
## Nonoperative
Almost all acute episodes of instability are managed nonoperatively with NSAIDs, early removal of any brace applied in the Emergency Department and referral to physiotherapy to regain range of movement and begin early quads and VMO rehabilitation. Rehabilitation of the trunk and hip girdle muscles help to stabilize the knee. Pes planus with overpronation of the feet, resulting in external tibial rotation, may respond to corrective orthoses (insoles).

## Operative
Surgery is indicated in the following situations:

- *Removal of loose bodies*, with potential for fixation of large osteochondral fragments

- *MPFL repair*, occasionally considered where there is a substantial bony fragment or for high-level athletes

- *MPFL reconstruction* for recurrent instability. Hamstring autograft is most commonly used to recreate a check-rein between the medial aspect of the patella and the isometric point on the femur, just distal and posterior to the medial epicondyle.

- *Tibial tuberosity transfer* can be considered where TT–TG is >20 mm, along with an MPFL reconstruction. The TT can also be moved distally to correct patella alta.

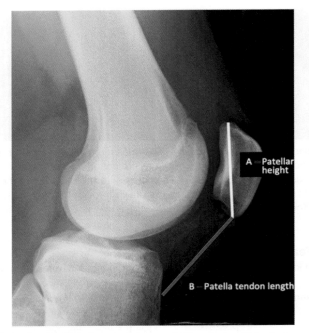

Fig. 3.17 Insall–Salvati ratio. This is calculated as A/B and should be between 0.8 and 1.2.

- *Lateral release* is not effective in isolation but may be used in combination with other surgeries.

- *Trochleoplasty* is occasionally offered for convex trochlear dysplasia but is technically highly demanding.

### Complications

- Recurrent instability occurs in 20%.

- Patellofemoral OA, causing PFJ pain and crepitus, is common.

## MENISCAL TEARS

Meniscal tears typically occur acutely in young patients after a twisting injury to a flexed, loaded knee, but they are more commonly sub-acute or chronic, presenting as a feature of osteoarthritic change.

## Classification

Meniscal tears are classified by their morphology (**Fig. 3.18**). The meniscus is vascular in its peripheral 25% (the red zone) but progressively more avascular toward the inner margin (white zone) (**Fig. 3.19**). Tears in the red zone have the capacity to heal, while those in the white zone generally do not.

## Assessment and Investigation
### Clinical Features
Meniscal tears may be accompanied by:

- *Swelling,* which is most commonly due to an effusion. Less commonly there may be a haemarthrosis after a tear in the red zone, although this is more commonly a sign of an ACL disruption.

- *Pain and tenderness,* localised specifically to the affected joint margin.

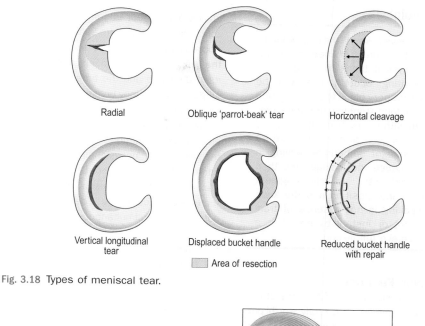

Radial

Oblique 'parrot-beak' tear

Horizontal cleavage

Vertical longitudinal tear

Displaced bucket handle

Reduced bucket handle with repair

Area of resection

Fig. 3.18 Types of meniscal tear.

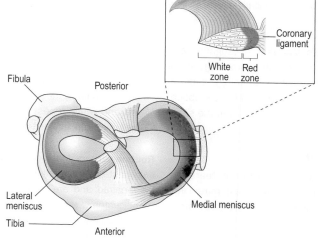

Coronary ligament

White zone    Red zone

Fibula

Posterior

Lateral meniscus

Tibia

Anterior

Medial meniscus

Fig. 3.19 Meniscal anatomy.

- *Clicking or catching*, where there is an unstable fragment. This is confirmed on McMurray's testing (refer to Examination section). The Thessaly test achieves the same provocation with the patient standing with 20 degrees of knee flexion, and the Apley test achieves the same with the patient prone and the examiner flexing and compressing the knee.

- *Locking*, the physical inability to straighten the knee, where there is a large fragment, for example, a bucket-handle tear (see Key Point box).

## ☑ Key Point

The term *'locked knee'* has a specific meaning in the context of knee injuries. It implies a physical block to knee extension. Presenting acutely, this will be evident as a rubbery block to passive knee extension. A long-standing unstable tear may present with intermittent locking, and the patient will complain of a recurrent 'click' or sense of something moving in the knee to cause the locking, and then another 'click' later as the fragment reduces back into position and the knee unlocks. Locking is not a sense of transient catching or instability, nor is it a failure to achieve full flexion.

### Radiographic Features

- Plain radiographs may show features of OA. If these are marked, it is rarely worth proceeding to MRI as meniscal tears are virtually guaranteed.

- MRI is the gold standard investigation and will confirm a tear and its morphology. It will also demonstrate other pathology, such as a parameniscal cyst or an ACL disruption, that may need to be considered at the same time.

## Management

While numerically most meniscal tears are treated nonoperatively, they are a common indication for knee surgery. There are three broad groups to consider:

**Urgent surgery.** Some tears can be repaired in the expectation of healing. A preserved meniscus retains the crucial shock absorption and load distribution function of the meniscus and protects against accelerated degeneration, and repair should therefore be undertaken wherever possible. The success of repair is time-critical, and these injuries should therefore be diagnosed and addressed within a time frame of days to weeks.

- *Bucket handle.* A complete or incomplete bucket handle tear is commonly in the red zone and is therefore often repairable. Success will relate to the exact location of the tear, whether the meniscal fragment is itself damaged and the time from injury to surgery. Surgery may be performed all-inside (using suture anchor devices) or inside-out (using sutures retrieved through a skin incision) or a combination of both. An outside-in technique is occasionally required to address the anterior horn. Success rates are ~80%, although this is much lower if there is a concurrent ACL deficiency that is not addressed simultaneously.

- *Root tears.* These usually occur at the posterior horns of the menisci, with detachment from the tibia. Although the meniscus itself remains intact, it subluxes out of the joint, and root tears are therefore functionally equivalent to a total meniscectomy. Surgery is performed by placing a suture through the posterior horn and bringing this out through a tunnel in the tibia. Again, early surgery is optimal.

- *Large radial tears.* There is increasing interest in repairing these tears, which span the red and white zones, although further data regarding efficacy are awaited.

**Routine surgery.** Meniscal tears with a mechanically unstable fragment in the white zone cannot be repaired and are usually treated by partial meniscectomy: excising that fragment with a meniscectomy shaver or radiofrequency ablation. The smallest amount of tissue possible is resected consistent with leaving a smooth and stable remnant. Excision is not urgent, although a large tear left untreated will cause progressive chondral injury. The most satisfactory results are achieved where the clinical and radiographic signs correlate closely, the tear is large and unstable and the joint is otherwise healthy.

**Nonoperative.** This is often the most difficult situation to explain to patients. An arthritic

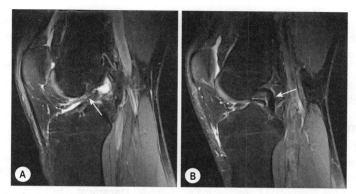

Fig. 3.20 Magnetic resonance imaging scan of the knee, sagittal reformats. A) The anterior cruciate ligament *(arrow)* is completely disrupted. B) The posterior cruciate ligament is intact but defunctioned.

knee will inevitably have degenerative meniscal tears as part of the overall arthritic picture. These are typically horizontal cleavage lesions (see **Fig. 3.18**). However, in the presence of degenerate articular chondral surfaces, meniscectomy often has little or no lasting beneficial effect. Management is as for early OA (see earlier).

**Meniscal transplant** surgery is being investigated for the small and specific group of young patients with a complete meniscal deficiency in an otherwise healthy knee.

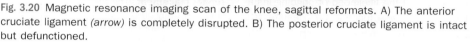

## THE ANTERIOR CRUCIATE LIGAMENT

Complex, multiligament knee injuries are covered in the Trauma companion volume to this book; however, ACL deficiency comprises a large component of a knee surgeon's elective practice and is described in further detail here.

## Assessment and Investigation

ACL disruption typically follows a torsional injury to the knee under load. The patient will often report feeling a 'pop' or 'snap' in the knee, followed by the rapid development of a tight, painful swelling within a couple of hours. This is a haemarthrosis and is almost pathognomonic of an ACL disruption, developing more rapidly than an effusion that is typically maximal more than 4 hours after injury. This gradually resolves, and a patient attending an outpatient consultation a few weeks later may have a surprisingly normal-looking knee. The cardinal symptom of ACL deficiency is recurrent instability, particularly with turning or pivoting, and a consequent loss of confidence in the knee.

## Radiological Features

- Plain radiographs are usually normal but may demonstrate an associated fracture, most commonly a Segond lesion – a flake avulsion of the anterolateral ligament (ALL) from the lateral tibial plateau.

- MRI (see **Fig. 3.20**) is the gold standard investigation, confirming disruption of the ACL and demonstrating any associated injuries, which may include:

  - Meniscal tears, typically bucket handle or meniscal root tears, which should prompt consideration of urgent surgery

  - Bone contusion, typically in a pivot shift pattern reflecting compression of the lateral compartment, which will cause pain and local tenderness for several weeks or months

- Chondral injury, particularly in chronic ACL deficiency

## Management

Management of ACL disruption is either nonoperative or surgical ACL reconstruction. Selection of patients suitable for surgery involves an assessment of the likelihood of ongoing instability. 'Copers', who function well despite ACL deficiency, are managed nonoperatively, whereas 'non-copers' are best managed surgically if they wish to return to activity, with pivoting activities usually most provocative. There is a linear relationship with age, with younger patients being less likely to cope with ACL deficiency. Patients over the age of 30 who do not wish to return to pivoting sports are often successfully managed conservatively.

### Nonoperative

Patients undergo a standardized ACL rehabilitation regime that aims to reduce swelling and restore comfort and range of movement in the first instance. Muscular training begins with closed-chain exercises (where the foot position is controlled by being on the floor or on an item of equipment), to open chain exercises (where the foot leaves the floor and greater proprioceptive control is needed), followed by sports-specific training. Increasingly provocative drills are added gradually. Recurrent effusions are not uncommon as load increases, but the development of instability symptoms requires a lowering of expectations or a reconsideration of surgery.

### Operative

Reconstructive surgery (see Box) involves securing a graft within tunnels in the femur and tibia. The correct placement of the tunnels is of the greatest importance. Other variables, including selection of graft material and method of fixation, remain areas of intense interest and research, which may be influenced by patient characteristics and surgeon preference. Rehabilitation is arduous and follows the same sequence as described for nonoperative management earlier. Return to sport follows the biological integration of the graft, and return of normal muscular control, at between 9 and 12 months.

---

### Considerations in ACL surgery

**Tunnel placement.** The tibial tunnel is most sited centrally on the plateau with the aid of a jig, just anterior to the PCL, using the anterior horn of the medial meniscus, the tibial spines or the intermeniscal ligament as a reference. The femoral tunnel is most commonly placed through an anteromedial portal, at the 10-o'clock position for a right knee (2-o'clock for the left), within a couple of millimetres of the back of the intercondylar notch. Femoral tunnels created via the tibial tunnel (transtibial drilling technique) result in a higher entry point and a more vertical graft. While satisfactory in controlling anterior translation, this position is biomechanically less satisfactory in controlling rotation (pivot). The double-bundle technique, with separate femoral and tibial tunnels for the anteromedial and posterolateral bundle reconstruction grafts, may result in more normal biomechanics at the expense of more complications. Neither drilling technique nor number of bundles has been shown to influence clinical outcome or patient satisfaction.

**Graft selection.** Autograft is most commonly used, with allograft having a risk of disease transmission and a higher failure rate, and usually reserved for revision or multiligament surgery. Hamstrings are the most commonly used graft internationally, but there is a preference for the middle-third patellar tendon for younger, more demanding patients returning to high-impact sports, and there is increasing interest in using the quads tendon. Synthetic the grafts have yet to show sufficient durability in this setting.

**Graft fixation.** Grafts are secured either with suspensory devices or aperture fixation (interference screws). Suspensory fixation can be via a static or adjustable loop, placed around a button that sits on the external tibial or femoral cortex.

**ALL repair.** The addition of a repair or reinforcement of the anterolateral ligament of the knee joint capsule is controversial but is reported to improve outcome in selected patient groups.

**ACL repair.** The ACL has no capacity to heal, and repair is therefore not usually attempted. One exception is an avulsion of the ACL (from either femoral origin or tibial insertion) in adolescents, where there is interest in suture repair through tunnels.

**Complications.** The overall success rate from reconstruction is around 95%. Structural failure is most commonly due to tunnel misplacement. *Infection* occurs in <1% and may be reduced by soaking the graft in vancomycin. *Arthrofibrosis* is most common where the knee has not regained a full range of movement prior to surgery. *Osteoarthritis* is a common late complication of the injury.

**Revision ACL reconstruction.** Revision of failed ACL reconstruction is challenging and requires an assessment of whether any elements of the primary surgery contributed to failure, including tunnel position, graft choice, fixation choice or patient rehabilitation protocol.

## SUBCHONDRAL INSUFFICIENCY FRACTURE OF THE KNEE

The subchondral insufficiency fracture of the knee (SIFK) is a stress fracture of the femoral condyle or tibial plateau occurring without trauma. The condition was previously known as **spontaneous osteonecrosis of the knee (SONK)** or **Ahlbäck disease** and is seen most often in women and those over 55 years of age.

- *Spontaneous* SIFK is most common. The subchondral insufficiency fractures lead to regional oedema, increased intraosseous pressure, bone infarction and necrosis.

- *Secondary* osteonecrosis arises following an identifiable insult such as alcohol misuse, corticosteroid therapy and sickle cell disease. Rarely, SIFK can occur following arthroscopic surgery.

## Assessment and Investigation

There is a sudden onset of severe knee pain, most often situated over the medial femoral condyle. After the acute episode, the symptoms are difficult to differentiate from those of OA or a degenerate medial meniscal tear with pain, which is worse on weight-bearing but is often constant in nature.

### Investigations

Plain radiographs may be completely normal. Following collapse of the articular surface, radiolucencies around, or flattening of, the joint surface may be visible.

MRI is the investigation of choice, typically demonstrating a unilateral subchondral fracture in the weight-bearing region of the medial femoral condyle on T2-weighted images (**Fig. 3.21**). There are often associated meniscal tears.

## Management

### Nonoperative Management

Protected weight-bearing, maintenance of range of movement and analgesics are advised. Necrotic bone will revascularize over time, but patients are advised that it can be difficult to predict whether the knee will be symptomatic in the long term.

### Surgical Treatment Includes

- *Core decompression* of the affected area with or without the use of bone substitute or grafting

- *Osteotomy* to offload the affected compartment

- *Arthroplasty* for salvage of joint destruction

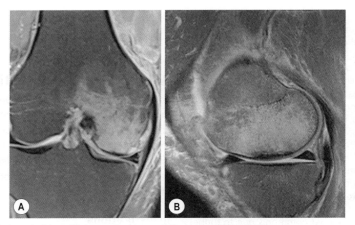

Fig. 3.21 Subchondral insufficiency fracture of the knee (SIFK). There is oedema and a subchondral fracture line.

## OSTEOCHONDRITIS DISSECANS

Osteochondritis dissecans (OCD) of the knee is an idiopathic, focal abnormality in which a fragment of subchondral bone and its overlying cartilage become separated (dissected) from the surrounding joint. The aetiology is uncertain, although traumatic and vascular insufficiency hypotheses are favoured.

### Assessment and Investigation

The condition may be entirely asymptomatic and diagnosed incidentally on radiographs. However, as the fragment becomes loose and mechanically unstable, it typically causes localised pain and recurrent effusions. If it dissects completely from its bed, it becomes a loose body, resulting in painful, intermittent locking.

#### Radiologic Features

- Plain radiographs typically show the lesion at the lateral aspect of the medial femoral condyle. A slightly posterior position may make the lesion clearer on a notch view (taken with the knee flexed).

- MRI is the gold standard investigation and may show synovial fluid dissecting around a mechanically loose lesion (**Fig. 3.22**).

## Management

While an asymptomatic lesion may be left alone, a painful, unstable lesion usually demands surgery. Surgery is usually arthroscopic and includes:

- *In situ fixation* of the OCD lesion, possible where the overlying cartilage remains intact.

- *Debridement and fixation,* usually required for unstable lesions as there is commonly fibrous tissue in the base of the defect. This is curetted out before fixation. Fixation devices depend on surgeon preference, but headless screws often fail to grasp adequately the small sliver of abnormal OCD bone, and headed screws compressing the subchondral bone may be preferred.

- *Excision of the fragment* may be all that is possible if it has been too badly damaged to salvage. This will leave a cartilage defect.

## CARTILAGE DEFECTS

Injury or OCD may result in a defect or ulcer in an otherwise intact articular surface, leaving

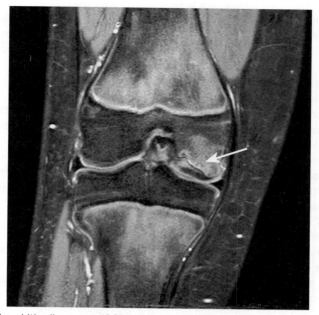

Fig. 3.22 Osteochondritis dissecans (OCD) of the medial femoral condyle (*arrow*).

exposed bone. The defect is a focus for further chondral damage at its margins and will typically enlarge over time, leading to irreversible OA. Articular cartilage does not, of course, regenerate, and despite being a common source of pain and a common finding at arthroscopy, there is no perfect treatment for full-thickness articular cartilage defects. Possible surgical options include:

- *Debridement* of any flaps of unstable articular cartilage at the margins, using mechanical punches and shavers, or radiofrequency ablation. This may result in a temporary respite from mechanical symptoms caused by catching and snagging.

- *Microfracture* of the base, a technique whereby small holes are created with a pick or drill, breaching the subchondral plate, which allows the movement of fibroblasts from the bone marrow into the defect. These create a fibrocartilaginous plug, which can improve the appearance of the defect. Unfortunately, fibrocartilage is far less robust than articular cartilage, and the contour of the plug rarely reaches a height where it contributes to structural load bearing.

- *Autologous chondrocyte implantation (ACI).* Chondrocytes can be harvested from the patient's knee, separated from their organic matrix and then cultured in vitro. The cultured cells can then be reimplanted, either under a roof of tissue (fascia lata is often used) or impregnated within a gelatinous matrix (MACI), which can be sutured or glued into place. Although this does replace the cellular component of the chondral defect, it does not replace the highly complex natural cartilage architecture, and the graft is thus less robust than the surrounding cartilage.

- *Mosaicplasty* or osteochondral autograft transfer surgery (OATS) is performed by taking a dowel of bone with an intact cartilage cap from a healthy part of the knee and implanting it into a defect in another part of the knee. The benefit is derived from taking the graft from a location of low mechanical load, usually the margin of the trochlea or intercondylar notch, and moving it to a position where there is high load. Mosaicplasty with a single dowel is the gold standard treatment for defects of up to 10 mm in diameter as it replaces both chondrocytes and matrix, albeit at the cost of possible donor site morbidity. Larger areas may be addressed with multiple dowels.

- *Osteochondral transplant* involves fresh cadaveric tissue that is harvested and prepared to fit larger chondral defects. It avoids the restrictions of donor site morbidity and can be used in far larger defects than mosaicplasty but is more expensive and complex and carries a small risk of the transmission of infection. The rejection problems associated with many other forms of tissue transplant are not encountered with osteochondral grafts.

## PATELLA TENDINOPATHY

Patella tendinopathy is a condition of chronic inflammation and the accumulation of micro-tears of the origin (enthesis) of the patella ligament at the inferior border of the patella. It is most commonly an overuse phenomenon, characterized by pain on loading, especially jumping, hence its common name *jumper's knee*.

## Assessment and Investigation

In the initial stages, the patient may complain of activity-related discomfort that settles with rest, ice, and anti-inflammatories. Pain may later become constant and restrictive. Examination reveals thickening and tenderness at the tendon origin.

### Radiologic Features

- Ultrasound will confirm thickening of the tendon with hypoechoic regions and neovascularization.

- MRI shows tendon thickening with increased signal on both T1- and T2-weighted images.

## Management

Management is usually nonoperative. Physiotherapy forms the mainstay of treatment, focussing on eccentric quadriceps strengthening exercises. Adjuvant treatment with extracorporeal shockwave therapy, ultrasound and injection of PRP has its proponents, although conclusive evidence is awaited. Intratendonous injection of corticosteroid risks tendon rupture and should be avoided.

Surgery is reserved for refractory cases and consists of decompression and debridement, possibly with radiofrequency ablation, of the tendon and the inferior pole of the patella.

## KNEE EXAMINATION

Knee examination follows the usual sequence of 'look, feel, move, special tests and neurovascular assessment', although modified slightly by first palpating the knee in extension, then assessing movement, and then palpating the knee at 90 degrees of flexion.

## Look

Expose both lower limbs completely. Stand at the end of the examination couch to compare the two sides and note:

- Alignment: Are the limbs straight, or is there a varus or valgus deformity?

- Deformity: There may be clear scars or deformity. The quadriceps may be wasted. The skin may be compromised (e.g., by induration, venous hypertension, or pitting oedema), and this may influence a decision on embarking on major surgery.

- Swelling: This may represent an effusion, synovitis or osteophytes.

**Feel** (knee extended)

- Heat: With the knee extended, palpate for generalized warmth and compare this to the other side.

- Effusion: A gross effusion will be obvious from inspection alone, but there are also two specific tests:

  - *Patellar tap* (**Fig. 3.23**): In a large effusion, press down on the patella and note that it descends through the fluid within the knee before coming to an abrupt stop as it meets the trochlea of the femur. Note that despite the term, no tapping is involved!

  - *Fluid sweep* (**Fig. 3.24**): A more subtle effusion can be demonstrated as a fluid sweep. With the flat of your hand, sweep the fluid from the medial aspect of the knee and up through the suprapatellar pouch; watch the fluid fill the normal concavity to the lateral aspect of the patella, making this region convex. Now empty this pouch of fluid, sweeping it up and through the suprapatellar pouch to fill the medial concavity.

- Patellar apprehension: Palpate the medial retinaculum just to the inner aspect of the patella, which will be tender after a dislocation. Grasp the patella and gently move it laterally. Excessive movement, discomfort or an expression of apprehension on the patient's face is suggestive of patellar instability.

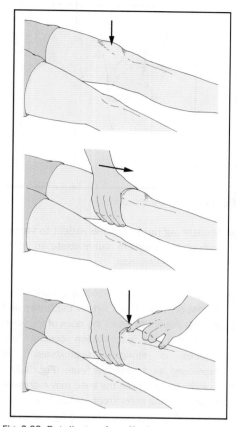

Fig. 3.23 Patella tap for effusion.

- Patellar grind: Compression and translation of the patella against the trochlea may demonstrate crepitus on movement, indicating OA of the PFJ.

## Move

Screen the hip and extensor mechanism, then establish the range of movement present, comparing this with the uninjured knee:

- Hip screening: Roll the limb gently from side to side, keeping the knee straight, and observe for any indication of groin or hip pain to exclude hip pathology presenting as referred pain at the knee.

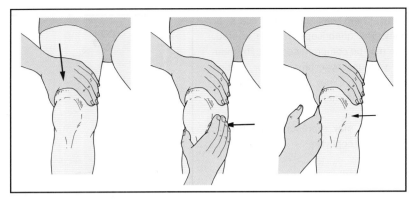

Fig. 3.24 Fluid sweep test.

- Straight leg raise: Ask the patient to lift the limb off the couch to demonstrate an intact extensor mechanism.

- Knee extension: Now allow the patient's heel to rest on your closed fist on the trolley and ask the patient to press the back of the knee down into the examination couch. Zero degrees is straight; hyperextension is expressed as a negative figure (**Fig. 3.25**). Inability to straighten the knee may represent a longstanding fixed-flexion deformity secondary to OA or may result from a tight effusion or haemarthrosis, pain inhibition or a mechanical block arising from a meniscal tear.

- Knee flexion: Finally, ask the patient to bend the knee fully. Inability to achieve full flexion is common, resulting from the presence of an effusion or simply the generalized irritability of an injured or arthritic knee. Comparison with the uninjured limb is often described in terms of how close the patient can bring the heel toward the buttock. Leave the knee flexed to 90 degrees.

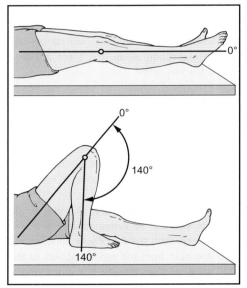

Fig. 3.25 Knee range of movement.

**Feel** (knee flexed)

- Tenderness: With the knee at 90 degrees, palpate the anatomical structures of the knee in an orderly manner. Start at the tibial tuberosity and work proximally along the patellar tendon, patella and quadriceps tendon, looking for tenderness or a defect. Now palpate along both the medial and the lateral joint margins. Localised tenderness here is suggestive of a meniscal injury, while generalized joint line tenderness in a degenerative knee is more suggestive of OA.

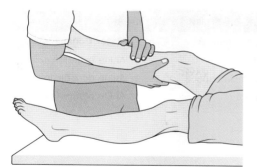

Fig. 3.26 Testing the collateral ligaments.

# Special Tests

Starting with the unaffected knee for comparison, assess:

1. Coronal stability and alignment with the varus and valgus stress tests

2. Cruciate ligaments

3. Menisci with McMurray test.

- Collateral ligaments: With the patient's ankle held firmly under your arm, place your hands around the proximal calf away from any areas of knee joint tenderness (**Fig. 3.26**). Is the limb straight? If there is varus or valgus malalignment, can this be corrected to bring the knee straight? Is the knee unstable? With the knee in full extension, push firmly medially and then laterally to stress first the MCL and then the LCL, and then repeat this at 30 degrees of knee flexion.

- Anterior and posterior cruciate ligaments: Assess for posterior sag or drawer, indicating PCL deficiency (**Fig. 3.27**). Perform the Lachman test for ACL insufficiency (**Fig. 3.28**). A detailed description of these, and of the assessment of the knee with multiple ligamentous injuries, including the pivot shift and dial tests, will be found in the *Orthopaedic Trauma* companion book.

- Menisci: Where you suspect an isolated meniscal instability, attempt to provoke this using McMurray test (see **Fig. 3.28**).

- Patella tracking: Where you suspect patellofemoral pain and instability, ask the patient to sit with the legs flexed over the edge of the examination couch, and then demonstrate active knee extension. Excessive lateral movement at terminal extension is termed the J-sign.

## Neurovascular Assessment

Palpate the dorsalis pedis and posterior tibial pulsations. Check for sensory and motor function in the distributions of the deep and superficial peroneal and posterior tibial nerves (**Table 3.6**).

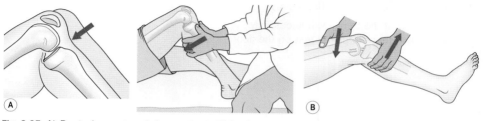

Fig. 3.27 A) Posterior sag and drawer test. B) Lachman test.

### Table 3.6    Sensory and motor innervation distal to the knee

| Nerve | Sensory Component | Motor Component |
|---|---|---|
| Superficial Peroneal Nerve | Lateral foot | Ankle eversion |
| Deep Peroneal Nerve | First dostal webspace | Ankle dorsiflexion |
| Tibial Nerve | Sole of foot | Ankle plantarflexion |

## Gait

Finally, ask the patient to stand and walk. Load bearing may reveal a previously unsuspected coronal plane deformity or insufficiency, such as a valgus thrust from a damaged MCL. Pain will result in an antalgic gait, with the patient attempting to minimize the stance phase on the painful knee. In the younger patient with a possible meniscal tear, ask the patient to adopt a deep squat and then shift the body weight from side to side (the duck waddle) (see **Fig. 3.28**).

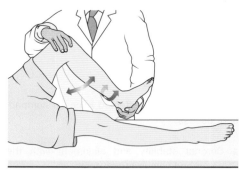

Fig. 3.28  McMurray test.

## Assessment of Hypermobility

Where you suspect that the patient is hypermobile, carry out an assessment according to the Beighton score (**Table 3.7**). Hypermobility may be simply part of benign joint hypermobility syndrome (BJHS) or part of a specific syndrome (e.g., Marfan or Ehlers–Danlos syndrome).

### Table 3.7    Beighton score: Points are allocated for each of the findings, up to a maximum of 9. A score ≥5 denotes hypermobility

| Joint/Finding | Negative | Unilateral | Bilateral |
|---|---|---|---|
| Passive extension of the little finger MCPJ >90° | 0 | 1 | 2 |
| Passive abduction of thumb to touch the forearm | 0 | 1 | 2 |
| Hyperextension of the elbows beyond 10° | 0 | 1 | 2 |
| Hyperextension of the knees beyond 10° | 0 | 1 | 2 |
| Forward flexion of the trunk, with knees fully extended, such that the palms rest on the floor | 0 | 1 | |

*MCPJ*, metacarpophalangeal joint.

## INTRODUCTION

The foot and ankle have evolved to provide stability in stance and efficient propulsion in gait. They can withstand up to eight times the body's weight when running.

The foot consists of 28 bones and 33 articulations. It is connected to the tibia and fibula of the lower leg via the ankle joint (**Figs 4.1** and **4.2**).

The true ankle joint, or tibiotalar joint, consists of the articular surfaces of the medial malleolus and distal tibia, lateral malleolus of the fibula, and the talar dome and its medial and lateral surfaces. The joint is supported and stabilized by the medial, lateral and syndesmotic ligament complexes (**Fig. 4.3**). The predominant axis of movement is dorsiflexion and plantarflexion around the intermalleolar axis between the tips of the medial and lateral malleoli, and the majority of movement of the foot and ankle complex in the sagittal plane occurs at the ankle. The talar dome is wider anteriorly. As a result, the ankle is more stable in dorsiflexion as the wider part of the talus engages. The ankle movements are coupled with hindfoot movements, contributing mainly to supination and pronation and slightly to inversion and eversion and internal/external rotation. The cartilage in the ankle is thinner than that in the knee or hip (2–3 mm); however, given the congruence and more limited range of movement, the surface is more resistant to wear than the hip or knee.

The hindfoot comprises three joints, the subtalar, talonavicular and calcaneocuboid joints. Alone, the subtalar joint inverts and everts the heel, but all three together allow supination and pronation. The interaction between these three joints allows the foot to have some flexibility in stance, allowing the foot to accommodate the surface of the ground for stability. When the heel lifts in preparation for toe-off, the resultant movement of the hindfoot 'locks' the foot to make it rigid, allowing push-off.

The midfoot joints, the naviculocuneiform joint and the tarsometatarsal joints, provide stability to the foot. They have little movement, but a degree of flexibility is present to help with shock absorption and for accommodation to the walking surface.

Finally, the forefoot comprises the highly mobile metatarsophalangeal joints (MTPJs) and the interphalangeal joints (IPJs) of the toes.

The aim of orthopaedic management of foot and ankle conditions is to maximize function by achieving a pain-free, stable, plantigrade foot while preserving normal motion and flexibility where possible.

## FOREFOOT

## FIRST RAY DISORDERS

### Introduction

The big toe, also referred to as the hallux, great toe or first toe, is the most crucial structure in the forefoot, bearing up to 50% of body weight while walking. The hallux includes the first metatarsal and the proximal and distal phalanges and is the terminal appendage of the medial column of the foot (**Fig. 4.4**). The MTPJ has a large arc of motion, with up to 90 degrees dorsiflexion and 40 degrees plantar flexion. The capsule, the collateral ligaments and the plantar plate are static stabilizers of the first MTPJ.

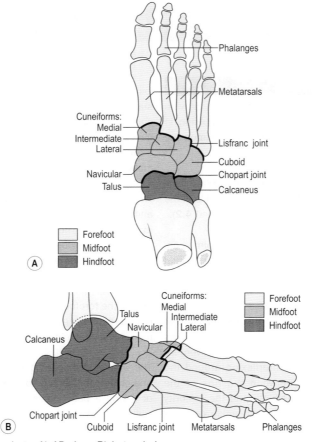

Fig. 4.1 Foot osteology: A) AP view. B) Lateral view.

Motor control of the hallux is provided by the flexor hallucis longus (FHL) and brevis (FHB), the extensor hallucis longus (EHL) and brevis (EHB), and the adductor and abductor hallucis. The two sesamoids, lying in the tendons of the FHB tendons, sit beneath the metatarsal head, and this mechanism plays a part in weight distribution and stability. The plantar fascia arises from the plantar surface of the calcaneal tuberosity and inserts onto each of the proximal phalanges, further supporting the first ray.

As the great toe is subject to large forces, abnormal loading through excessive physical activity and neuromuscular disease, poor footwear or loss of sensation (e.g., diabetes) can lead to progressive joint luxation (hallux valgus (HV)) or accelerated osteoarthritis (hallux rigidus).

## HALLUX VALGUS

### Background

Hallux valgus (HV) is a common deformity characterized by medial deviation of the metatarsal and lateral (valgus) orientation of the toe. It can lead to a prominence medially over the first MTPJ (**Fig. 4.5**). HV is also called a bunion. As the condition progresses, the great toe pronates due to a change in the orientation of pull from the surrounding tendons. The long tendons are displaced lateral to the MTPJ,

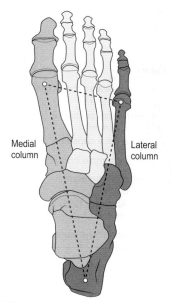

Fig. 4.2 The foot comprises the medial and lateral column. These are the longitudinal arches. There is a third 'transverse' arch under the MTPJs. The three posts of the first metatarsal head, fifth metatarsal head and heel together comprise a 'tripod'.

increasing the deforming forces (**Fig. 4.6**). When the deformity is severe, the great toe will begin to push the lesser toes laterally, overriding or underriding the second toe. Predisposing factors include family history, female gender,

joint laxity and flat foot deformities. Regular use of footwear which is too narrow across the toe box or with excessive heel height can contribute to the risk of developing a deformity.

## Symptoms

- **Pain**: Patients often present due to discomfort and pain in the forefoot. The pain may be derived from the first metatarsal joint itself or from the prominent metatarsal head, causing problems with footwear fitting and inflammation of the metatarsal bursa. It may also be mediated by pressure on the cutaneous nerve. As HV develops the first ray becomes less functional, which can also lead to symptoms of pain or pressure under the lesser metatarsal heads, known as transfer metatarsalgia.

- **Functional limitation**: Pain may limit walking.

- **Aesthetic concerns**: Patients may complain about the look of their foot and have difficulty wearing certain items of footwear.

## Signs

- Deformity
  - Valgus orientation of the first MTPJ
  - Possible hammer deformity of the lesser toes
- Erythema
  - Skin inflammation may occur over the medial first MTPJ.

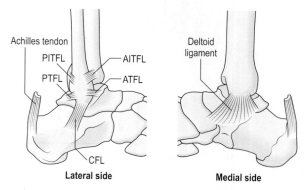

Fig. 4.3 Osseoligamentous anatomy. *AITFL*, anterior inferior tibiofibular ligament; *ATFL*, anterior talofibular ligament; *CFL*, calcaneofibular ligament; *PITFL*, posterior inferior tibiofibular ligament; *PTFL*, posterior talofibular ligament.

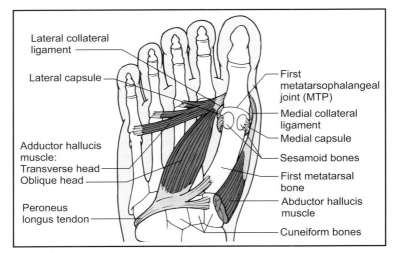

Fig. 4.4 Anatomy of first ray from the plantar aspect.

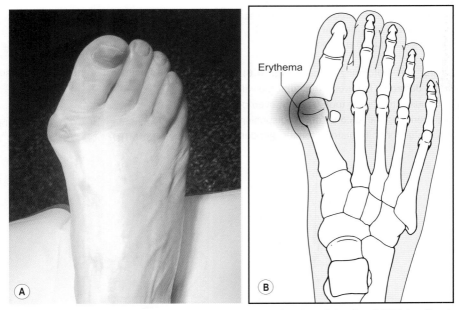

Fig. 4.5 Hallux valgus. (a bunion) A) There is a valgus deformity of the first MTPJ, leading to prominence, rubbing and erythema of the skin overlying the medial aspect of the joint. B) Schematic.

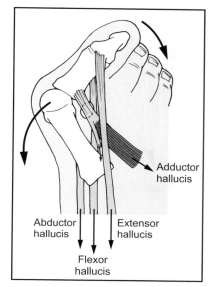

Fig. 4.6 Anatomical changes in HV: There is progressive lateralization of the pull of the long tendons and adductor to the great toe, accentuating deformity.

## Investigation

The initial diagnosis is a clinical one; however, plain weight-bearing anterior–posterior (AP), oblique and lateral foot X-rays provide key information for treatment planning.

Radiological assessment (**Fig. 4.7**)

- The metatarsal head will have moved medially in relation to the sesamoid bones.
- Any loss of congruence of the joints should be noted.
- The presence of coexisting osteoarthritis and the presence of underlying deformity such as pes planus or metatarsus adductus can be detected.
- The **HV angle (HVA)** is the angle subtended by lines drawn along the mid axis of the proximal phalanx and first metatarsal (normally <15 degrees).

- The **intermetatarsal angle (IMA)** is the angle created between the longitudinal axis of the first and second metatarsals (normally <9 degrees).
- The **interphalangeal angle** is the angle across the IPJ of the hallux (normally <10 degrees).
- The **distal metatarsal articular angle (DMAA)** measures the relationship of the articular surface with the long axis of the metatarsal. A case of adult-onset HV is more likely to be incongruent with a normal range DMAA, whereas a case of juvenile HV is more likely to have developed as a congruent deformity with an abnormal DMAA (normally <10 degrees).

## Treatment

Initial nonoperative management should include education, analgesia and appropriate footwear with sufficient breadth and height to accommodate the forefoot. Podiatry/orthotic support can be enlisted for custom footwear and management of pressure areas/skin.

When nonoperative measures fail adequately to relieve symptoms, surgery can be considered. It should be offered only in the presence of significant functional or pain symptoms and not as a cosmetic procedure. Caution should be exercised in young patients and men as there are higher rates of unsatisfactory results and revision surgery.

Multiple surgical options are available (**Fig. 4.8**). Their aim is to reposition the metatarsal head over the sesamoids and realign the toe so that the deformity is corrected on weight-bearing structures and pain is relieved. Where the joint has become incongruent, the correction should include restoration of joint congruence. Care must be taken in a congruent deformity so that the congruence is not lost during the correction. Flexible deformities are often suitable for joint-preserving surgery, with a combination of osteotomies and soft tissue balancing. Generally, the greater the magnitude of the deformity,

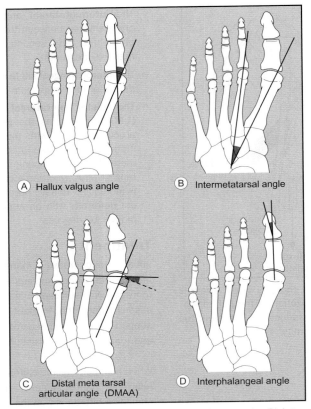

Fig. 4.7 Angles used to assess hallux valgus. A) Hallux valgus angle. B) Intermetatarsal angle. C) Distal metatarsal articular angle. D) Interphalangeal angle.

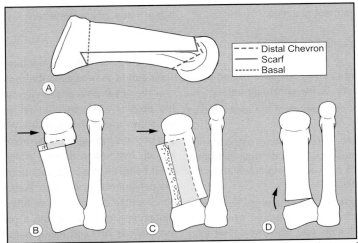

Fig. 4.8 First Metatarsal Osteotomies. A) Lateral view B) AP view of distal chevron C) AP view of scarf D) AP view of basal.

the more proximal an osteotomy is required. Currently, the scarf osteotomy is commonly used to achieve reproducible correction. It is often coupled with an Akin osteotomy of the proximal phalanx of the hallux. Where more proximal deformity occurs (increased IMA) or where significant instability or arthritis of the tarsometatarsal joint (TMTJ) is present, corrective fusion of the tarsometatarsal joint (Lapidus procedure) is indicated. If there is arthritis at the first MTPJ, corrective fusion of this joint is recommended.

## Procedure: First Metatarsal Osteotomy

Surgical correction of HV (bunion) is a common surgical procedure usually performed as day surgery under general or regional anaesthesia. A number of operative techniques have been described, and many variations exist; however, the most common procedures are the scarf, basal and distal (e.g., chevron) osteotomies of the first metatarsal. Joint-preserving techniques are generally preferred, but first ray arthrodesis procedures may be used in severe, hypermobile or revision situations. There is little need for excisional metacarpophalangeal arthroplasty (Keller), except in very low-demand patients or certain salvage situations. The versatile scarf osteotomy can be used to correct the HV deformity in several planes. For this reason it is one of the most commonly performed first metatarsal osteotomies. In some patients addition of an Akin osteotomy of the proximal phalanx is required to achieve full correction.

The type of osteotomy is decided based upon the nature of the deformity in conjunction with patient factors (such as activity profile, age and gender).

The skin is incised along the medial border of the foot over the first metatarsal and proximal phalanx. If an Akin osteotomy is anticipated, the wound can be extended distally. Care is taken to protect the dorsal cutaneous nerve, and a full-thickness incision through the MTPJ

capsule is performed to expose the joint. Capsulotomy is undertaken and will require retensioning and repair to restore joint stability after the osteotomy is performed. The shaft of the metatarsal is exposed. Subperiosteal dissection can then be employed to elevate the capsule and soft tissues dorsally. On the plantar surface, soft tissue stripping is minimized to avoid devascularization of the metatarsal head. Lateral release of the suspensory ligament, adductor tendon and lateral first MTPJ capsule is also needed when the deformity is not fully passively correctable.

The medial eminence is resected with the saw in line with the medial border of the metatarsal shaft, leaving the groove for the medial sesamoid intact. The scarf osteotomy is Z-shaped and performed using a power saw with a small blade width. Once the desired correction has been made, it is fixed with two headless compression screws (**Fig. 4.9**).

The scarf osteotomy can correct the IMA and HVA and can improve the DMAA. If there is further deformity present in the toe, an Akin osteotomy of the proximal phalanx can be performed to complete the correction.

## HALLUX VARUS

### Introduction

In contrast to HV, a primary varus deformity of the hallux is rare. It most commonly occurs as a result of overcorrection of a HV deformity. It may also be found congenitally, and if correctable, is likely due to abductor hallucis overactivity and settles when children begin walking; otherwise, it can be part of a more complex syndrome (e.g., cerebral palsy, Marfan syndrome, Ehler–Danlos syndrome and Down syndrome). The incidence is higher in populations where walking barefoot is common.

### Signs

Examination reveals medial deviation of the toe at the MTPJ (**Fig. 4.10**). A gap between the first and second toes and dorsal contracture of the great toe may be present, although the lesser toes may

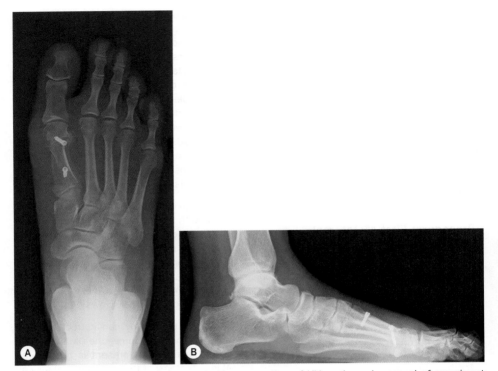

Fig. 4.9 Scarf osteotomy X-rays demonstrating correction of HV angle and removal of prominent medial bump. A) AP. B) Lateral.

also be deviated medially. The EHL tendon may be visible and subluxed medially, pulling the phalanx into deformity. There may be associated deformities. A flexible deformity may be well tolerated, but as the toe becomes stiffer, symptoms are more likely, particularly in footwear. Management should include evaluation of the underlying cause, symptomatic management with analgesia, well-fitting footwear and podiatry input. Surgery may be indicated when nonoperative measures fail and is often on a bespoke basis and aims to address tendon, soft tissue and bony deformities. Reconstruction of the lateral collateral ligament using the extensor digitorum brevis or part of the extensor digitorum longus tendon has been described, although artificial ligament devices are showing some promise. Once the deformity is fixed, fusion of the first MTPJ is indicated.

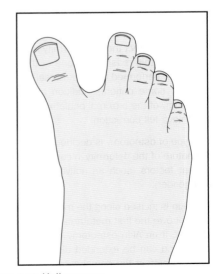

Fig. 4.10 Hallux varus.

## HALLUX RIGIDUS

## Introduction

Arthritis of the great toe, known as hallux rigidus, is a degenerative condition of the MTPJ. This small joint is vulnerable due to its wide arc of motion compared to the remaining great toe joints and being subjected to large forces estimated at twice the body's weight. Heavy use (e.g., kneeling with hyperextension), changes in mechanics (pes planus), genetics and trauma have been implicated as causative factors.

## Symptoms

- **Pain** from the first MTPJ is the primary presenting complaint. In the early stages this is mild and experienced at the extremes of motion. Pain on dorsiflexion is classic. Later the pain becomes more generalized and associated with motion.

- **Stiffness** of the first MTPJ.

- **Tenderness** from the pressure of footwear over prominent dorsal osteophytes can be particularly troublesome.

- **Deformity**: In more severe cases, joint erosions can cause deviation of the toe toward the lesser toes.

## Signs

- A bulky first MTPJ which is stiff and painful to move.

- Skin changes dorsally where footwear has been rubbing.

- Deviation toward the second toe may develop.

- The arc of movement is reduced, with pain at the ends of this range or throughout the arc of movement.

## Investigation

Weight-bearing AP, oblique and lateral X-rays should be performed and will show the extent of the first MTPJ disease, alignment of the toe and overall shape of the foot (**Fig. 4.11**).

## Treatment
### Nonoperative

- Initial treatment should be symptomatic and include analgesia and footwear optimization.

- Stiff-soled shoes act to splint the joint, and rocker bottom shoes may help to reduce the requirement of MTPJ dorsiflexion. Many off-the-shelf shoes, particularly running shoes, will have some of these features, and prescription footwear is not always necessary.

- Joint injection with a steroid may offer a temporary relief of pain but does not slow disease progression.

### Surgical

Surgery is considered when nonoperative means are ineffective.

- A **dorsal cheilectomy** (excision of osteophytes and up to 30% of the dorsal metatarsal articular surface) can be performed if focal irritation from the dorsal osteophyte is the primary problem, and in 75% of cases the deformity does not return.

- Surgery to fuse the joint (**MTPJ arthrodesis**) (**Fig. 4.12**) is indicated for patients who have pain throughout the range of movement of the joint and where a cheilectomy will not suffice. Range of movement is sacrificed for a pain-free but immobile joint. In the majority of patients, the joint is already significantly stiff prior to the procedure. Patients should be advised that footwear options will be reduced, primarily in terms of heel height, thereafter.

- If range of movement is required, **replacement** or **interposition arthroplasty** can be performed (hemiarthroplasty or total MTPJ replacement), although results of surgery are less certain. More recently, hydrogel polymer interposition implants have shown promising early results and may become more widespread if long-term results are maintained.

- **Excision arthroplasty** (Keller procedure) is now rarely used in modern foot surgery; however, there may be an occasional role in very low-demand patients.

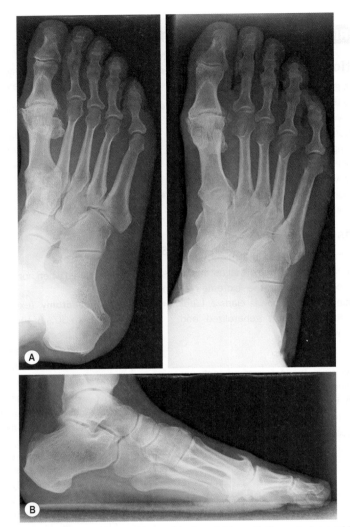

Fig. 4.11 Weight-bearing AP and oblique X-ray of hallux rigidus. A) There is loss of joint space of the first MTPJ. B) Lateral view demonstrating dorsal osteophyte.

## Clinical Technique

### First MTPJ Fusion (Arthrodesis)

Indicated for end-stage arthritis or severe valgus deformity of the joint. The aim is to achieve a stable, pain-free fusion, with sufficient dorsiflexion to allow the foot to roll forward in gait but still allow the toe to contact the ground for push-off.

The joint surfaces are prepared to congruent bleeding bone to allow optimal positioning prior to fixation. The joint should be fixed with 5–10 degrees of valgus, neutral rotation and dorsiflexion such that the pulp of the toe rests on the 'ground' during simulated weight-bearing positioning. Variation in arch height between individuals means this is a more reliable method than using the first metatarsal as

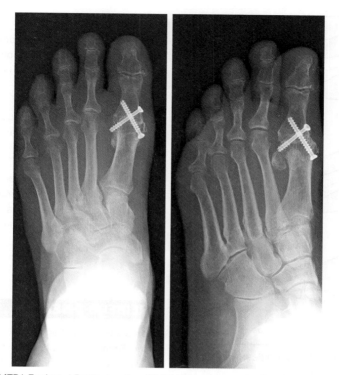

Fig. 4.12 First MTPJ Fusion – Postoperative AP/Oblique demonstrating successful fusion.

the reference. Many methods of fixation are described, including crossed screws, specific anatomical locking plates, memory staples and combinations of the above (**Fig. 4.12**).

## LESSER TOE DEFORMITY

## Background

The lesser toes play an important role in lower limb function, aiding in stability as they accommodate the surface of the ground and spreading load across the forefoot. The lesser toes each have three phalanges.

Lesser toe deformities are generally the result of chronic abnormal forces placed upon the toes, resulting in muscle imbalance or weakening of ligaments and capsule.

**Hammer, mallet and claw toe** are deformities in the sagittal (flexion/extension) plane and are due to imbalance of the intrinsic and extrinsic muscles (**Fig. 4.13**). These deformities are usually due to repetitive use, inappropriate footwear (causing repeated forced hyperextension), underlying neurological conditions, other foot deformity (pes cavus) following trauma (i.e., secondary to compartment syndrome) or inflammatory joint disease. Due to its prominent length, the second toe is most commonly affected.

A **bunionette** (also known as a tailor bunion) is a common condition caused by prominence of the fifth metatarsal head on the lateral border of the foot. This is commonly associated with varus deviation of the fifth toe at the MTPJ. This varus toe may overlap, underride or rub against the fourth toe, and rotational changes may

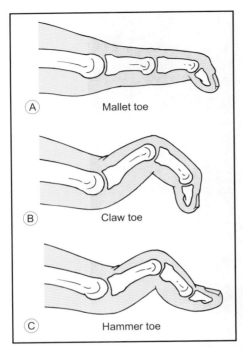

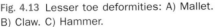

Fig. 4.13 Lesser toe deformities: A) Mallet. B) Claw. C) Hammer.

occur. The prevalence increases with age, and women are five times more likely to develop the deformity than men.

**Crossover toe** is a complex deformity which results in medial displacement of the second toe over the great toe with associated hyperextension and supination. It is thought to be due to excessive mechanical pressure on the second MTPJ, forcing the toe dorsally, often in the presence of HV, long second toe, unstable arch or tight Achilles complex.

## Symptoms

Symptoms of lesser toe deformities include difficulties with fitting footwear, rubbing and callosities and pain, often under the metatarsal heads, known as metatarsalgia. Patients may also complain about the aesthetic appearance of their foot.

## Signs

The pattern of deformity is noted (**Fig. 4.13**). The presence or absence of other signs of a wider neurological disorder is noted.

## Management

Nonoperative management encompasses analgesia, accommodating footwear, pressure relief and splinting.

Operative management is employed when nonoperative management fails and can augment the biomechanics of the toes (tendon transfers, osteotomies) or correct deformities (osteotomies, arthrodesis).

## FREIBERG DISEASE

Spontaneous infarction of the metatarsal head, called Freiberg disease, predominantly affects the second metatarsal, occasionally the third metatarsal, but rarely the remainder. It is most frequent in female adolescents and is associated with increased athletic activity and long second metatarsals.

## Symptoms

Presentation includes symptoms of pain and stiffness around the affected MTPJ which is worse upon activity and can be replicated upon examination.

## Signs

Palpable enlargement of the joint, along with tenderness or pain upon motion, may be seen upon examination.

## Investigation

X-rays may show no changes in early disease, but appearances of avascular necrosis can be observed: subchondral sclerosis, fragmentation and flattening of metatarsal head and joint destruction (**Fig. 4.14A**).

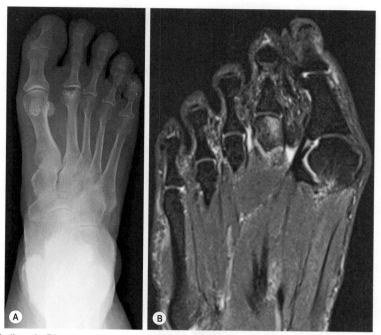

Fig. 4.14 Freiberg's Disease. A) AP X-ray demonstrating AVN of second metatarsal head. B) MRI with inflammation demonstrated in the second metatarsal head (white – high signal) on this T2 view of the forefoot in the early stages of the disease.

Magnetic resonance imaging (MRI) can show oedematous change in the metatarsal head in early disease (**Fig. 4.14B**).

## Management

Nonoperative treatment is often effective for symptomatic relief with activity modification, nonsteroidal anti-inflammatory drugs (NSAIDs) and orthoses designed to immobilize or offload the area, such as stiff soles or metatarsal bars.

When symptoms fail to respond, surgical options can be considered. For mild disease, debridement and cheilectomy of the metatarsal head may be sufficient. A shortening osteotomy may relieve excess joint pressure. With localised disease, a closing wedge osteotomy to rotate an area of healthy articular cartilage (often from the plantar aspect) into the joint is effective (**Fig. 4.15**). Removal of loose bodies, drilling of

exposed subchondral bone and interposition arthroplasty are options for more advanced disease.

## MORTON'S NEUROMA

## Background

Intermetatarsal neuritis, or Morton's neuroma, is not a true neuroma, but a thickening of the intermetatarsal nerve where it passes deep to the intermetatarsal ligament between the metatarsal heads prior to bifurcating to form the digital nerves. The cause is not fully understood; however, it is thought to be the result of repetitive compression and microtrauma of the nerve as it passes through this space, causing perineural fibrosis. Women are affected nine times as often as men, and the condition becomes more common with age.

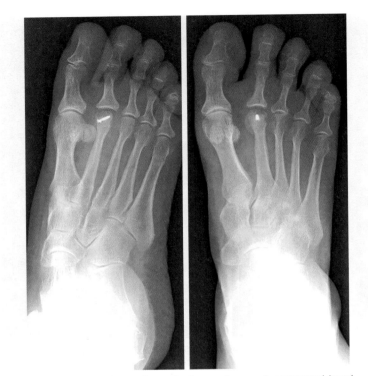

Fig. 4.15 Postoperative X-ray of shortening osteotomy of second metatarsal head.

The nerve of the 3/4 intermetatarsal space is the most frequently affected, possibly due to the fact that it receives fibres from both the medial and lateral plantar nerves. Patients complain of burning pain in the forefoot which worsens in weight-bearing positions (particularly in narrow-toed shoes or high heels).

## Symptoms

The patient may complain of pain, paraesthesia or numbness of the skin between the two toes.

## Signs

Examination may reveal tenderness in the intermetatarsal space or reduced sensation between the toes. Squeezing the foot across its width while palpating the intermetatarsal space may provoke symptoms or demonstrate a palpable Mulder's click (**Fig. 4.16**).

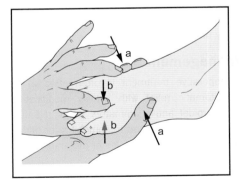

Fig. 4.16 Mulder's Click – Grasp the space between the metatarsal heads where the neuroma is suspected to be between thumb and forefinger. At the same time, the metatarsal heads are squeezed together. If a neuroma is present, it may be squeezed out with a palpable click. This can cause discomfort, so it should be performed carefully.

## Investigation

Diagnosis may be made clinically; however, ultrasound scanning will confirm the diagnosis and be used to evaluate the size of the lesion (**Fig. 4.17**). MRI is also useful and will help exclude alternative diagnoses.

## Treatment

Nonoperative treatments include shoes with adequate width. A metatarsal pad may help spread the metatarsals and ease symptoms. Local anaesthetic and steroid injection into the intermetatarsal space may also relieve symptoms, although the effects may not be lasting, and patients should be counselled regarding the risks. Some evidence suggests ultrasound-guided injection may be more effective.

Surgical treatment consists of resection of the nerve and division of the intermetatarsal ligament. This is usually performed via a dorsal incision to avoid a painful plantar scar.

## ANKLE DISORDERS

## CHRONIC ANKLE INSTABILITY

### Background

Sprains of the ankle are a common injury, most frequently injuring the lateral ligament complex via an inversion-type mechanism. There is often a rotational component to these injuries, and the anterior talofibular ligament (ATFL) is usually injured first, followed by the calcaneofibular ligament (CFL). The posterior talofibular ligament is rarely injured. The CFL can be injured in isolation with a purely varus injury mechanism.

The majority of ankle sprains fully resolve with nonoperative measures, but a few patients go on to experience chronic lateral ankle instability. There are many differential diagnoses for chronic ankle pain and mechanical symptoms (**Table 4.1**).

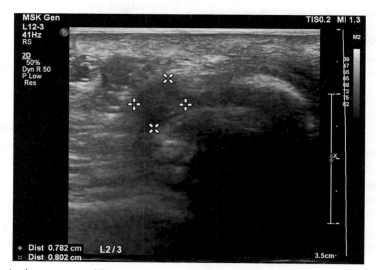

Fig. 4.17 Morton's neuroma – Ultrasound demonstrating hypoechoic lesion between the plantar aspect of the metatarsal heads.

| Table 4.1 Differential Diagnosis of Chronic Ankle Pain and/or Mechanical Symptoms | |
|---|---|
| Tendon pathology | Peroneal tendon tear |
| | Subluxing peroneal tendons |
| | Posterior tibial tendon injury |
| Bone | Weber A fracture or avulsion of the lateral malleolus |
| | Fracture/nonunion of the anterior process of the calcaneum |
| | Fracture/nonunion of the lateral process of the talus (snowboarder's fracture) |
| | Osteochondral injury to the talar dome |
| | Fracture/nonunion of the fifth metatarsal |
| | Tarsal coalition |
| Ligament injuries | Lateral ankle ligament sprain (ATFL +/– CFL) |
| | High ankle sprain: sprain of the syndesmotic ligaments |
| | Deltoid ligament sprain |
| | Subtalar instability |
| Intra-articular pathology | Osteochondral lesion of talar dome |
| | Anterior impingement |

Chronic lateral ankle instability results from attenuation of the ligaments following injury. This can be accentuated by underlying deformity such as a varus hindfoot alignment in a cavus foot. A similar chronic medial ligament attenuation is seen in the later stages of an adult-acquired flat foot deformity.

## Symptoms

- **Mechanical instability**: This is reported as repeated 'going over on the ankle' or 'twisting' it. In more minor cases it only occurs on uneven ground. As symptoms progress it can occur at any point, even on flat surfaces.

- **Pain**: There may be discomfort due to recurrent stretching and recurrent inflammation of the ligamentous complex.

- **Swelling**: Swelling and effusion may occur following an episode of instability.

## Signs

The ankle may appear normal in between episodes.

- **Swelling** and **bruising** may be observed around the lateral ligamentous complex if there has been recent episodic instability.

- Difficulty may be observed during single-limb stance due to impaired proprioception.

- **Instability** may be demonstrated via the anterior draw and talar tilt tests during examination (**Fig. 4.37**).

## Investigation

### X-rays

- Weight-bearing radiographs AP and lateral of the ankle. This may detect tilting at the tibiotalar joint line or an underlying tibial or hindfoot deformity.

- Weight-bearing radiographs AP and oblique and lateral of the foot if an associated deformity is suspected (such as a cavus foot)

- Stress X-rays can reveal talar tilt but may be challenging and painful to perform.

### MRI

MRI can demonstrate an attenuated or damaged lateral ligament but cannot fully inform on dynamic function and mechanical properties. Up to 60% of patients with ankle instability have associated pathology, such as an osteochondral or peroneal tendon injury, and MRI is useful for preoperative planning.

# Management

## Nonoperative Management

The aims are to aid stability, promote proprioceptive function and prevent further sprains. In the chronic setting functional treatment is preferred; however, a short period of cast or boot immobilization can help settle severe symptoms. Physiotherapy is advised to maximize normal range of movement and strengthen the dynamic stabilizers and proprioception. Bracing may be useful, particularly during sports or other provocative movements. Orthotic insoles can reduce the impact of associated hindfoot valgus.

## Operative Management

Surgery is indicated when conservative measures fail to control symptoms adequately control symptoms. The ligaments are usually found to be in continuity but lax. Techniques comprise anatomical ligament repair versus ligament reconstruction.

- **Broström repair** is the most commonly utilized anatomical repair. It re-tensions the ATFL and CFL ligaments (**Fig. 4.18**). The extensor retinaculum is commonly used to augment the repair (Gould modification). This increases the mechanical stability and is also thought to aid in the restoration of proprioceptive feedback through the stretch receptors in the ligament. Recent developments of these techniques have sought to augment anatomical repair with synthetic suture and fixation screw devices. More research is required to examine the long-term outcome of such techniques in terms of function and complications.

- **Chrisman–Snook** ligament reconstruction is the most commonly used biological ligament reconstruction technique. In this technique half of the peroneus brevis tendon is routed through the fibula and the lateral wall of the os calcis before being tensioned and sewn back on itself. This reconstruction aims to replace both the ATFL and CFL; however, it sacrifices a portion of the dynamic stabilizers. Modifications of this technique using

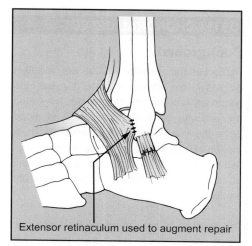

Extensor retinaculum used to augment repair

Fig. 4.18 Broström–Gould (anatomical) Ligament Repair. The residual ligaments are divided, tensioned and re-sutured. The Gould modification described adds additional reinforcement to the extensor retinaculum. This can be secured to the fibula through tunnels or using anchors.

hamstring graft and synthetic augments have been developed by some surgeons to avoid this problem.

Traditionally, these patients are immobilized for 6 weeks before beginning functional rehabilitation. In selected patients, early mobilization using a splint to limit inversion has shown a faster return to activity.

---

## Surgery Technique: Broström Repair

The ligaments are divided, leaving a small cuff on the fibula. The distal ends of the ligaments are then tensioned and repaired back onto the fibula and the proximal cuff is oversewn– 'pants over vest' (**Fig. 4.18**). In the Gould modification, the inferior extensor retinaculum is also incorporated into the repair for reinforcement. In most patients the success rate for an anatomical repair is >85%. Augmentation or reconstruction may be required for revision or in a patient with hypermobility.

## OSTEOCHONDRAL DEFECT

### Background

Osteochondral defects (OCDs) are localised defects in the articular surface that are most commonly found on the talar dome. They affect the articular cartilage and underlying bone. While the true incidence is unknown (as these may be asymptomatic and some are only identified as incidental findings) they can be a cause of considerable symptoms including pain and swelling.

The aetiology is not well understood, but most cases are thought to result from trauma, with acute injury, or repetitive loading. Symptomatic OCDs are said to develop after 5% of ankle sprains.

Defects tend to be located at the 'shoulders' of the talus, with medial defects being more common. Medial defects tend to be deeper and posterior while lateral defects are more likely to have a definite history of trauma. Lateral defects are also shallower and anterior and are more likely to require surgical treatment.

Osteochondral lesions at the ankle can also occur at the distal tibia. Assessment and management are the same as those for talar lesions; however, outcomes and prognosis are poorer.

### Symptoms

Patients experience deep pain within the ankle. This is often activity-related and may be associated with swelling or a sensation of instability. They may recall a sprain or specific injury.

### Signs

- Joint line tenderness
- There may be signs of swelling or an effusion.
- Associated disorder of alignment or ligamentous instability

### Investigation

- **X-rays:** Weight-bearing AP and lateral ankle radiographs may identify larger lesions (**Fig. 4.19**). Subtle or early OCD may not be clearly seen.

- **Cross-sectional imaging** will show the OCD more clearly, as well as allow for evaluation of the dimensions of the lesion (**Fig. 4.20**). It can be used to classify the defect (**Table 4.2**). MRI or computed tomography (CT) scanning could be selected. The choice may depend on local expertise. MRI will provide further information regarding the surrounding ligaments and tendons, allowing for full surgical planning.

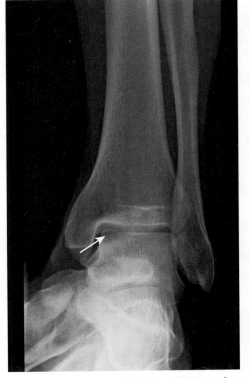

Fig. 4.19 Osteochondral defect – AP X-ray of ankle demonstrating abnormality in talus.

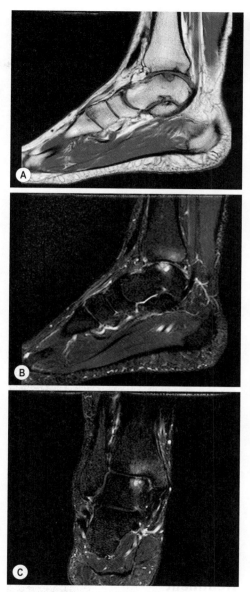

**Table 4.2   MRI Classification (Anderson)**

| Stage | Finding |
| --- | --- |
| Stage I | Subchondral trabecular compression |
| Stage II | Incomplete separation of fragment |
| Stage IIA | Formation of subchondral cyst |
| Stage III | Presence of unattached and undisplaced fragment with synovial fluid undermining the lesion |
| Stage IV | Displaced osteochondral fragment |

There is no evidence that asymptomatic lesions progress into more severe pathology such as ankle arthritis, and no treatment is required.

### Nonoperative Treatment

A period of rest in a boot or cast may be beneficial in acute presentations. Physiotherapy may be useful if there is symptomatic instability.

### Operative Treatment

Surgery is usually required in stage III and IV lesions. The aims are to remove loose unstable fragments and restore the joint surface.

- Ligamentous instability and malalignment and associated pathology should be addressed at the same time.
- Arthroscopic techniques are usually used to address the lesion.
- Acute unstable fragments may benefit from acute fixation.

Chronic lesions should be debrided to stabilize cartilage edges, and the bony crater should be drilled, microfractured or curetted to healthy bleeding bone. Bone grafting may be required for a deep defect. This bone stimulation allows mesenchymal cells from the bone marrow to enter the defect, where they can differentiate and produce a fibrocartilage cap to the lesion.

Fig. 4.20 MRI of ankle OCD. The area is represented by inflammation and high signal on T2 weighted images: A) T1 weighted lateral. B) T2 weighted lateral. C) T2 weighted coronal.

## Treatment

Patient factors, the size of the lesion and associated pathology or malalignment will all be relevant in planning treatment management.

This produces a moderately durable surface, although the properties are biomechanically inferior to hyaline cartilage.

Overall results of treatment are good; 80% of patients report good or excellent results from an arthroscopic debridement. Outcomes are best in younger patients and where the lesion is less than 1.5 cm in diameter.

When surgery is not successful, more complex techniques with an evolving evidence-base such as osteochondral autologous transplantation (OATS or mosaicplasty), autologous chondrocyte implantation (ACI) or matrix-induced autologous chondrocyte implantation (MACI) can be helpful.

## ANKLE ARTHRITIS

### Background

Ankle arthritis most commonly (>65%) occurs after trauma and is associated with both fractures and ligamentous instability. Cartilage loss is due to irreversible damage occurring at the time of trauma or abnormal loading due to chronic incongruence or instability. Only 10% of cases are attributed to primary osteoarthritis, and the remainder are due to inflammatory arthritis, osteonecrosis, dysplasia or neuropathy. While less common than end-stage hip or knee arthritis, its impact on quality of life is equally severe. It may occur in isolation, but adjacent deformity or arthritis should be identified and addressed as part of the management. In the absence of gross deformity, the pattern of degeneration in primary osteoarthritis forms a predictable pattern, beginning with osteophyte formation, then joint space loss and sclerosis.

### Symptoms

- **Pain** is the most common symptom. Ankle pain is typically experienced deep within the joint. The patient will usually indicate the anterior joint line when asked to localise their pain. It is usually aggravated with movement and weight-bearing positioning.

- **Stiffness**
- **Functional limitation**

### Signs

- Deformity
- Antalgic gait
- Effusion
- Pain along joint line
- Bulky/tender anterior osteophyte
- Reduced range of movement (dorsiflexion and plantar flexion)

### Investigation

#### X-rays

- Standard weight-bearing AP, lateral and oblique X-rays should be performed. These demonstrate loss of joint space, osteophyte and cyst formation, along with subchondral sclerosis. There may also be joint incongruity (**Fig. 4.21**). If complex deformities are associated (e.g., tibial malunion), then long leg X-rays should be obtained.

- CT scanning is useful for assessing deformity, patterns of osteophytes and bone stock.

#### Injection

If examination and X-rays are insufficient, a diagnostic injection (often image guided) with local anaesthetic can help localise the painful pathology. This can be useful where other potential surgical targets exist (i.e., subtalar joint).

### Treatment

#### Nonoperative

- Weight loss/walking aids
- Analgesia (NSAIDs)
- Activity modification (reduce impact)
- Steroid injection
- Footwear adaptations/orthoses/ankle brace to absorb impact and limit painful ranges of movement

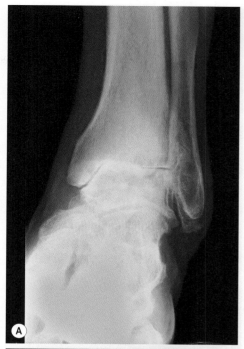

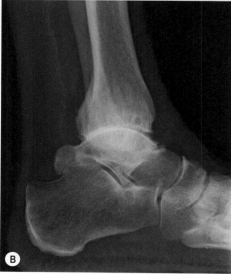

Fig. 4.21 Ankle osteoarthritis – A) AP. B) Lateral X-rays.

## Operative Treatment

Associated deformities of the foot and ankle should also be addressed.

- **Debridement** (cheilectomy): When symptoms are localised to a specific area such as an anterior osteophyte, localised surgical debridement of the area can reduce symptoms and delay more invasive procedures.

- **Distraction arthroplasty**: The indication for this technique is younger patients with end-stage ankle arthritis. The joint is distracted through application of an articulated circular frame. This treatment remains controversial, and reported success rates are roughly 50%.

- **Periarticular osteotomy** (supramalleolar or calcaneal): In the presence of extra-articular deformity, patients can develop unicompartmental disease in the lateral or medial half of the tibiotalar joint. Patients with early degenerative change, minimal intra-articular deformity and a good range of motion may be suitable for realignment osteotomy.

- **Ankle arthrodesis:** This approach remains the gold standard for treatment of ankle arthritis. Fusion of the tibia to the talus eliminates pain at the expense of any remaining ankle joint movement. It is a robust and lasting treatment, suitable for younger patients and those with high levels of physiwwcal activity. Following ankle fusion, there may still be up to 25% of sagittal plane motion through the midfoot and forefoot. There may be a reduction in stride length, but this is often not perceptible to others.

## Surgical Technique: Ankle Arthrodesis

A wide range of surgical techniques are described for ankle fusion which can be performed either arthroscopically or open and via

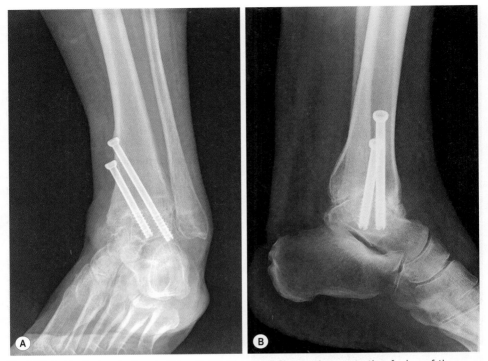

Fig. 4.22 Ankle fusion (arthrodesis) – A) AP. B) Lateral X-rays, demonstrating fusion of the tibiotalar joint with a cannulated screws.

a range of approaches. The principle is to remove any residual cartilage on the joint surfaces and prepare the bone to congruent bleeding bone surfaces. The joint is then aligned such that the physiological hindfoot valgus of 5 degrees is achieved, the foot is plantigrade, and the normal foot progression angle of 10 degrees is recreated with external rotation. Fixation is commonly performed with compression screws and/or a specialist plate (**Fig. 4.22**). Fusion of the ankle with or without additional subtalar fusion can also be performed using an intramedullary hindfoot nail inserted via the sole of the foot.

**Total ankle arthroplasty**: Modern designs have improved survival rates, which approach 80% at 10 years (**Fig. 4.23**). Wear and failure rates are higher in the younger, more active patients due to the increased forces to which

the joints are exposed, and arthroplasty is generally reserved for lower demand patients. Successful total ankle arthroplasty requires minimal deformity, adequate bone stock and a soft tissue envelope.

## HINDFOOT AND MIDFOOT ARTHRITIS

## HINDFOOT ARTHRITIS

### Background

Hindfoot arthritis is loss of cartilage and osteophytosis of the hindfoot joints (**Fig. 4.1**):

- Talonavicular
- Subtalar (talocalcaneal)
- Calcaneocuboid

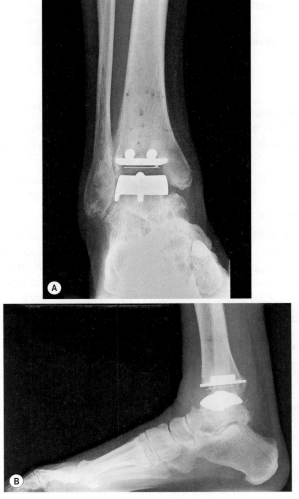

Fig. 4.23 Total ankle replacement – A) AP. B) Lateral X-rays.

These joints supplement the movement of the tibiotalar joint with supination and pronation of the foot in reference to the long axis of the leg. Degenerative disease is most often a consequence of trauma or osteoarthritis and less frequently due to rheumatoid, psoriatic or spondyloarthropathies. It can occur in isolation but frequently occurs in conjunction with tibiotalar arthritis, and up to five to seven times the body's weight is transmitted through these joints in gait.

## Symptoms

There may be a sustained period of subclinical arthritis and tolerable pain. By the time patients present they predominantly complain of the following:

- Stiffness and pain around the heel, particularly in weight-bearing positions

- Increased symptoms when walking over uneven ground

Swelling around the hindfoot and ankle joint

Loss of flexibility

Difficulty in fitting footwear: (rubbing around the heel)

## Signs

The patient will often indicate the lateral aspect or back of the hindfoot as the site of pain when subtalar arthritis is present.

- Inspection:
  - Antalgic gait
  - Swelling
  - Widening of the heel
  - Skin changes (calluses, ulceration)
- Palpation
  - Localised tenderness over the talonavicular or calcaneocuboid joints
- Movement
  - Reduced and/or painful inversion and eversion of the heel or pronation/supination of the foot

## Investigation

### X-rays

- Standard weight-bearing AP, oblique and lateral X-rays of the foot and ankle are usually adequate to visualize alignment and identify degeneration.

- If extra-articular deformities are identified (e.g., tibial malunion), then long leg standing X-rays should be obtained.

### Cross-sectional Imaging

- CT scans are more sensitive and specific if X-rays are insufficient and are useful for assessing complex deformities and bone stock.

- MRI may be helpful in identifying inflammatory change, ligament or tendon pathology, stress or insufficiency fractures, or osteochondral damage.

### Diagnostic Injection

If examination and X-rays are inconclusive or multiple areas of interest are identified, a diagnostic injection (often image-guided) with local anaesthetic can help to localise the symptomatic joints.

## Management

### Nonoperative

- Weight loss/walking aids

- Analgesia (NSAIDs)

- Activity modification (reduce impact)

- Steroid injection

- Footwear adaptations/orthoses to absorb impact and limit painful ranges of movement

### Operative

Given the limited range of movement required in the hindfoot, fusion remains the mainstay of surgical management. This can be subtalar, talonavicular, calcaneocuboid or a combination. Fusion of all three joints is known as a '**triple fusion**' (Fig. 4.24).

- Deformity correction can be achieved during the fusion to achieve a stable plantigrade foot, with restoration of a normal hindfoot alignment and arch.

- Less commonly, an additional realignment osteotomy of the calcaneus may be added.

- Combination arthrodesis may be necessary, along with tibiotalar fusion (tibio-talar-calcaneal), pantalar fusion or ankle arthroplasty.

## MIDFOOT ARTHRITIS

## Introduction

The midfoot joints include the naviculocuneiform (NC) joint complex, which has three facets, medial, middle and lateral, and the tarsometatarsal joints (**Fig. 4.1**). The NC joint and the second and third TMTJs have little movement and form the stable complement of the midfoot. The first, fourth and fifth TMTJs also have little range of motion in the normal foot but are more flexible, allowing the foot to accommodate to the surface of the ground.

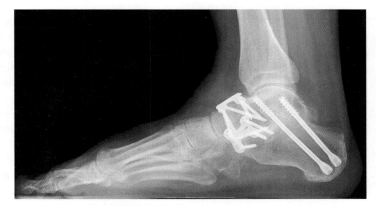

Fig. 4.24 Triple Fusions – Lateral X-ray.

## Background

Midfoot arthritis is loss of cartilage and osteo-phytosis of the joints between the midfoot bones (navicular, cuboid, medial, intermediate and lateral cuneiform).

The osteoarthritic process can be either be primary, idiopathic or secondary to trauma (e.g., following a Lisfranc injury). Degeneration may also occur secondary to autoimmune rheu-matological arthroses. As degeneration pro-gresses, repetitive loading can eventually lead to failure of these static restraints and midfoot collapse.

## Symptoms

- Pain in the midfoot area, particularly in the longitudinal arch during the push-off phase of gait. Swelling and deformity
- Footwear issues (fitting and rubbing) from prominence of dorsal osteophytes
- Gait instability (tripping up due to alteration in foot biomechanics)

## Signs

### Inspection
- Loss of longitudinal arch (initially only in weight-bearing positions)
- Forefoot abduction and hindfoot valgus
- Midfoot collapse
- Achilles tendon contracture

### Palpation
- Tenderness particularly on the plantar aspect of the midfoot
- Correctable deformity in early disease

### Movement
- There is minimal movement in these joints in a normally functioning foot.
- Dynamic loss of arch height may be seen during gait.

## Investigation
### X-rays
- AP and lateral X-rays of the foot
- Arthritic picture (loss of join space, sclero-sis, and osteophytes
- Midfoot collapse and disruption of Meary's angle (**Fig. 4.25**)

### Cross-sectional Imaging
- MRI is more sensitive and specific if X-rays are insufficient. It can confirm dysfunction in associated structures such as the tibialis posterior tendon.

### Diagnostic Injection (Image-Guided)
- May be useful to differentiate which degen-erative area is the source of pain.

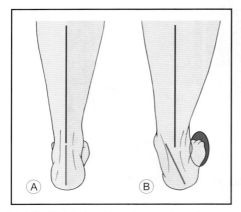

Fig. 4.25 Weight-bearing stance, viewed posteriorly. The hindfoot is in valgus. More of the lateral border of the foot can be seen, the "too many toes sign".

## Management

### Nonoperative

- Weight loss/walking aids
- Analgesia (NSAIDs)
- Activity modification (reduce impact)
- Steroid injection
- Footwear adaptations/orthoses: cushioned heel, longitudinal arch support, stiff sole, and rocker bottom.

### Operative

- Midfoot arthrodesis of affected joint(s) can result in near to normal function (**Fig. 4.26**).
- Can be supplemented with a hindfoot realignment (e.g., calcaneal osteotomy) and/or an Achilles tendon lengthening procedure.

## FOOT DEFORMITY

### Introduction

This section describes conditions associated with abnormality of the height of the arch of the foot. The foot naturally has three main arches: the medial and lateral longitudinal arches and the transverse arch (**Fig. 4.2**). These arches are used as shock absorption while in weight-bearing positions, but they also provide a mechanical advantage in propulsion during walking and running. The main determinant of foot shape is the medial longitudinal arch.

Decreased (pes planus) and increased (pes cavus) concavity of the medial longitudinal arch are common foot deformities.

A change in the medial longitudinal arch can be either dynamic or static and flexible or fixed. In the tripod model, there is balance between the three posts of the first metatarsal head, the fifth metatarsal head and the heel in the normal foot. When the medial column is elevated or deficient (flattening of the longitudinal medial arch), maintaining ground contact with all three posts drives the hindfoot into valgus. When the medial post of the first ray is plantar flexed (in the cavus foot), the hindfoot tilts into varus on stance.

## PES PLANOVALGUS

### Introduction

Despite public perception, pes planus (flat foot or fallen arches) is common and physiologically normal in the majority of patients, particularly in children. A pathological flat foot is defined as the loss of the medial longitudinal arch associated with pain.

Loss of the longitudinal medial arch when in weight-bearing positions is associated with forefoot abduction and valgus position of the hindfoot (thus, it is often called pes planovalgus).

It is important to differentiate between constitutional flat foot and adult-acquired flatfoot deformity.

Pathological causes of flat foot include the following:

- Congenital

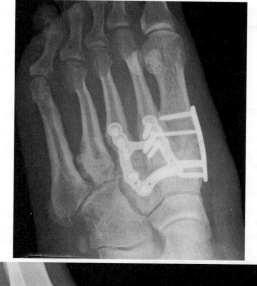

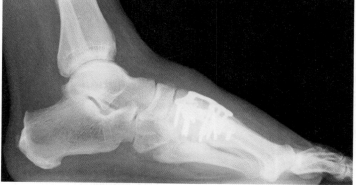

Fig. 4.26 Midfoot fusion (TMT joints) – Postoperative X-rays.

- **Tarsal coalition** (calcaneonavicular or talocalcaneal), which can be fibrous or ossified
- **Congenital vertical talus**
- **Hypermobile** (usually bilateral), either familial or as part of a syndrome:
  - Marfan
  - Ehlers–Danlos
  - Down
  - Morquio
  - Fragile X

- **Acquired**
  - **Posterior tibial tendon (PTT) insufficiency**
    - Most common cause of adult-acquired flat foot deformity
    - Most commonly found in women in their 50s
    - Associated with hypertension, diabetes, obesity and steroid use
    - The tibialis posterior functions as a dynamic arch support that decreases due to tendinopathy, and then static constraints gradually fail.

- **Inflammatory joint disease**
- **Degenerative midfoot disease (idiopathic or post-trauma)**
- **Neuropathic**

## Information: Posterior Tibial Tendon Disorder

Posterior tibial tendon disorder (PTTD) is the most common cause of symptomatic flat foot presenting in adults (**Table 4.3**). The tibialis posterior tendon initiates heel raise in gait and is the primary muscle supporting the arch. It is at risk of tendinopathy, particularly when under increased stresses due to the biomechanical environment, such as increased levels of physical activity, tight Achilles tendon/gastrocnemius, preexisting flat foot deformity or elevated body mass index (BMI). It can also be affected by inflammatory disorders. There is a relatively avascular zone in the tendon 2–6 cm proximal to its distal insertion which restricts the healing capacity.

## Symptoms

- Pain
  - Arch pain
  - Medial ankle pain or pain radiating up medial lower leg
  - Lateral hindfoot pain: subfibular or sinus tarsi impingement
  - Other pain attributed to flat foot (knee pain, hip pain, lower back pain)
- Difficulty with footwear
- Awareness of a change in foot shape, either acutely or over a period of time
- Difficulty in walking/standing on one foot

## Signs

### Inspection
- Flattened arch in weight-bearing positions (unilateral or bilateral)
- Valgus hindfoot position (**Fig. 4.26**)

- Supinated midfoot/first ray relative to the hindfoot
- Abducted midfoot (more than 1.5 toes visible laterally when viewed from behind = 'too many toes' sign) (**Fig. 4.26**).

### Palpation
- Tenderness in the arch
- Tenderness along the PTT
- Swelling along the course of the PTT
- Sensation

### Movement
- Associated tight gastrocnemius (Silverskiöld test: improvement in passive ankle dorsiflexion when the knee moves from extension to flexion)
- Flexibility/correction
- Hindfoot
- Subtalar
- Transverse tarsal joint

## Investigation
- Painless and insensate pes planus may require investigation for diabetes.
- Multiple joint pain may prompt testing for inflammatory arthropathy.
- Hypermobility may be investigated for genetic syndromes detailed above.
- PTT insufficiency may be confirmed with ultrasound scanning or MRI.

### Weight-bearing X-rays (AP, Lateral, Oblique)
- Meary's angle (**Fig. 4.27**)
- Reduced calcaneal pitch
- Midfoot abduction
- Tarsal coalition, accessory navicular, congenital vertical talus

## Treatment

Painless asymptomatic flat foot deformity with intact tibialis posterior and no gastrocnemius contracture does not need intervention.

**Table 4.3    Classification of Posterior Tibial Tendon Disorder (Modified Johnson and Strom)**

Stage I: Posterior tibial synovitis without underlying deformity
Stage II: Flexible flat foot deformity, posterior tibial tendon diseased and nonfunctional
IIA: Hindfoot valgus without forefoot abduction
IIB: Hindfoot valgus with forefoot abduction
IIC: Hindfoot valgus with fixed forefoot supination
Stage III: Rigid flat foot deformity
Stage IV: Flat foot with incompetence of deltoid ligament of the ankle, valgus talar tilt

## Nonoperative Treatment

- Analgesia
- Anti-inflammatory drugs
- Resting (walking boot 3 months) may help settle acute symptoms.
- Physiotherapy to help PTTD and Achilles tendon/gastrocnemius tightness
- Orthoses: Use device such as a UCBL foot orthosis to help support heel position and medial arch. In more advanced disease a hinged ankle brace incorporating a foot orthosis such as a Richie Brace may be effective. By supporting the foot, strain in the medial tissues is reduced, and some improvement in lateral impingement may also be achieved.

## Operative Treatment

Persistent severe symptoms are considered for surgery. There are a range of techniques, and the extent of the deformity and associated degenerative changes will guide treatment. These treatment options are based primarily on tibialis posterior deficiency.

- Stage I disease
  - Tibialis posterior debridement
- Stage II disease: Flexible deformity
  - Tendon transfer flexor digitorum longus into navicular to reconstruct tibialis posterior
  - Medial displacement calcaneal osteotomy
  - Lateral column lengthening (Evans).
  - Lateral opening wedge osteotomy of the anterior process of the calcaneus to correct midfoot abduction

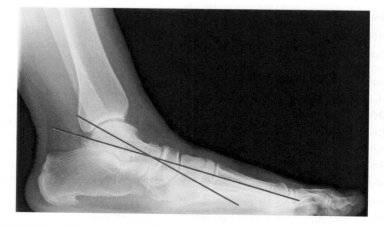

Fig. 4.27 Lateral foot X-ray in pes planus – Meary's angle is the angle between the longitudinal axis of the talus, and the axis of the first metatarsal, and should be 0 degrees +/- 5 degrees. In this case of pes planus, it is apex inferior and >10 degrees.

- Gastrocnemius lengthening, if contracture present
- Stage III: Rigid deformity
  - Corrective triple arthrodesis (subtalar, talonavicular, calcaneocuboid)
  - Gastrocnemius lengthening, if contracture present
- Stage IV: Valgus ankle instability
  - Tibiotalocalcaneal arthrodesis

## PES CAVOVARUS

## Background

Unlike flat foot, pes cavus (or cavovarus) is rarely physiologically normal, and the majority of cases are associated with neurological pathologies or follow trauma. It is characterized by increased height of the longitudinal arches, hindfoot varus, forefoot adduction, pronation of the forefoot and flexion of the first ray. It is frequently driven by muscular imbalance between intrinsic and extrinsic muscles or by complementary muscle groups. Commonly, tibialis posterior and peroneus longus function is preserved while the tibialis anterior, peroneus brevis and intrinsic foot muscles become weak.

### Causes

- Neuromuscular
  - Spinal disease: spinal dysraphism, diastematomyelia, syringomyelia, tumour or tethering (often **unilateral** cavovarus)
  - Hereditary motor and sensory neuropathies (HMSNs): Charcot–Marie–Tooth disease
  - Central nervous system disorder: Friedreich ataxia, cerebral palsy
  - Poliomyelitis
  - Muscular dystrophy
- Post-traumatic
  - Post compartment or crush syndrome
  - Hindfoot/midfoot malunion
- Idiopathic: variant of normal, mild and usually bilateral
- Congenital: residual clubfoot, arthrogryposis

Unless the cause is known, a patient presenting with pes cavus, particularly with progressive disease, should be fully examined with MRI of the spine, neurophysiological testing and consideration of neurological referral.

## Information: Charcot–Marie–Tooth

- Most common inherited neuromuscular disorder (incidence of 40 per 100,000)
- Falls under Hereditary Motor Sensory Neuropathies (HMSNs), which are neuromuscular degenerative conditions in the absence of metabolic disorders
- Usually autosomal dominant (chromosome 17), but can be recessive or X-linked
- Results in abnormal sensation and motor dysfunction/imbalance and can manifest with pes cavovarus, scoliosis, muscle wasting (particularly hand), hammer toes and hip dysplasia
- Four types:
  - Type 1 (65%): Demyelination due to mutated myelin protein-22. Affects myelinated cells (however, pain and temperature sensation are preserved as these fibres are unmyelinated). Schwann cells then remyelinate repeatedly, causing an 'onion bulb' deformity with reduced nerve conduction.
  - Type 2: Axonal loss and Wallerian degeneration
  - Type 3: Like type 1 but infantile onset, with severe and rapid demyelination with delayed motor development
  - Type 4 and X-linked Charcot–Marie–Tooth: Also demyelinating and more severe than type 1, but recessive with multiple further subtypes based on genetics

## Symptoms

- Foot deformity
- Recurrent ankle sprains (from varus hindfoot position)
- Lateral foot pain

- Metatarsalgia
- Calluses on base of first and fifth metatarsal heads or along lateral border of foot
- Clawing of toes

## Signs

- Accentuated medial longitudinal arch (**Fig. 4.28**)
- Plantarflexed first ray
- Hindfoot varus
- Clawed toes
- Unstable gait (poor base)
- Muscle wasting and weakness
- Possible sensory loss
- Other associated deformities (e.g., scoliosis or hand signs in Charcot–Marie–Tooth)
- Tendoachilles contracture

## Investigations

- Weight-bearing X-rays (AP, lateral, oblique) (**Fig. 4.29**)
  - Meary's angle increased apex dorsal (>10 degrees)
  - Increased calcaneal pitch (> 30 degrees)
  - Hindfoot varus
- Neurological diagnostic investigations
  - MRI of the spine
  - Electrodiagnostic studies (electromyography/nerve conduction)
  - Genetic testing
  - Neurology referral

## Treatment

### Nonoperative

- Physiotherapy to stretch a tight Achilles or gastrocnemius tendon and maximize strength and balance
- Orthoses. Functional foot orthosis to accommodate plantarflexed first ray and stabilize varus heel. Ankle foot orthoses may be required if significant weakness is present.
- Accommodative footwear (mild deformity)

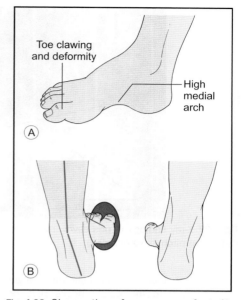

Fig. 4.28 Observation of a pes cavus foot. A) high medial arch and toe deformities. B) hindfoot varus, with sight to medial border of foot and hallux (peek-a-boo toe sign).

### Operative

Surgical treatment should be considered when nonoperative treatments have failed. A combination of procedures is usually selected to target the specific issues in patients. These include joint-preserving techniques in flexible deformity and fusion in more severe and rigid deformity.

- Soft tissue procedures
  - Achilles tendon lengthening
  - Plantar fascia release
  - Tibialis posterior transfer to dorsum of foot for foot drop
  - Tibialis anterior transfer to lateral cuneiform to neutralize dynamic supination
  - Peroneus longus to brevis transfer to maximize eversion power
  - Jones transfer: Fusion of first IPJ and transfer of EHL to the first metatarsal neck to reduce cavus and clawing and improve dorsiflexion.

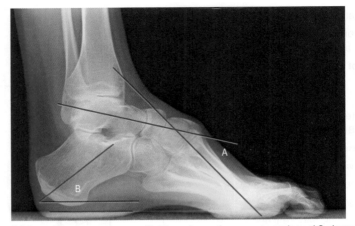

Fig. 4.29 X-ray findings in pes cavovarus. A) Meary's angle apex superior >10 degrees. B) Calcaneal pitch (>30 degrees).

- Lesser toe extensor digitorum longus transfer to metatarsal necks plus IPJ fusions (addresses clawing), analogous to Jones transfer
- Lateral ankle ligament repair or reconstruction, for instability
- Bone procedures
  - First ray elevation osteotomy (rarely, lesser rays may also require elevation)
  - Lateralizing or lateral closing wedge calcaneal osteotomy (for rigid varus hindfoot deformity)
  - Corrective triple arthrodesis: reserve for severe deformity and degenerative change

## DISORDERS OF TENDONS AND FASCIA

## ACHILLES TENDINOPATHY

### Background

The Achilles tendon is the conjoined tendon of the gastrocnemius and soleus muscles. The pathophysiology behind tendinopathy is outlined in [chapter 1], and the principles translate into the common diagnosis of Achilles tendinopathy. This disease can be categorized by the location of symptoms along the gastrocnemius–soleus complex: insertional, midsubstance (noninsertional) and musculotendinous junction (rare and self-limiting). Persistent tendinopathy may be a risk factor in Achilles tendon rupture.

- **Midsubstance Achilles tendinopathy** typically occurs in middle-aged patients. It occurs between 2 and 6 cm proximal to the insertion. It often results from repetitive strain (exercise and/or obesity) on a background of poor vascular supply. This area of the tendon has a natural vascular watershed, and factors such as smoking, diabetes and genetics contribute. It is thought to represent a degeneration of the tendon, with a loss of the natural balance between microtrauma and repair. In a proportion of cases there is a recent history of fluoroquinolone antibiotics. The natural history is thought to be self-limiting, with 80% of cases improved by 2 years. However, cases resistant to nonoperative treatment may require surgery.
- **Insertional Achilles tendinopathy** occurs within 2 cm of the calcaneal insertion. This condition is most common amongst middle-age and elderly patients, particularly in those who have a tight Achilles tendon or gastrocnemius. Repetitive trauma causes

inflammation, and the relatively good local blood supply causes cell mediated inflammation, mucoid degeneration and metaplasia in cartilaginous and bony/calcific tissue. It is often associated with a Haglund deformity (a posterosuperior prominence in the calcaneus).

## Symptoms

- Pain with weight-bearing positions and activity, particularly repetitive or impact such as running
- Swelling
- Irritating lump
- Acute rupture

## Clinical Examination

- Visible fusiform swelling
- Tenderness
- Fusiform thickening or swelling of the tendon
- Pain on tiptoe standing or heel dips
- Tight Achilles tendon or gastrocnemius

## Investigation

- Ultrasound scanning may demonstrate thickening, partial/total chronic rupture and/or calcific changes
- MRI may demonstrate high intensity disorganised tissue, thickening, partial/total chronic rupture and calcific changes

## Treatment

### Nonoperative
- Activity modification
- Physiotherapy-guided eccentric and isometric therapy (particularly effective for midsubstance)
- Footwear modification: A heel lift may reduce strain and improve symptoms.
- NSAIDs
- Transcutaneous nitrates: Application of glyceryl trinitrate patch over the symptomatic area
- Extracorporeal shock wave therapy

- Intra-tendonous steroid... Steroid injection is **contraindicated** due to risk of rupture

## Surgical Treatment

Surgery may be considered for cases refractory to over 6 months of nonoperative therapy.

Noninsertional Achilles tendinopathy:
- Radiofrequency coblation of diseased tendon
- Proximal medial head of gastrocnemius release
- Debridement and excision of degenerative tendon (moderate–severe disease)
  - FHL transfer if >50% of the Achilles tendon is diseased or ruptured

Insertional Achilles tendinopathy
- Debridement of tendon insertion +/– Haglund deformity or calcification resection (for insertional cases)
- The tendon will need to be reattached if the insertion is found to be unstable or becomes so after debridement.

## PLANTAR FASCIITIS

## Background

The plantar fascia (or aponeurosis) is a thick layer of connective tissue originating in the proximal calcaneus fanning out to the metatarsal heads and inserting on the phalanges. It forms the windlass mechanism of the foot and is a passive support of the longitudinal medial arch (**Fig. 4.30**).

The most common pathology of the plantar fascia is plantar fasciitis. Chronic tensile loads and microtrauma result in degeneration of the plantar fascia. Symptoms usually begin at the posteromedial heel caused by inflammation and periostitis at the shared origin with small

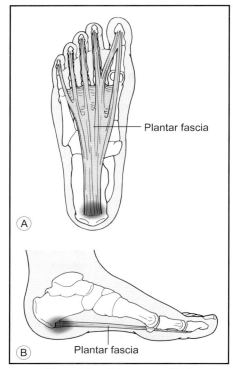

Fig. 4.30 Plantar fascia anatomy. A) View from plantar aspect. B) Lateral aspect. The location of pathology is usually around the origin on the medial/plantar calcaneum.

muscles of the foot (quadratus plantae, flexor digitorum brevis and abductor hallucis).

Risk factors for the condition include biomechanical factors such as a tight Achilles tendon or gastrocnemius causing increased strain in the plantar tissues, repetitive stresses such as regular running, increased BMI or occupations involving long periods of standing. Biological causes include recent quinolone antibiotics and reactive arthritis.

The differential diagnosis includes other causes of pain in the plantar fascia or heel such as plantar fibromatosis or insertional Achilles tendinopathy. It can also occur as part of a triad along with PTTD and tarsal tunnel syndrome (compression of tibial nerve behind the medial malleolus).

## Symptoms
- Dull constant heel pain with aggravation on heel strike during gait, particularly first thing in the morning (as the Achilles tendon/calf muscle tends to shorten during sleep)
- Pain worsens with weight-bearing activity through the day.

## Signs
- Antalgic gait
- Pes planus (due to attrition of fascia)
- Tiptoe gait (avoiding heel strike)
- Point tenderness at the medial calcaneal tubercle
- Diffuse tenderness throughout the plantar fascia
- Tibial nerve dysfunction (Tinel test, sensory disturbance in the sole/digits)
- Gastrocnemius/soleus contracture

## Investigation
- Laboratory tests: In young patients with multiple sites of pain, inflammatory rheumatological conditions should be excluded.
- X-rays
  - Saddle sign lucency at medial calcaneal tuberosity on lateral view
  - Calcaneal spurs (arising at short flexor apophyses)
- MRI
  - Fascial thickening
  - Visualizes extent of disease
  - Will indicate other diagnoses, e.g., stress fracture of the calcaneum
- Electromyography
  - Aids tarsal tunnel syndrome diagnosis

## Treatment
### Nonoperative
- Reduce load through weight loss, cessation of impact activity and reduced duration on feet
- Tendoachilles and plantar fascia stretching (most effective intervention)
- Casting to aid Achilles stretching

- Night splints +/− great toe wedge
- NSAIDs
- Extra corporeal shockwave therapy
- Steroid injection (risk of recurrent pain, fascial rupture and heel fat pad atrophy)
- Orthoses

## Operative (>9–12 Months Nonoperative Treatment)

Surgery is only necessary in <5% of cases, and only after 12 months of nonoperative treatment.

- Radiofrequency coblation
- Plantar fascial release (controversial and may result in arch destabilization)

## THE DIABETIC FOOT

## Introduction

The World Health Organization estimates 1 in 11 adults have diabetes, and worldwide, a person loses a leg every 20 seconds due to diabetic complications.

Diabetes mellitus affects multiple body systems through dysfunction of the body's ability to produce or respond to insulin. The management of diabetes involves a multidisciplinary team approach. Good glycaemic control can prevent the complications associated with the disease; however, this is difficult to achieve in many patients.

Diabetic foot disease develops in up to 15% of diabetic patients and can significantly impact on their quality of life. The three main manifestations of diabetic foot disease are infection, ulceration and Charcot arthropathy.

The two main causes of diabetic foot disease are **diabetic vascular disease** and **neuropathy**. Approximately two-thirds of diabetic patients will have some form of neuropathy, which may affect sensory, motor and autonomic pathways.

In the lower limbs, sensory loss affects touch and pain sensation and presents in a stocking distribution, reducing the awareness and protective responses to excessive pressure or repetitive minor trauma. Motor neuropathy can affect the intrinsic foot muscles, leading to clawing of the toes and increased forefoot pressures. Autonomic dysfunction can leave the skin thick, dry and at risk of cracking. Diabetic vascular disease can affect the peripheral arterial supply, although autonomic dysfunction can lead to vasodilatation masking the vascular insufficiencies unless regular screening is performed. This combination of factors contributes to the risk of developing infection through unrecognized trauma, diabetic foot ulceration or, in some patients, developing Charcot arthropathy.

## DIABETIC FOOT SCREENING

Diabetic patients should be screened and monitored for diabetic foot disease. Those at low risk can be educated in foot care and monitoring and managed in the community setting with annual screening, but for higher risk patients, regular multidisciplinary clinic visits are required.

The components of screening are:

- Optimization of glycaemic control
- Patient education on diabetic control, footwear, avoidance of barefoot walking and regular foot checks
- Examination for skin lesions/infections/nail disease/deformity, e.g., claw toes which might lead to risk of skin breach or infection
- Podiatry input for nail care/callus debridement where appropriate
- Screening for peripheral neuropathy: Failure to feel a 10 g monofilament defines loss of protective sensation
- Detection of peripheral arterial disease (PAD)

- Palpate and record dorsalis pedis and posterior tibial pulses
- Ankle-brachial pressure index (ABPI) measurement is the ratio of systolic pressure at the ankle to that of the arm. Ratio of <0.9 indicates peripheral arterial disease. ABPI can be normal or raised in the presence of calcified arterial disease.
- Footwear referral: Orthotic footwear may be used to avoid or offload pressure areas in an at-risk foot.
- Escalation of care in presence of infection, ulceration, critical ischaemia or suspicion of Charcot arthropathy.

### Table 4.4    Wagner Classification of Diabetic Foot Ulcers

- Grade 0 – intact skin
- Grade 1 – superficial ulcer of skin or subcutaneous tissue
- Grade 2 – ulcers extend into tendon, bone or capsule
- Grade 3 – deep ulcer with osteomyelitis or abscess
- Grade 4 – partial foot gangrene
- Grade 5 – whole foot gangrene

## DIABETIC FOOT ULCERS

Despite preventative measures, foot ulcers are common in patients with diabetic neuropathy. The International Working Group for the Diabetic Foot (IWGDF) estimates a lifetime risk of foot ulcers in diabetic patients of 20-30%. Recurrence rates are high, and diabetic ulcers are an underlying factor in up to 85% of lower extremity amputations.

Diabetic ulcers commonly occur in areas of skin which are under increased pressure, such as over a bony prominence. Shear and stress within the tissues lead to damage.

Ulcers can be described as neuropathic, ischaemic or mixed. Neuropathic ulcers tend to have an area of clean granulation tissue under an area of necrotic skin. Ischaemic ulcers are often painful, with necrotic tissue extending down into the base.

### Classification

Multiple classification systems have been developed and can be used for assessment and to monitor progress. The Wagner system is in wide usage, is simple and has been shown to have some value in predicting the foot at risk of amputation (**Table 4.4**). The IWGDF currently recommends the Site, Ischaemia, Neuropathy, Bacterial infection, Area, Depth (SINBAD) classification for monitoring of diabetic foot ulcers (**Table 4.5**).

### Treatment

- Optimization of glycaemic control
- Local wound care and debridement
- Manage infection with surgical debridement/antibiotic therapy
- Offload pressure areas
  - External: Total contact cast or insoles to distribute pressures and avoid point loading, rest, elevation and restriction of weight-bearing activity
  - Internal: Resection of bony prominences/ correction of deformity
- Achilles tendon lengthening to reduce forefoot pressures
- Amputation: Partial or whole foot amputation (below knee) may become necessary in severe infection, gangrene or critical ischaemia.

## CHARCOT ARTHROPATHY

### Background

This is a progressive destructive arthropathy seen in individuals with peripheral neuropathy.

**Table 4.5 Site, Ischaemia, Neuropathy, Bacterial Infection, Area, Depth (SINBAD) Classification of Diabetic Foot Ulcers (Maximum Score 6)**

| Clinical Feature | Score = 0 | Score = 1 |
|---|---|---|
| Site | Forefoot | Midfoot or hindfoot |
| Ischaemia | Pedal blood flow intact; at least one pulse palpable | Clinical evidence of reduced pedal blood flow |
| Neuropathy | Protective sensation intact | Protective sensation lost |
| Bacterial infection | None | Present |
| Area | Less than 1 cm$^2$ | Greater than 1 cm$^2$ |
| Depth | Skin and subcutaneous tissue | Reaching muscle, tendon or deeper |

Initially described in patients suffering from syphilis, diabetes mellitus is now the most common underlying cause. The underlying pathophysiology is multifactorial. In the neurotraumatic theory the process is triggered by trauma (acute or repetitive microtrauma) in the absence of normal protective sensation. In the neurovascular theory autonomic neuropathy leads to hyperaemia, causing impairment of venous outflow and capillary leakage. An inflammatory cascade is initiated, and with ongoing mobilization, failure of bones, ligaments and tendons will lead to progressive deformity and collapse. The age of onset is typically between 30 and 50 years old with a history of diabetes of over 10 years.

## Symptoms

- Acute-onset of red, hot and swollen limb that is typically **not** painful.

## Signs

- Systemically well (except in the presence of secondary infection)
- Palpable pulses and prompt capillary refill
- Skin temperature difference of >2°C to the unaffected limb
- Bilateral disease is seen in up to 30% of patients
- Deformity may be present in established disease
- Concurrent manifestations of diabetic foot disease

## Investigations

### X-rays

- May be normal in early disease
- Useful for monitoring disease progression and assessing deformity (**Fig. 4.31**)

### MRI

- Useful in early disease, detects soft tissue changes, bone marrow oedema and joint effusions
- May aid differentiation between Charcot and infection

### CT Scanning

- Useful for evaluating deformity and operative planning

### Bone Scan

- Detects increased bone activity but may not differentiate Charcot arthropathy from osteomyelitis

The disease stage and anatomical location can be used to classify the progression of the disease (**Tables 4.6 and 4.7**)

## Management

The aim of treatment is to prevent deformity and reach the consolidation stage of the disease with a stable, plantigrade foot. Nonoperative treatment is the basis for this, but operative intervention is sometimes required.

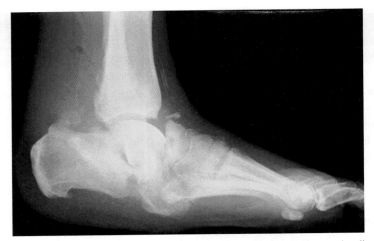

Fig. 4.31 End-stage Charcot arthropathy. X-ray demonstrates fragmentation and collapse of the talus and midfoot.

## Nonoperative Management

- **Weight bearing**: Non-weight-bearing activity was traditionally recommended for the acute phase of the disease, but it is now thought most patients can be allowed to bear weight in an appropriate support.

- **Total contact cast/insole**: Total contact casting avoids localised pressure over any prominences and helps to prevent progressive foot deformity. In the early phase of treatment, swelling rapidly recedes, and regular cast changes are necessary to ensure the cast remains well fitting and to prevent rubbing or ulceration beneath the cast. Once a stable situation is achieved, a total contact insole can be fashioned for use in a removable boot or shoe.

- **Bisphosphonate therapy:** Bisphosphonate therapy may reduce osteoclastic activity; however, the overall time to reach the consolidation phase may be extended, and the evidence is not currently conclusive.

**Table 4.6   Eichenholtz Staging**

| Stage | Stage Description | Clinical Presentation | Radiographic Findings |
|-------|-------------------|----------------------|----------------------|
| 0 | Patient at risk. Neuropathy with history of trauma | | No destructive change |
| 1 | Development/ fragmentation | Erythema, swelling, warmth. Clinical similarity to infection | Subchondral fragmentation, joint subluxation or dislocation |
| 2 | Coalescence | Decreasing erythema, swelling and warmth | New bone formation |
| 3 | Consolidation/remodelling | Inflammatory signs resolved. Residual deformity | Bone healing and remodelling |

## Table 4.7   Anatomical Classification

| Type | Anatomical Location | Clinical Relevance |
|------|---------------------|--------------------|
| 1 | Midfoot (tarsometatarsal) | Most common. Relatively stable. Risk of rocker bottom foot and plantar prominence. |
| 2 | Hindfoot | Unstable. Collapse of arch and rocker bottom sole may result. Ongoing instability. |
| 3A | Ankle | Unstable and high risk of deformity. |
| 3B | Posterior calcaneus | May lead to pes planus. |
| 4 | Multiple sites | |
| 5 | Forefoot | High risk of ulceration and infection. |

## Operative Treatment

Nonoperative treatment is effective in many patients. Operative treatment is usually delayed until after the fragmentation stage of the disease to minimize provoking or exacerbating increased Charcot activity.

- Exostectomy
- Prevention of deformity
- Achilles tendon lengthening
- Arthrodesis in situ of affected regions
- Deformity correction with corrective arthrodesis (**Fig. 4.32**)
- Amputation

## CLINICAL EXAMINATION OF THE FOOT AND ANKLE

Assessment of a patient with foot and ankle symptoms requires detailed history-taking, focused clinical examination and selection of the most appropriate investigations.

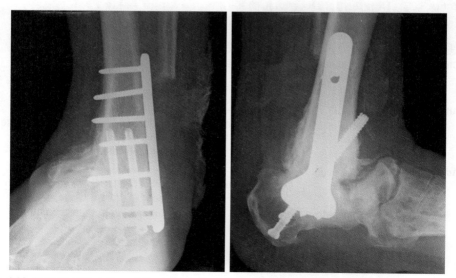

Fig. 4.32 Post-operative X-ray following hindfoot fusion for Charcot arthropathy.

## History-Taking

The history should include the patient's age, occupation, duration of symptoms, nature and severity of symptoms and any relevant underlying conditions.

Pain should be assessed in terms of its location, quality, pattern and severity. The relation to activities such as walking and sport should be elicited. From the pattern of pain, the differential diagnosis can start to be narrowed down (**Table 4.8**).

## Examination

During examination of the foot and ankle, both lower limbs should be exposed from the knee down. Inspection of the lower limbs should include standing, walking and sitting evaluations. The patient's footwear should be examined, looking for stretching and wear patterns. The use of any orthoses or walking aids should be noted.

The generic components of the musculoskeletal examination are applied with **Look-Feel-Move**, followed by appropriate selection of special tests. In the foot and ankle, these components more naturally fall into **standing**, **walking** and **sitting** sections.

If signs of pathology affecting other joints or neurological signs are elicited, examination of those joints or the spine may be indicated following the foot and ankle assessment.

## Look

- Appraisal of coronal and sagittal alignment and posture
- Accentuation or absence of arches
- Observation of intrinsic or proximal muscle loss
- Observation of deformity in the hindfoot or forefoot
- Observation of great and lesser toe deformities
- Observation of dorsal and plantar skin for evidence of rubbing, callosities or ulceration
- Gait should be assessed, particularly the main foot and ankle components of heel strike and toe-off.

### Table 4.8   Differential Diagnosis Based on Foot and Ankle Pain

| Age Group | Heel | Location of Pain | | |
|---|---|---|---|---|
| | | Medial/Dorsal Foot | Hallux | Forefoot |
| **Children** | Sever's disease | Köhler disease | Tight shoes/ socks<br>Ingrown toenail | Verruca pedis |
| **Adolescents** | Calcaneal exostosis<br>Bursitis | Cuneiform exostosis<br>Peroneal flat foot | Early hallux rigidus<br>Hallux valgus<br>Nail problems | March fracture<br>Freiberg disease<br>Pes cavovarus<br>Verruca pedis |
| **Adults** | Plantar fasciitis<br>Insertional Achilles tendinopathy | Flat foot<br>Osteoarthritis<br>Inflammatory arthritis | Hallux valgus<br>Hallux rigidus<br>Gout<br>Nail problems | Metatarsalgia<br>Morton's neuroma<br>Pes cavus<br>Inflammatory arthritis<br>Gout<br>Verruca pedis<br>Tarsal tunnel syndrome |

## Feel

- The joints and structures of the hindfoot, midfoot and forefoot are sequentially and logically palpated to detect and locate pain.
- Assessment of the lower limb sensation, pulses and capillary refill can also be performed at this point.

## Move

- Move is split into assessment of both active and passive joint motion, along with eliciting instability. Each joint should be isolated, where possible, and compared with the other side, starting at the ankle and working distally (**Fig. 4.33**).

## Special Tests

Special tests are applied to confirm or refute a specific diagnostic hypothesis. There is a large selection of tests, and this list is not exhaustive.

**Double Heel Raise**. The double heel raise looks for hindfoot flexibility in an individual with a valgus abnormality of the hindfoot. In a flexible deformity the heel will move from a position of valgus in stance to a varus alignment on tiptoe. If there is associated pes planus, the arch may also reform in a flexible foot. If the deformity is fixed the heel valgus will not correct.

**Tiptoe Stance (Single Heel Raise)**. The tiptoe stance is used to examine tibialis posterior function when pes planus is present. The patient is asked to stand on one leg and then go up onto their tiptoes to show whether the tibialis posterior tendon has sufficient strength to initiate the heel raise. In a flexible foot the arch will reform, and the heel will move from valgus to varus.

**Coleman Block Test**. The Coleman block test is indicated when there is a cavus deformity of

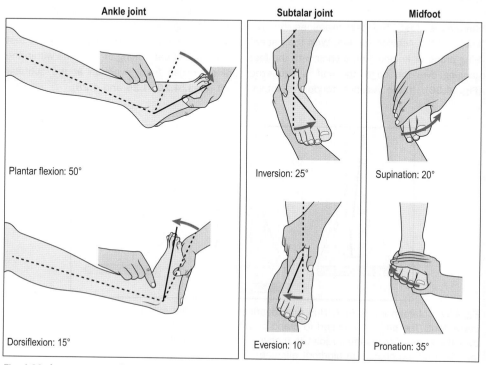

| Ankle joint | Subtalar joint | Midfoot |
|---|---|---|
| Plantar flexion: 50° | Inversion: 25° | Supination: 20° |
| Dorsiflexion: 15° | Eversion: 10° | Pronation: 35° |

Fig. 4.33 Assessment of ankle motion.

the hindfoot. It demonstrates if hindfoot varus is a flexible deformity driven by plantarflexion of the first ray. The patient is asked to stand on a flat block approximately 2 cm high with the heel and lateral rays resting on the block and the medial border of foot over the edge. If the hindfoot corrects from varus to valgus, then the hindfoot deformity is correctable and driven by the forefoot deformity (**Fig. 4.34**).

**Silverskiöld Test**. The Silverskiöld test differentiates between a tight Achilles tendon and tight gastrocnemius muscle in patients with a tight calf (limited dorsiflexion or equinus deformity). Ankle dorsiflexion is measured with knee extended and then with the knee flexed (**Fig. 4.35**). If the limitation is present with both the knee flexed and extended the tightness is within the Achilles tendon or ankle joint capsule. If the range of movement improves with knee flexion (gastrocnemius relaxed), then a tight gastrocnemius muscle is present.

**Simmonds' Test**. This test examines the continuity of the Achilles tendon. With the patient lying prone or kneeling on a chair with the feet hanging over the edge, the calf is squeezed (**Fig. 4.36**). If the Achilles tendon is intact,

plantarflexion of the foot will be seen. In this position the resting posture of the limb can be seen. With an Achilles rupture, the affected foot will rest in a position of increased dorsiflexion in comparison to the unaffected side. The tendon can also be palpated for any gaps or swelling.

**Anterior Drawer and Talar Tilt Tests** (**Fig. 4.37**). The anterior drawer test assesses the ATFL. With the knee flexed to relax the gastrocnemius, the distal tibia is grasped with one hand and the heel with the other. The upper hand can be positioned to allow a finger to rest on the anterolateral joint line. With the tibia stabilized, the heel is drawn anteriorly. In a slender individual, a sulcus sign at the joint line may be visible. If not, the motion of the talus may be felt with the finger positioned at the joint line.

The talar tilt test assesses the CFL. The gastrocnemius is relaxed with knee flexion. The hindfoot is gripped, and the talus is tilted into varus. Palpation of the joint line during the test helps differentiate tilting of the talus within the ankle mortise from inversion at the subtalar joint (**Figs. 4.20**, **4.26** and **4.28**).

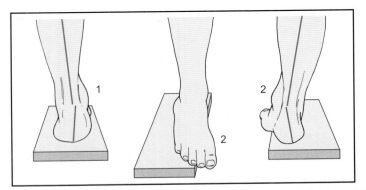

Fig. 4.34 Coleman Block Test: This test identifies whether the subtalar joint is mobile in a cavus foot. The patient is asked to stand on a block positioned to allow the first ray to hang over the edge. If the subtalar joint is mobile, the hindfoot will move into valgus. If the subtalar joint is fixed, no change in hindfoot alignment will occur.

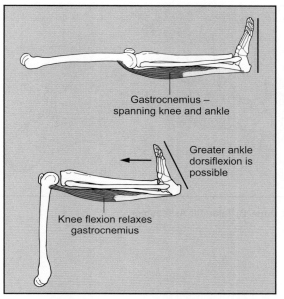

Gastrocnemius –
spanning knee and ankle

Greater ankle
dorsiflexion is
possible

Knee flexion relaxes
gastrocnemius

Fig. 4.35 Silverskiöld Test. As the gastrocnemius crosses both the knee and ankle joint, knee flexion will relax tension and allow further foot dorsiflexion. If there is no improvement with knee flexion, the contracture is at the level of the soleus and/or joint capsule.

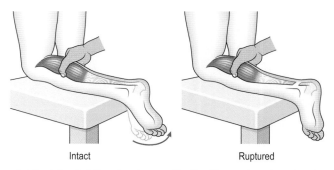

Intact                                    Ruptured

Fig. 4.36 Simmonds' Test for Achilles tendon continuity. The patient kneels on a chair with the affected leg, allowing the foot to hang freely. If a rupture is present, the foot will not plantar-flex when the calf muscle is squeezed.

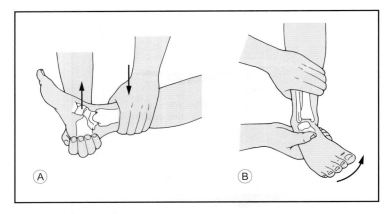

Fig. 4.37  A) Anterior Draw. B) Talar Tilt Assessment.

## ROTATOR CUFF TENDINOPATHY

### Background

Shoulder pain affects approximately 7% of the population at any one time, and this number increases to approximately 25% for the elderly population. Rotator cuff tendinopathy is a common cause of shoulder pain and functional limitation. Traditionally, overhead activities and mechanical impingement were thought to result in direct damage to the tendon and secondary changes in the subacromial space. Impingement resulted from anatomical structures, including the acromion, acromioclavicular (AC) joint and coracoacromial (CA) ligament. Anatomical variants, such as a hooked acromion, were thought to increase the risk of impingement. More recently, rotator cuff tendinopathy has been recognized as part of the normal ageing processes. Blood flow in the rotator cuff has been observed to decrease with age, and some parts of the rotator cuff, mainly around the insertion points, have been found to be relatively hypovascular and at risk of degeneration. Subsequent pain reduces rotator cuff activation and leads to secondary scapular dysfunction.

The rotator cuff cable and crescent play important roles in determining the functional significance of a rotator cuff tear (**Fig. 5.1**). Imaging findings often do not correlate with clinical findings. In many cases evidence of rotator cuff tendinopathy can be seen in patients without symptoms. The use of terms such as 'tears' reinforces a focus on repair as the main and only way of treating this condition. In most cases, nonoperative management will likely be successful.

Rotator cuff tears can progress over time. Symptomatic tears are likely to increase in size, while asymptomatic tears may progress and result in pain and weakness. Over time,

a torn rotator cuff may retract and become scarred. The muscle bellies can be replaced by fat, which is thought to be irreversible.

The subscapularis tendon can also demonstrate degeneration and tearing. The subscapularis is the sole rotator cuff muscle that inserts into the lesser tuberosity and is primarily an internal rotator of the shoulder. Pathology here can lead to anterior shoulder pain, weakness of internal rotation and difficulties reaching behind the back.

In most cases, rotator cuff tears represent the end point of a degenerative process. Partial tears may also be evident, and this is

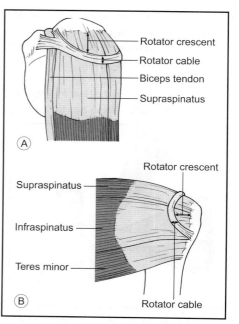

Fig. 5.1 Rotator cuff anatomy: A) Superior view of supraspinatus insertion demonstrating rotator cuff cable and crescent. B) Posterior view demonstrating confluence of cuff tendons.

caused by a portion of the tendon insertion pulling away. These tears are classified as either articular- or bursal-sided.

In rare cases, in younger patients, a rotator cuff tear may be caused by acute high-energy trauma. In older populations, rotator cuff tears may occur following a shoulder dislocation. It is important that patients over the age of 40 with a shoulder dislocation are assessed for the possibility of a rotator cuff tear when their initial symptoms have subsided. This is usually possible around two weeks after injury.

## Symptoms

- Lateral shoulder and upper arm pain

- Pain aggravated by overhead activities

- Weakness

## Signs

- Painful arc: Active movement in the middle range of the arc may be painful. When this movement is replicated passively, the pain is often reduced (**Fig. 5.2**).

- Eliciting Signs such as the Neer Impingement Sign may be useful. These aim to "trap" the

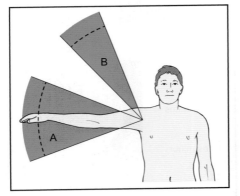

Fig. 5.2 The painful arc (A) is thought to occur at the point where the damaged portion of the rotator cuff and associated inflamed bursa are trapped by "impinging" structures. Pain in the higher range (B) is more likely to arise from the acromioclavicular joint.

inflamed portion of the tendon between the acromion and greater tuberosity.

## Investigation

- Plain radiographs should be obtained to exclude another differential diagnosis such as AC joint osteoarthritis and glenohumeral joint osteoarthritis (GHJOA) or a rare condition such as a tumour. Occasionally, some changes such as sclerosis or cyst formation may be seen around the greater tuberosity or under-surface of the acromion, indicative of long-standing impingement and cuff deficiency.

- Ultrasound scanning can be used to assess the rotator cuff and long head of the biceps (**Fig. 5.3**).

- Magnetic resonance imaging (MRI) is useful to assess the rotator cuff, including determining if there are any tears (**Fig. 5.4A**), retraction or fatty infiltration (**Fig. 5.4B**) of the cuff muscles. This approach can be used as a predictor of outcome in cases of repair of rotator cuff tears.

## Treatment

**Physiotherapy:** The aim of physiotherapy treatment is to re-establish rotator cuff strength and balance. There is often a benefit to core muscle training and recruitment of the deltoid and periscapular musculature.

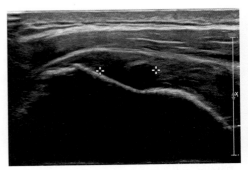

Fig. 5.3 Ultrasound image of tear of supraspinatus. It is retracted. The gap is between the two markers, measuring approximately 1 cm, resulting in retraction to the humeral head.

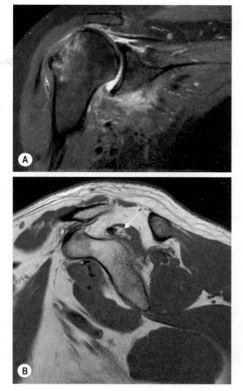

Fig. 5.4 MRI scan: A) Coronal plane showing rotator cuff tear and superior translation of humeral head. B) Sagittal plane through scapula showing fatty atrophy of supraspinatus (arrow).

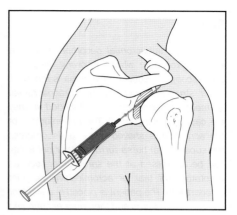

Fig. 5.5 The posterior approach is commonly used when injecting corticosteroid into the subacromial space.

support widespread use of other agents such as platelet-rich plasma (PRP).

**Surgery:** If there has not been a sustained response to a nonoperative management programme (up to 1 year of therapy and two steroid injections), surgery may be considered. This most commonly consists of repair or debridement of the rotator cuff +/− arthroscopic subacromial decompression (**Fig. 5.6**). Evidence does not support early surgical intervention.

**Corticosteroid injection:** Corticosteroid injection may be a useful adjunct to treatment and aims to reduce inflammation (**Fig. 5.5**). Anatomical landmark-based techniques should be used initially, and ultrasound scanning can be considered if there is a failure to respond. Common approaches are either posterior or lateral. The aim is to inject corticosteroid and local anaesthetic into the subacromial bursa, which will then provide a therapeutic window where physiotherapy can be more effectively accomplished. It is important not to give repeated corticosteroid injections where there is only a short-term response. There is a risk of long-term tendon damage with multiple injections, and they should only be considered to facilitate a rehabilitation programme. There is no evidence as yet to

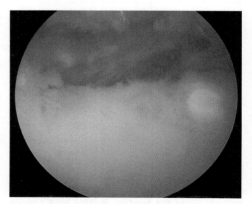

Fig. 5.6 Arthroscopic view of subacromial space. The inflamed bursa has been removed, and the inferior surface of the acromion has been shaved to reduce impingement (incidental calcific deposit noted to right side of cuff).

## Surgery

*Arthroscopic subacromial decompression is a keyhole procedure where, following diagnostic arthroscopy, the subacromial bursa is removed. Other structures such as the coracoacromial ligament are assessed and debrided if they are causing impingement. The undersurface of the acromion is shaved away to decompress the subacromial bursa further. Other pathology can be addressed at the same time, such as a rotator cuff tear or acromioclavicular joint osteoarthritis. The patient is placed in a sling for comfort for 24 hours and thereafter encouraged to move their arm with early physiotherapy.*

*When a rotator cuff tear has been detected pre-operatively, repair is planned. This is often accomplished with a double-row technique (*__Fig. 5.7__*), although a variety of techniques have been described. In some cases, primary repair is not possible. In these cases, the tendon edges can be debrided and the long head of the biceps tenotomized or tenodesed (if degenerate).*

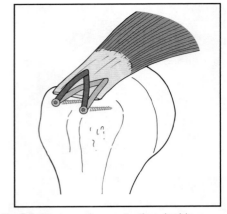

Fig. 5.7 Diagram demonstrating double-row repair of a torn supraspinatus tendon

### CALCIFIC TENDONITIS

## Background

Although calcific tendonitis can affect many tendons, the most common site of deposition is the rotator cuff. The calcific deposit is associated with inflammation in the adjacent tendon and subacromial bursa. Although it can occur asymptomatically, in most cases calcific deposit causes acute-onset severe pain. It occurs bilaterally (with staged disease more common than simultaneous) in 10% to 20% of cases. The supraspinatus is most commonly affected, with the subscapularis least affected.

It is hypothesized that a metaplastic change occurs within the tendon, leading to a change of tenocytes to chondrocytes, and subsequent deposition of calcification that may be triggered by tissue hypoxia, among other factors.

Three stages have been described (Uhthoff):

1. Precalcific: transition of tendon tissue to fibrocartilage

2. Calcific: deposition of calcium. This stage is characterized by formation followed by resorption. The resorptive phase is mostly like to lead to symptoms and functional impairment.

3. Postcalcific: remodelling and healing of the tendon

The most common outcome is spontaneous resolution, with healing of the tendon. It is not commonly associated with the onset of a rotator cuff tear where the lesion occurred.

## Symptoms
- Pain

  - Often severe

  - Nocturnal

  - Can be refractory to common analgesics

- Loss of function

## Signs

- The signs are similar to that of shoulder impingement and rotator cuff tendinopathy. They are caused by impingement of the inflamed calcific deposit during shoulder movements

- Painful arc (**Fig. 5.2**)

## Investigation

Plain radiographs are diagnostic in identifying the calcific deposit (**Fig. 5.8**). They can usually be seen on an anterior–posterior (AP) view in internal and external rotation. In some cases, an axillary and/or supraspinatus outlet view can be used to identify a deposit in a more unusual location. These can be classified using the Gartner classification (**Fig. 5.9**)

Ultrasound scanning may be used to confirm the diagnosis, although this is usually unnecessary. It is more commonly used to deliver image-guided aspiration and injection.

MRI is less useful in the evaluation of calcific deposits. The low number of resonating protons in a deposit make it difficult to see with this modality. Surrounding oedema can lead to a false-positive result for a rotator cuff tear.

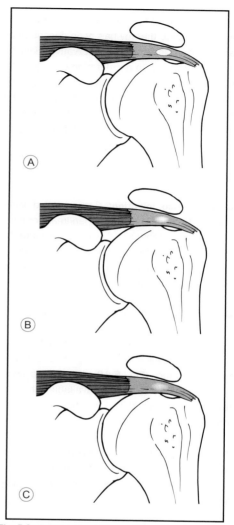

Fig. 5.9 Gartner and Heyer Classification. A) Clearly circumscribed and dense (during formation). B) Clearly circumscribed, translucent, cloudy and dense. C) Cloudy and translucent, resorptive.

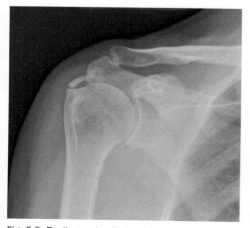

Fig. 5.8 Radiograph of shoulder with calcific deposit in supraspinatus tendon.

## Treatment

**Physiotherapy:** Initial treatment is rest, antiinflammatory medication and physiotherapy. The aim of physiotherapy treatment is to reestablish rotator cuff strength and balance and support the patient through the healing phase. There can often be a secondary capsulitis causing restriction in movement. Extracorporeal shock wave therapy has been described as an option in addition to conservative management. It may lead to acceleration of fragmentation of the deposit and assist in reabsorption and healing. The evidence is equivocal, and it may be beneficial when combined with another modality such as needling. It is less likely to be effective in the treatment of a patient with acute onset of shoulder pain due to a calcific deposit.

**Corticosteroid injection:** Corticosteroid injection can be under taken via a landmark or ultrasound guided approach. It is performed into the subacromial space and can provide temporary or permanent relief of symptoms. It should be considered the first line management.

**Ultrasound-guided barbotage:** Ultrasound-guided barbotage (percutaneous aspiration) is effective and recommended if symptoms do not respond to a simple subacromial corticosteroid injection. (**Fig. 5.10**). Ultrasound scanning is safe and readily available. It does require a clinician skilled in ultrasound-guided intervention.

**Dry needling:** This technique is also performed with ultrasound guidance, with multiple perforations of the deposit, to promote local bleeding and resorption.

**Arthroscopic excision:** This approach is often considered the last resort, given the efficacy of conservative and ultrasound-guided techniques (**Fig. 5.11**).

---

## Technique

### Ultrasound-Guided Aspiration/Barbotage

A needle is placed into the deposit under guidance (**Fig. 5.10**). The contents are then aspirated. Some deposits are quite fluid-based and aspirated as a white, chalky liquid.

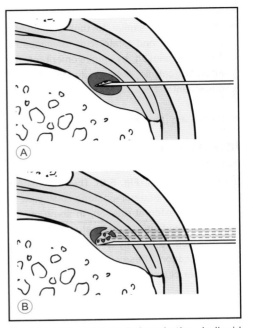

Fig. 5.10 Ultrasound-guided aspiration. In liquid deposits, simple aspiration may decompress the lesion. In harder deposits, they may need to be broken up by passing the needle backwards and forwards several times, with injection of saline to dissolve the deposit.

In other cases, local anaesthetic or saline can be injected to dissolve a more solid deposit. Two needles can be placed to allow irrigation and wash through. Percutaneous treatment is not indicated in very small deposits (<5 mm).

### Arthroscopic Excision of Calcific Deposit

The patient is positioned for shoulder arthroscopy in the position most familiar to the surgeon (beach chair or lateral). A standard posterior view portal is created. The glenohumeral joint is assessed as usual, paying attention to the undersurface of the rotator cuff. The camera is then inserted into the subacromial bursa. The deposit can usually be identified bulging up through the superior aspect of the supraspinatus tendon (**Fig. 5.11**). The deposit is incised and debrided. An arthroscopic shaver is useful as it usually has a suction portal incorporated

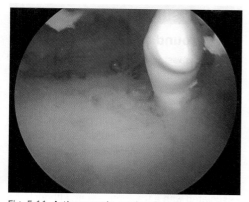

Fig. 5.11 Arthroscopic evaluation and debridement of calcific deposit. The white material is the deposit being expressed superiorly from the supraspinatus tendon.

into the end. Other procedures can also be performed, such as a more extensive subacromial decompression, although there is evidence that acromioplasty is unnecessary and that bursectomy alone is effective.

## SHOULDER INSTABILITY

### Background

Shoulder instability can occur with or without a history of trauma. Chronic instability can present as full recurrent glenohumeral joint dislocations or as a more subtle feeling of instability or apprehension on certain manoeuvres.

The shoulder joint is inherently unstable because of the relative mismatch between the size of the humeral head and glenoid. The glenoid is deepened by the labrum.

### Atraumatic Instability

Atraumatic instability can result from the following:

- **Abnormal soft tissue (hyperlaxity):** Patients may exhibit features of hyperlaxity or have a collagen disorder, such as Ehlers–Danlos syndrome.

- **Abnormal joint (glenoid dysplasia):** Patients may have a developmental deficiency of the glenoid and labral structures.

- **Abnormal muscle patterning:** These patients have a relative dominance of large extrinsic shoulder muscles such as pectoralis major and latissimus dorsi. These muscles overpower the relatively weaker rotator cuff muscle because of abnormalities in neural function and sequencing of movements.

### Posttraumatic Instability

A previously structurally normal shoulder may develop chronic instability after traumatic glenohumeral dislocation. During the initial injury there are several components:

- Capsular tear: These can include more complex lesions such as humeral avulsion of glenohumeral ligament (HAGL)

- Labral tear/detachment (Bankart lesion)

- Glenoid rim attrition/fracture

- Hill Sach's defect (Hatchet): This is a defect on the posterior humeral head. Depending on its location, it can engage on the glenoid rim during abduction and external rotation, leading to instability.

In addition, there can also be cartilaginous lesions such as glenolabral articular disruption (GLAD). The labrum can also detach in continuity with the periosteum on the front of the glenoid neck (anterior labral periosteal sleeve avulsion (ALPSA)). The risk of recurrent instability is greater in patients who are younger at the time of their first dislocation, patients undertaking contact sport and shoulders with boney defects (humeral or glenoid).

### Investigations

Plain X-rays (AP and axillary) are used to determine if there is deficiency of the glenoid

+/− humeral head, along with any evidence of secondary osteoarthritis.

**MRI arthrography:** An MRI scan with contrast (MR arthrogram) is useful to define the extent of the labral injury and associated injuries such as HAGL, ALSPA and GLAD. The shape of the glenoid, anterior glenoid attrition and glenoid track can be measured.

**Computer tomography (CT) scanning:** A CT scan may also be also required in cases of more complex bony defects.

## Management

**Atraumatic instability:** Patients should be managed with physiotherapy to address muscle balance.

**Posttrauma instability:** Patients should undergo initial physiotherapy to address any secondary muscle patterning issues.

- Arthroscopic stabilization: The labrum is reattached to suture anchors placed arthroscopically in the glenoid rim.

- Open stabilization: The labrum and the anterior capsule are repaired.

- Remplissage: Capsule is anchored into a surface defect of the humeral head (Hill-Sachs).

- Bone-block procedures: Where there is loss of bone at the front of the glenoid, the glenoid can be augmented using several techniques. The most commonly used technique is the Bristow–Latarjet technique, where the coracoid tip is transferred and fixed to the front of the glenoid with screws. The short head of the biceps is left attached to the coronoid tip and acts as a sling to prevent dislocation. Other options involve the use of autograft (iliac crest) bone blocks.

# FROZEN SHOULDER

## Background

Adhesive capsulitis of the shoulder is commonly referred to as a 'frozen shoulder'. It usually occurs with an insidious onset of significant shoulder pain that is followed by profound stiffness. The pathological description of it as adhesive capsulitis is related to the microscopic features of inflammation and fibrosis that are observed in the glenohumeral joint and bursa (**Fig. 5.12**). In some cases it can be associated with a traumatic event, although the trauma is usually minor and not associated with significant structural damage. Where there has been an episode of trauma, or another issue such as a seizure, radiographs should be obtained to exclude a fracture or dislocation. There is a peak incidence in women in the 40 to 60 year age group, with a lifetime prevalence of up to 5%. It is seen more commonly in patients who also suffer from diabetes mellitus, with a relative risk that is five to ten times that of the general population. In approximately 40% of cases, it can affect the contralateral

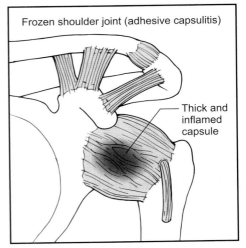

Frozen shoulder joint (adhesive capsulitis)

Thick and inflamed capsule

Fig. 5.12 The glenohumeral joint in adhesive capsulitis (frozen shoulder) demonstrating capsular inflammation and fibrosis, leading to pain and stiffness.

side, either simultaneously or, more commonly, at a later point. It is described as following three phases: freezing (6 months), frozen (6 months) and thawing (6 to 12 months). The natural history of a frozen shoulder is resolution over a period of approximately 18 to 24 months. In some cases, it can result in more prolonged pain and stiffness.

## Symptoms

- General shoulder pain, usually preceding the onset of stiffness

- Pain radiating to the neck and down the arm

- Subtle altered sensation in nondermatomal pattern in the arm because of shoulder protraction and pressure in the subcoracoid area

- Stiffness, including the loss of passive movement, with a firm end point, most commonly in external rotation

- Difficulty with functional and occupational tasks

## Investigation

Investigations are useful to exclude other pathology in the shoulder. In particular, plain radiographs (two views) should be obtained to exclude osteoarthritis or a posterior shoulder dislocation. Both of these conditions can mimic a frozen shoulder and may be missed in the initial assessment. Other investigations are usually not specific.

## Treatment

- Physiotherapy consists of a simple home-exercise programme working within the range of comfort. Terminal, painful and passive stretching are avoided.

- Analgesia and anti-inflammatory medication may be useful in the initial stage.

- A glenohumeral joint corticosteroid injection may be useful in the early stage. This can be accomplished using a posterior approach, aiming towards the coracoid. It can also be performed using ultrasound scanning or fluoroscopic guidance which landmark-based techniques have failed. It is most effective during the freezing phase where the inflammatory process is at a peak.

Further treatment should be considered where there is significant pain and functional limitation persisting at 6 months. In cases that are refractory to injection and physiotherapy, more invasive treatment may be considered.

- Manipulation under anaesthesia (MUA): A general anaesthetic is administered, and the shoulder is gently stretched in abduction and then external rotation. Care must be taken not to apply too much force, as there is a small risk of humeral fracture with the procedure. A glenohumeral joint corticosteroid injection is often also administered to reduce recurrence. Physiotherapy is also started immediately afterwards to maintain the improved range of movement.

- Hydrodilation (distension arthrogram): This is a procedure usually carried out by interventional radiologists, although some orthopaedic consultants have received training and perform this with ultrasound guidance. Under fluoroscopic or ultrasound guidance, a large volume of sterile saline is injected into the glenohumeral joint. This achieves a capsular stretch and, in many cases, rupture of the tight capsule, while avoiding the risk of fracture that comes with MUA. Corticosteroid and local anaesthetic are then instilled to provide analgesia and reduce the risk of recurrence. It is important that physiotherapy is commenced immediately to work on the restored range of movement.

- Arthroscopic capsular release: This is an arthroscopic procedure where the thickened, scarred capsule is debrided and divided with a radiofrequency ablation probe. Adhesions around the subscapularis are released. Care is required at the lower part of the anteroinferior capsule, where the axillary nerve can be closely adhered to the inflamed capsule. Completion of the release is usually achieved with a final MUA. Addition of an arthroscopic posterior capsule release has not been shown to produce superior functional outcomes.

## Glenohumeral Joint Corticosteroid Injection (Anatomical Landmark-Based)

*The skin is prepared using alcohol or another appropriate antiseptic agent. A corticosteroid agent such as 40 mg of methylprednisolone acetate (Depo-Medrone) or triamcinolone can be mixed with a local anaesthetic such as 10 ml of 0.5% levobupivacaine. A green needle (21G) is used. These can been obtained in longer lengths, which can be useful to ensure penetration of the joint. The needle is inserted from the posterior aspect of the shoulder, approximately 1 cm below and medial to the posterolateral edge of the acromion, aiming anteriorly, towards the coracoid.*

## ARTHRITIS AROUND THE SHOULDER

## ACROMIOCLAVICULAR JOINT OSTEOARTHRITIS

## Background

The synovial joint between the distal clavicle and acromion withstands significant loading through the upper limb. Although the anatomy is variable, a fibrocartilaginous disc is often found that helps to dissipate these forces.

The AC joint is most commonly acutely injured through damage to the AC and coracoclavicular ligaments, leading to AC joint separation and dislocation. AC joint osteoarthritis is also commonly observed, particularly in the over 50-year age group. The condition often commences with degeneration of the intraarticular disc. It is also more common in men and those undertaking heavier lifting, such as weightlifting. It may also occur secondary to previous injury, such as AC joint dislocation.

While degeneration is common, it is often an asymptomatic process that is incidentally detected on imaging for other reasons, such as a chest X-ray. Care must be taken not to wrongly attribute symptoms to an otherwise asymptomatic process.

## Symptoms
- Pain localised to the AC joint

- Firm swelling around the AC joint

- Pain on abduction to a high arc (**Fig. 5.2**)

## Signs
- Pain on palpation

## Investigation
- X-rays of the shoulder are important to exclude other causes of shoulder pain such as calcific tendonitis (**Fig. 5.8** & **Fig. 5.13**).

- An AP view of the AC joint may be helpful to observe the AC joint more fully.

- Plain radiographs are often adequate to make the diagnosis. Occasionally, other investigations may be necessary to look for alternative or associated pathology such as rotator cuff tendinopathy. In this case consideration should be given to either ultrasound scanning or MRI. Both of these modalities are capable of demonstrating capsular thickening and degeneration around the AC joint.

- Local anaesthetic injection may be undertaken as a diagnostic test. Abolition of pain confirms the diagnosis.

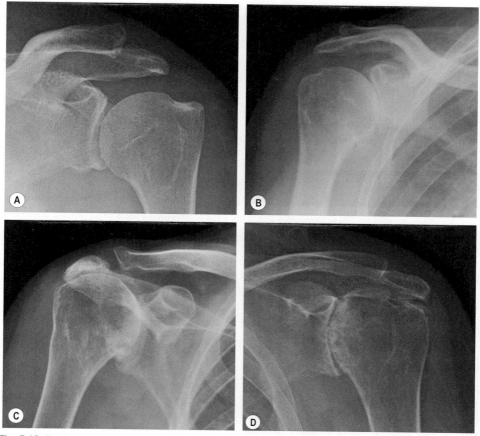

Fig. 5.13 Radiographs of different forms of arthritis around the shoulder: A) Acromioclavicular osteoarthritis. B) Glenohumeral osteoarthritis. C) Rotator cuff arthropathy. D) Rheumatoid arthritis.

# Treatment

## Nonoperative

- Lifestyle advice should be considered to reduce abnormal forces going through the upper limb.

- Analgesia and intermittent anti-inflammatory medication.

- Corticosteroid injection is possible via a landmark and palpation approach or with ultrasound guidance. Ultrasound guidance is helpful in patients in whom it is difficult to palpate the AC joint.

## Operative

AC joint excision can be achieved via an arthroscopic or open approach:

- Arthroscopic: The AC joint is shaved away from its inferior aspect, working upwards towards the top of the joint. This is usually performed at the same time as a subacromial decompression and is known as the Mumford procedure. This technique is useful if there is evidence of coexisting impingement (subacromial bursitis/rotator cuff tendinopathy). Care should be taken to fully excise the area as it can be difficult fully to visualize the most posterior aspect of the joint arthroscopically.

- Open AC joint excision: A direct incision is made over the AC joint, and the articular surface and the disc are excised. This approach is useful in patients with specific isolated symptoms, as there is a higher probability of complete excision.

## GLENOHUMERAL JOINT OSTEOARTHRITIS

### Background

Glenohumeral joint OA (GHJOA) results in loss of cartilage on the glenoid or humeral articular surfaces. It can occur as a primary process (with no obvious cause), or as a result of trauma (fracture or dislocation), avascular necrosis or upper limb neuropathy (Charcot). The pathological process is similar to other osteoarthritic processes. Arthritis resulting from rotator cuff disease and tears is termed rotator cuff arthropathy (RCA) and has a different pattern of radiological changes.

GHJOA may also be the end result of rarer pathologies, such as crystal arthropathies. Milwaukee shoulder is a rapidly destructive process that affects the shoulder due to deposition of calcium pyrophosphate dihydrate (CPPD) deposition. Neuropathic (Charcot) shoulder can result in similarly progressive joint destruction. This most commonly results from spinal cord abnormalities such as syringomyelia.

GHJOA is more common in female patients, and the incidence increases with increasing age.

The predominant symptoms are pain and stiffness. It is important to distinguish between other forms of arthritis such as RCA or inflammatory arthritis. It is also important to exclude other causes of stiffness such as a frozen shoulder or locked posterior dislocation.

### Symptoms

- Pain

- Stiffness, leading to loss of function

### Signs

- Pain on palpation

- Restricted active and passive range of movement

### Investigation

- **X-rays** to distinguish from other traumatic or nontraumatic causes of stiffness. There are signs of loss of joint space, and an inferomedial osteophyte is commonly seen on the humeral head. The head is usually congruently centred in the glenoid, with no superior migration (**Fig. 5.13**).

- **Ultrasound scanning/MRI** may be useful to assess cuff integrity if arthroplasty is being considered.

- **CT scanning** may be a useful adjunct to surgical planning for arthroplasty to examine glenoid version and bone stock.

### Treatment

- Activity modification

- Corticosteroid injection

- Arthroscopic debridement: This treatment may give short- to medium-term relief of symptoms in younger patients. Capsular release is coupled with debridement of degenerative chondral tissue and subacromial decompression.

- Arthroplasty: When patients have significant pain and functional limitation, arthroplasty may be offered. If the rotator cuff is intact, anatomical total shoulder replacement may be undertaken.

## ROTATOR CUFF ARTHROPATHY

### Background

RCA is a particular pattern of osteoarthritis that results from altered joint biomechanics that occurs when there is rotator cuff insufficiency. Cuff deficiency, particularly in the superior portion, allows the humeral head to rise (and to become translate anteriorly) over time. The change in force across the glenohumeral joint causes articular cartilage loss. As the disease progresses, the humeral head can come into contact with the inferior surface of the acromion. It results in pain and stiffness. It is more common in women, with the incidence increasing from age 60 onwards. Disease progression is commonly classified using the Hamada classification (**Table 5.1**).

### Symptoms

● Pain

● Stiffness, leading to loss of function

### Signs

● Passive stiffness

● Rotator cuff weakness

### Investigation

● **X-rays** can distinguish from other traumatic or nontraumatic causes of stiffness. These will demonstrate a characteristic superior migration of the humeral head, along with loss of joint space. Subchondral sclerosis can be seen around the glenohumeral joint and the acromion (**Fig. 5.13**). Rounding off of the undersurface is termed 'acetabularization'.

● **Ultrasound scanning/MRI** may be useful to assess cuff integrity in early cases, where superior migration is not apparent.

● **CT scanning** may be a useful adjunct to surgical planning for arthroplasty to examine the glenoid version and bone stock.

### Treatment

● Activity modification

● Corticosteroid injection

● Arthroplasty may be offered to patients in the older age group with significant pain and functional limitation. As the rotator cuff is deficient, the most reproducible functional results are achieved from reverse total shoulder arthroplasty.

| Table 5.1:  Hamada Classification of RCA | |
|---|---|
| Grade 1 | Acromiohumeral interval >6 mm |
| Grade 2 | Acromiohumeral interval <6 mm |
| Grade 3 | Acromiohumeral interval <6 mm with acetabularization of the acromion |
| Grade 4 | 4A) GH narrowing without acetabularization<br>4B) GH narrowing with acetabularization |
| Grade 5 | Humeral head collapse with avascular necrosis |

## INFLAMMATORY ARTHRITIS OF THE SHOULDER

The shoulder can be affected in inflammatory arthritides such as rheumatoid arthritis.

### Symptoms

● Pain

● Joint swelling and synovitis

● Stiffness, particularly prolonged in the morning

● Other extra articular features such as nodules

## Signs

- Stiffness

- Rotator cuff weakness

## Investigation

- **X-rays:** Classical features of inflammatory arthritis can be seen, including loss of joint space, periarticular erosions and osteopaenia (**Fig. 5.13**). In the modern era, treatment with disease-modifying antirheumatic drugs (DMARDs) can reduce the prominence of these changes, and patterns can appear more osteoarthritic in nature.

- **Ultrasound scanning/MRI** may be useful to assess cuff integrity as the cuff may be thinned or deficient.

- **CT scanning** may be a useful adjunct to surgical planning for arthroplasty to examine glenoid version and bone stock. Bone may be weaker due to osteopaenia, and this can lead to challenges during arthroplasty.

## Treatment

- Activity modification

- DMARDs and corticosteroids under care of rheumatologist

- Arthroplasty: When patients have significant pain and functional limitation, arthroplasty may be offered. Care must be taken to select an appropriate arthroplasty based on the rotator cuff status and residual bone stock. This can include resurfacing arthroplasty, anatomical total shoulder replacement or reverse geometry shoulder replacement.

## SHOULDER ARTHROPLASTY

Shoulder arthroplasty encompasses a range of joint replacement procedures, from resurfacing to hemiarthroplasty to total shoulder replacement (**Fig. 5.14** & **Fig. 5.16**).

**Resurfacing:** The humeral head is resurfaced with a metal implant. Although more bone is preserved, this procedure can be associated with difficulties in sizing, leading to overstuffing and poor function.

**Hemiarthroplasty:** The humeral head articular surface is replaced, with the addition of a humeral stem. Fixation is with uncemented or cemented techniques. This technique has been used most commonly in trauma situations, but it can be used in cases of GHJOA and RCA provided there is no significant bone loss in the glenoid. The advent of reverse shoulder replacement has reduced the use of hemiarthroplasty. In younger patients, pyrocarbon has been postulated as potentially beneficial bearing surface when coupled with the native cartilage of the glenoid.

**Total shoulder replacement (anatomical):** In addition to the humeral replacement, the glenoid is also resurfaced. The most commonly used implant is a polyethylene component, which is secured with cement. On the humeral side, there are stemmed and stemless options, along with cemented or uncemented fixation techniques. This procedure is mainly undertaken for patients with GHJOA with an intact rotator cuff. If the cuff is deficient, there is a risk of instability.

**Total shoulder replacement (reverse geometry):** This technique involves placing a baseplate and convex glenosphere on the glenoid surface. This articulates with a concave tray that is placed on a stem that is inserted into the humerus. This increases tension in the deltoid and allows it to initiate and control flexion and abduction (**Fig. 5.15**). This approach is ideal for rotator cuff–deficient shoulders and fracture situations where tuberosity healing is not assured. Medializing the centre of rotation contributes to the optimization of movements of deltoid force, along with reducing stress at the implant–bone interface (**Fig. 5.15**).

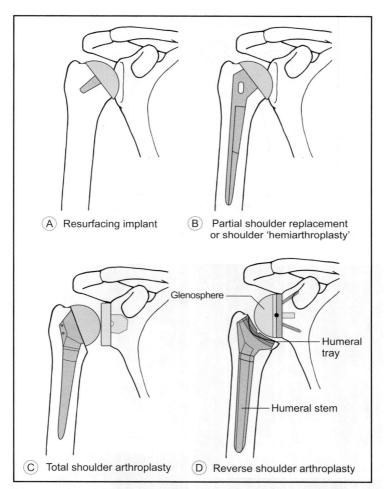

Fig. 5.14 Types of shoulder arthroplasty: A) Resurfacing. B) Hemiarthroplasty. C) Anatomic total shoulder replacement. D) Reverse geometry total shoulder replacement.

# Indications for Arthroplasty

- Osteoarthritis

  - GHJOA

  - RCA

- Inflammatory arthritis

- Complication of trauma

- Acute trauma

  - Avascular necrosis

  - Nonunion

  - Osteoarthritis with deficient rotator cuff

  - Chronic instability with degenerative changes

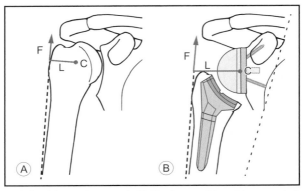

Fig. 5.15 Reverse total shoulder replacement: A) The humeral head is moved distally (increased, (F). The moment of force of the deltoid is increased (L). The centre of rotation (C) is medialized. B) Deltoid is recruited to flex and abduct the shoulder, replacing the deficient rotator cuff.

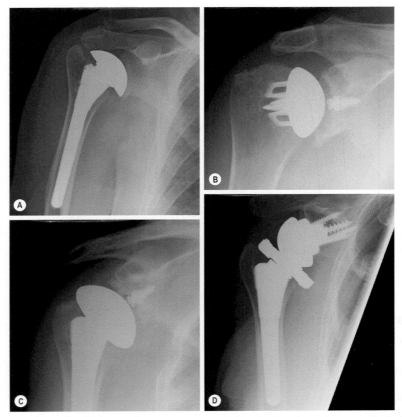

Fig. 5.16 Arthroplasty options around the shoulder: A) Hemiarthroplasty (uncemented). B) Total shoulder replacement with stemless surface hemi-replacement. C) Total shoulder replacement (hybrid cemented glenoid and uncemented stem). D) Reverse geometry total shoulder replacement (uncemented).

## Reverse Geometry Total Shoulder Replacement

The procedure can be performed through a deltopectoral approach (**Fig. 5.17**) which provides good exposure to the glenohumeral joint. The superolateral approach offers the advantage of a more direct view and exposure of the glenoid, but specialized retractors are required to ensure the optimal view. Poor exposure can result in component malposition. This can lead to instability, notching and early loosening.

The humeral head is cut to allow access to the glenoid. The glenoid is then prepared with residual cartilage being removed. A baseplate is attached with and usually secured with a combination of a coated post and/or screws. A glenosphere is then secured to the baseplate. The humeral canal is prepared to accept a stemmed implant. Fixation can be cemented or uncemented. A humeral tray is placed on the stem and this articulates with glenosphere.

## Complications

### Early
- Infection
- Instability and dislocation
- Neurovascular injury (including traction from lengthening of arm)

### Late
- Infection
- Instability and dislocation
- Loosening of humeral component
- Loosening of glenoid component
- Scapular notching (**Fig. 5.18**)
- Polyethylene wear
- Fracture

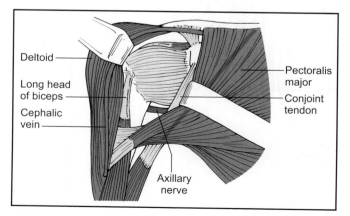

Fig. 5.17 Deltopectoral approach: The superficial plane between deltoid and pectoralis major is identified containing the cephalic vein. The vein is usually taken laterally. The clavipectoral fascia is then incised lateral to the conjoint tendon. Care is taken to avoid damage to the axillary nerve.

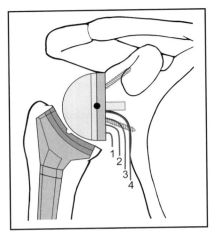

Fig. 5.18 Scapular notching: This complication is unique to reverse shoulder replacement. The most medial aspect of the humerus impinges on the scapular underneath the glenosphere resulting in bone loss (categorised into 4 stages). In severe cases it can threaten the stability of the glenoid component. It is reduced by implants that lateralize the humeral shaft to reduce impingement in adduction.

## Shoulder Examination

### Introduction

The shoulder girdle is complex – the osseous anatomy is shown in (**Fig. 5.19**). Movement occurs at the glenohumeral and scapulothoracic articulations. The brachial plexus pass nearby and axilliary artery are in close proximity. The standard examination technique of 'look, feel, move' is be applied. It is important to have knowledge of the underlying anatomical features to relate examination findings to potential pathology.

### Look

The patient should have their torso exposed, and routine inspection for muscle wasting, scars (**Fig. 5.20**), swelling, erythema and deformities should be performed. A common pitfall is to examine the shoulder only from the front; however, the majority of muscles controlling the shoulder are located around the scapula posteriorly. Therefore inspection from behind is essential. The resting positions of

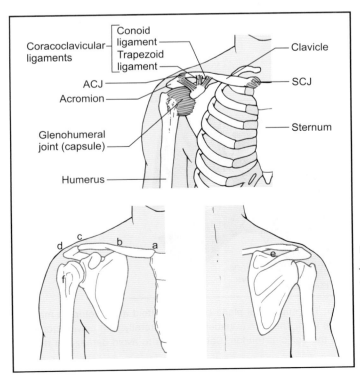

Fig. 5.19 Bones and joints of the shoulder girdle: palpate the sternoclavicular joint (a) clavicle (b) to the ACJ (c), and acromion (d) scapula spine (e) humeral head (f) biceps tendon.

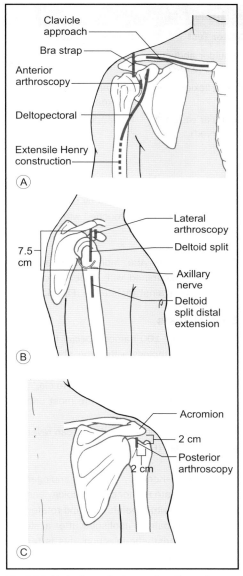

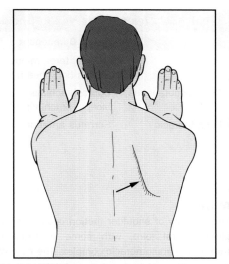

Fig. 5.21 Winging of the scapula can be demonstrated by asking the patient to pushing against a wall. This can be caused by paralysis of serratus anterior (medial winging-long thoracic nerve palsy) or the rhomboids (lateral winging-drosal scapular/spinal accessory nerve palsy).

Fig. 5.20 Typical surgical scar locations from shoulder surgery when observed from the font A), side B) and rear C).

the shoulder and scapula should be compared to the opposite side and noted. If the patient pushes against a wall, scapular asymmetry and dyskinesia can be demonstrated (**Fig. 5.21** scapula)

## Feel

Patients will often describe poorly localised pain over their shoulder which can be localised further by palpation. Palpation should be undertaken in a systematic manner beginning with the sternoclavicular joint, working along the clavicle to the AC joint onto the acromion following it posteriorly along the spine of the scapula. The humeral head, shaft and biceps tendon in the bicipital groove can then be assessed for tenderness. Muscle bulk, particularly of the deltoid and periscapular muscles (rotator cuff and latissimus dorsi), should be assessed, in which global loss is indicative of disuse or a massive rotator cuff insufficiency, whereas isolated atrophy may indicate focal cuff disease or neurological lesions. Finally, nerve function is assessed by motor and sensory testing, with the axillary nerve and musculocutaneous nerves being relevant to shoulder function (**Table 5.2**).

| Table 5.2 | Relevant Nerves in Shoulder Girdle Examination | | |
|---|---|---|---|
| **Nerve** | **Motor Component** | **Motor Test** | **Sensory Component** |
| Axillary | Deltoid, teres minor, triceps (long head) | Shoulder abduction | Regimental badge patch |
| Musculocutaneous | Coracobrachialis, biceps, brachialis | Elbow flexion | Lateral cutaneous nerve of forearm |
| Long thoracic | Serratus anterior | Scapular winging (observed) | Not applicable |

## Move

The majority of shoulder motion occurs at the glenohumeral joint, with some contribution from the scapulothoracic complex. The ratio of movement of the glenohumeral joint to the scapulothoracic joint is approximately 2:1.

Initial active screening movements can quickly and effectively exclude a limitation to range of movement and function. The patient should be asked to reach up behind their head, and then to reach as far as they can behind their back (**Fig. 5.22**). Rotator cuff strength is examined in each domain of supraspinatus (arm abducted and internally rotated), infraspinatus (external rotation with arm at side) and subscapularis (hand on belly and elbow pushed forward) (**Fig. 5.24**).

If these screening movements are limited, individual movements should be examined actively then passively and compared between sides. A lack of passive correction indicates articular stiffness within the joint(s), whereas limited active movement with full passive correction is more likely due to muscle, tendon or neurological dysfunction. Movement can also be limited by pain, and any improvement following injection of local anaesthetic should be noted.

Active movements should measured in degrees, with the exception of internal rotation, which is measured by the anatomical position which can be touched with the thumb (**Fig. 5.23**).

The strength of the individual rotator cuff tendons is examined with a series of active movements against resistance (**Fig. 5.24**).

## Special Tests

There are over 100 named special tests used to localise pathology within the shoulder with generally poor reported sensitivity and specificity for the pathologies they purport to diagnose. There are a few tests which are most useful.

Cross-body adduction (scarf test) can reveal AC joint pathology (**Fig. 5.25**).

The Hawkins–Kennedy test for impingement can demonstrate rotator cuff pathology and can often coexist with a painful arc and rotator cuff weakness. If pain is abolished after a steroid and local anaesthetic injection, this is termed a positive Hawkins test (**Fig. 5.26**).

The Speed and O'Brien tests can help to differentiate between the superior labral and long head of biceps pathology (**Fig. 5.27**).

Anterior instability can be examined by looking for the sulcus sign and anterior apprehension (**Fig. 5.28**).

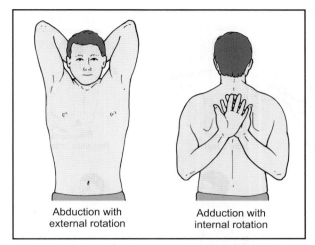

Abduction with
external rotation

Adduction with
internal rotation

Fig. 5.22 Screening movements: these mirror functional requirements of shoulder motion – reaching to the top of the head and behind the back.

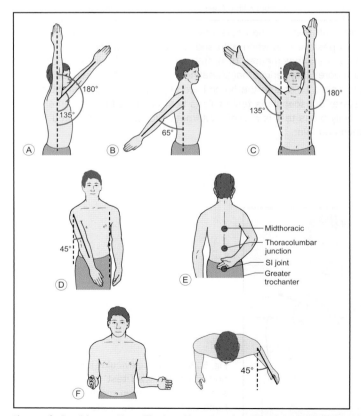

Fig. 5.23 Directions of shoulder motion. Flexion A), extension B), abduction C), adduction demonstrating restriction of the right shoulder) D), internal rotation E), external rotation F).

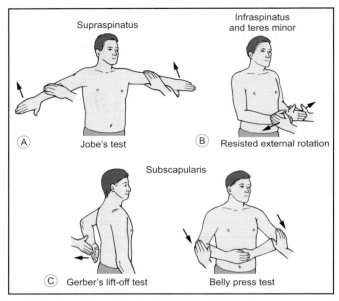

Fig. 5.24 Rotator cuff testing. The active tests indicated by black arrows and resisted by the examiner with a positive sign when pain and/or weakness is identified. Jobe's test A) ('empty-can') can be supplemented by a 'full-can' (thumbs up) variation engaging the deltoid which should theoretically reduce pain/weakness. When testing resisted external rotation B) care should be taken to ensure the humeri are slightly abducted from the torso as a levering 'trick' manoeuvre. Subscapularis testing C) is best assessed using Gerber's 'lift-off test'; however, the belly press test is a useful alternative for those with limited internation rotation of the glenohumeral joint.

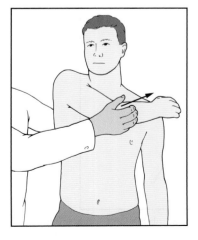

Fig. 5.25 Acromioclavicular joint (ACJ). The cross chest adduction, or 'scarf test' is performed by flexing the shoulder to 90°, then moving it into adduction until the hand rests on the opposite side. A positive test will result in pain the AC joint.

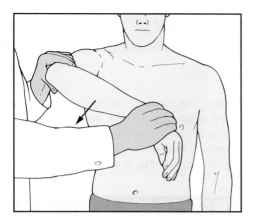

Fig. 5.26 Hawkins Test. The arm is placed into 90° of shoulder flexion, the elbow flexed and the arm internally rotated. Pain on internal rotation is suggestive of rotator cuff pathology.

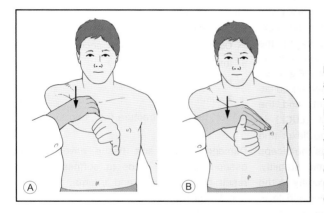

Fig. 5.27 Resisted flexion with arm rotated: A) O'Brien's Test – the arm is internally rotated. Reproduction of pain may suggest superior labral pathology, while B) Speed's Test pain on resisted flexion with the arm externally rotated may localise pathology around the long head of biceps.

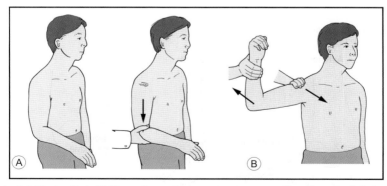

Fig. 5.28 Instability testing. A) The sulcus sign may appear on pulling the arm inferiorly, B) Anterior apprehension sign. The examiner places abducts the shoulder and eternally rotates the arm. If the patient develops apprehension that the shoulder may dislocate the test is positive. The finding is confirmed by the examiner placing their hand on the front of the shoulder and pushing back. This should alleviate the patient's concern.

## ANATOMY

The elbow is a hinge joint that also incorporates forearm rotation through the linked proximal and distal radioulnar joints (**Fig. 6.1**). There is close congruity of the articular surface of the trochlea and ulna, which comprise the humeroulnar articulation. In flexion, the coronoid fits snugly into the coronoid fossa and in extension, the olecranon moves into the olecranon fossa (**Fig. 6.2**). Laterally, the radial head provides stability through its contact with the capitellum. Together, these osseous constraints give considerable stability to the elbow. In addition, further static constraint is provided by the collateral ligaments (**Fig. 6.3**). On the medial side, the ulnar (medial) collateral ligament is most important, and the lateral ulnar collateral ligament (LUCL) is important on the lateral side. The flexor and extensor muscle groups as well as the biceps and triceps contribute to dynamic stability. The ulnar nerve lies in close proximity to the posterior aspect of the medial epicondyle in the cubital tunnel. The radial nerve travels through the lateral intermuscular septum before crossing the elbow between the brachioradialis and brachialis dividing into the posterior interosseous nerve and the superficial radial nerve (**Fig. 6.4**).

## THE STIFF ELBOW

### Clinical Summary

Elbow stiffness can result from several different pathological processes:

- Osteoarthritis (primary or secondary)
- Inflammatory arthropathy
- Haemophilic arthropathy
- Trauma
- Soft tissue contracture (i.e., burns)

Damage to the soft tissue envelope and osseous anatomy leads to stiffness. It can result from arthrosis and trauma. The functional range of elbow flexion is 30 to 130 degrees (**Fig. 6.5**). A loss of extension reduces

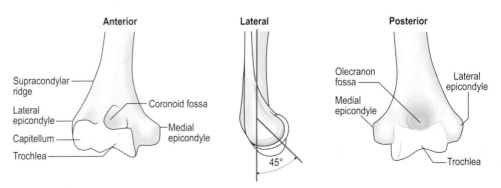

Fig. 6.1 Distal humerus: osteology.

Anterior

- Supracondylar ridge
- Lateral epicondyle
- Capitellum
- Trochlea
- Coronoid fossa
- Medial epicondyle

Lateral

45°

Posterior

- Olecranon fossa
- Medial epicondyle
- Lateral epicondyle
- Trochlea

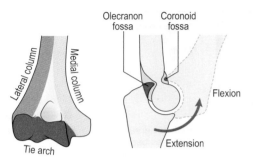

Fig. 6.2 Distal humerus: functional anatomy.

how far the arm can reach. Minor loss of extension does not limit function. It is far more difficult to compensate for loss of flexion. The elbow flexes to bring the hand closer to the body and head, and restriction can result in difficulty undertaking personal hygiene and feeding. Forearm rotation can be restricted by incongruity or synostosis around the proximal radioulnar articulation.

Stiffness results from damage to a variety of anatomical structures (**Fig. 6.6**):

- Extrinsic (outside the joint)
  - Arthrofibrosis of the capsule
  - Contracture of collateral ligaments
  - Muscle contractures (brachialis, triceps and biceps)
  - Bony malunion
  - Heterotrophic ossification
- Intrinsic (within the joint)
  - Osteophytes
  - Intra-articular malunion
  - Loose bodies
  - Articular incongruity
  - Intra-articular adhesions
- Mixed
  - It is extremely common to see a combination of both intrinsic and extrinsic pathology.

## Symptoms

Patients with stiffness commonly complain of the following:

Loss of Function: difficulty positioning the hand in space, particularly bringing it close to the body for eating and personal hygiene.

Pain: Pain may arise from capsular inflammation or impingement of osteophytes in terminal

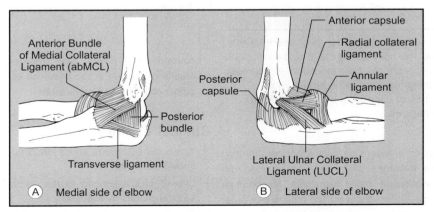

Fig. 6.3 Elbow: collateral ligaments and stability. A) The anterior band of the medial collateral provides stability throughout the range of motion, with the posterior band only tensioning in deep flexion. B) Similarly, the lateral ulnar collateral ligament is the crucial ligamentous restraint on the lateral (radial) side of the elbow.

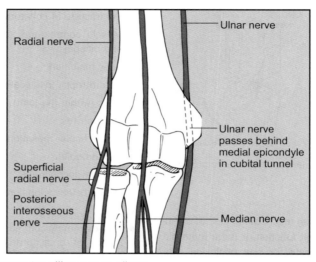

Fig. 6.4 Elbow: nerves travelling across elbow.

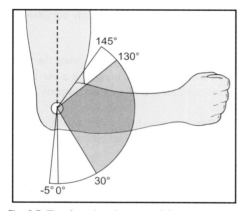

Fig. 6.5 The functional range of flexion of the elbow. The normal range is 0 to 145 degrees (some people can hyperextend to –5 degrees). The range required to undertake most activities of daily living and work is 30 to 130 degrees.

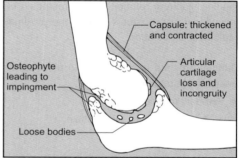

Fig. 6.6 Causes of elbow stiffness.

possibility of a chronic pain syndrome. The results of surgery in the presence of neuropathic pain are less predictable.

## Clinical Examination

flexion or extension. Significant pain through the midrange of motion should raise the question of more significant humeroulnar degenerative changes. The presence of other types of pain such as allodynia and hyperalgesia should alert the clinician to the

- Scars from previous injuries and surgeries should be noted.
- Overall joint alignment in the coronal and sagittal planes is assessed.
- The flexion arc and forearm rotation are measured with a goniometer.

- The presence of impingement pain at the end of flexion and extension is noted, along with any midflexion and forearm rotation pain.

- The sensory and motor function of the ulnar nerve is assessed. Elbow stiffness can contribute to positional compression of the nerve in the cubital tunnel. Planned release may aggravate any underlying ulnar neuropathy if compression is not addressed at the same time as release.

## Investigation

Plain radiographs are most important when assessing the following:

- Bony structure and possible previous malunion

- Osteophytes, particularly in the coronoid and olecranon fossa

- Heterotopic ossification

- Degenerative changes

- Existing metalwork

Computed tomography (CT) scanning may be useful if the pattern of osteophytes is unclear, particular if an arthroscopic approach to arthrolysis is being considered.

## Treatment

### Nonoperative

- A reasonable period of time after the acute trauma should elapse to allow for the possibility of spontaneous improvement and maturation of arthrofibrosis and scar tissue. Range of motion continues to improve after elbow trauma for up to 12 months and intervention should not usually be considered earlier.

- While physiotherapy can be useful passive stretching should be avoided as it can lead to aggravation of capsular inflammation and the development of HO. Physiotherapy should focus on encouraging the use of the elbow for the activities of daily living. Augmenting proprioception is important with the use of single layers compression bandage.

- Progressive static splintage is not thought to be of significant benefit in the long term and is not commonly used.

### Operative

- Surgery should only be considered in the case of prolonged stiffness and if the patient is unresponsive to nonoperative treatment.

- Surgical management of the stiff elbow consists of release and debridement of the structures that are restricting motion.

## Surgical Procedure: Arthrolysis of the Elbow

Arthrolysis is a surgical procedure that addresses elbow stiffness resulting from trauma or arthritis. It is a bespoke procedure that address the unique combination of problems that result in an individual's stiffness. Perioperative analgesia is very important and can be accomplished with a regional nerve block infusion catheter. This allows for prolonged analgesia for 24 to 48 hours.

### Approach

Arthroscopic: In milder cases, capsulectomy and debridement of impingement can be performed arthroscopically.

Open: This approach is used for patients with retained metalwork, greater stiffness and where there has been previous surgery. The elbow can be approached from either posterior or lateral incisions.

### Surgical Steps

Restriction of extension is addressed by dividing the anterior capsule and releasing it from the anterior humerus (**Fig. 6.7**). Posterior osteophytes on the olecranon and in the olecranon fossa are debrided.

Restriction of flexion is addressed by elevating the posterior capsule and triceps from the posterior humerus. Such anterior and posterior elevation is termed the 'column procedure'. Impinging anterior structures (coronoid and coronoid fossa) are debrided.

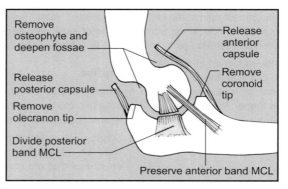

Fig. 6.7 Elbow arthrolysis – surgical steps required to achieve full release (MCL = medial/ulnar collateral ligament).

Residual restriction of flexion can be caused by contraction of the posterior band of the medial collateral ligament (MCL). This structure can be divided, protecting the ulnar nerve and the anterior band.

The radial head may cause impingement in flexion and restrict forearm rotation. Radial head excision is simple, safe and effective.

When there has been a significant extension contracture (inability to flex), the ulnar nerve should also be prophylactically decompressed to avoid traction neuropathy when motion is restored.

**Postoperative Care**

Continuous passive motion can be considered for the flexion arc for 48 hours, while there is anaesthetic blockade. Passive stretching is avoided. The patient is encouraged to use their arm actively for activities of daily living. Overhead range of motion exercises are particularly beneficial as they reduce the potentially negative impact of the triceps and biceps (**Fig. 6.8**).

## ELBOW OSTEOARTHRITIS

## Clinical Summary

Primary elbow osteoarthritis is uncommon. As with all primary idiopathic osteoarthritis,

the disease progress is characterized by loss of articular cartilage. Osteophytes form in the periarticular region. In the elbow, because of its highly congruent articulation, osteophytes can quickly lead to reduction in range of movement and pain **Fig. 6.9** and **6.10**. Many factors have been implicated, including genetics, joint alignment and trauma. Some studies have reported higher rates of disease in patients with occupational histories that include strenuous manual work.

Osteoarthritis generally appears in the lateral aspect of the elbow initially, around the radiocapitellar joint, with loose bodies and osteophytes. It tends to affect the dominant arm and principally affects men.

## Symptoms

- Pain occuring at the terminal ranges of movement, resulting from impingement of osteophytes in extension and flexion.
- Stiffness with reduction in extension, flexion and forearm rotation
- Occasionally there are associated neurological symptoms from secondary ulnar nerve impingement

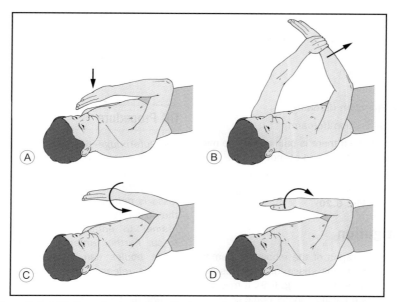

Fig. 6.8 Elbow Rehabilitation: Supine elbow flexion and extension A and B) exercises can improve range of motion by reducing triceps and biceps tone and increasing elbow stability. Forearm rotation is improved with active assisted pronation C) and supination D).

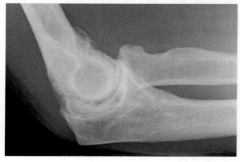

Fig. 6.9 Lateral Elbow X-ray: osteophyte in olecranon fossa

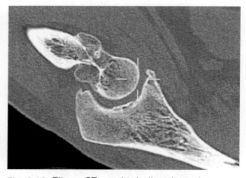

Fig. 6.10 Elbow CT: sagittal slice through humeroulnar joint, with osteophytes in the olecranon and coronoid fossae, leading to impingement pain and reduced range of motion.

- **Inspect**
  - Scars, skin changes and muscle bulk
  - Coronal valgus or varus malalignment
  - Inspect hand distally for signs of ulnar neuropathy

- **Palpate**
  - Palpate epicondyles and the olecranon, along with lateral and medial joint lines
  - Perform Tinel test over cubital tunnel

- **Move**
  - Examine active and passive range of movement
    - Extension
    - Flexion
    - Pronation (forearm)
    - Supination (forearm)
  - Determine if there is pain during the mid-range or at the end of movement
  - Determine if there is pain up on forearm rotation with a clenched fist (grip and grind) (**Fig. 6.20**)

## Investigation

- Plain radiographs of the elbow will demonstrate loss of joint space, osteophytes and subchondral sclerosis (**Fig. 6.9**). It may also demonstrate calcified loose bodies.
- CT scanning may be helpful to determine the pattern of osteophytes (**Fig. 6.10**). It can be useful when planning surgery such as debridement +/− arthrolysis.

## Treatment

- Nonoperative: This is the mainstay of treatment, with activity and occupational modification, along with intermittent analgesia with anti-inflammatory medication.
- Operative treatment should be considered if the range of movement is less than the functional arc of 30 to 130 degrees (**Fig. 6.5**).
  - **Debridement and arthrolysis:** These procedures can be performed arthroscopically or open. The aim of the procedure is to remove impinging loose bodies and osteophytes. Thickened, contracted capsule is also released to regain movement. The radial head may be excised during this procedure if it is impinging on flexion or preventing forearm rotation.
  - **Arthroplasty:** In select cases total elbow replacement may be considered. It should not be performed in young patients who still perform significant manual tasks; arthroplasty in these cases leads to early failure and complex revision requirements.

## OK Procedure

*The Outerbridge–Kashiwagi (OK) procedure is a form of arthrolysis. The elbow is entered posteriorly through a triceps split. The olecranon tip is removed, and the fossa is debrided (**Fig. 6.11**). The floor of the fossa is then removed with a small reamer to enter the anterior coronoid fossa. Further anterior osteophytes and loose bodies can be removed and the capsule released through this approach. The radial head may also be removed by extending the posterior midline approach with a lateral flap.*

## INFLAMMATORY ARTHROPATHY OF THE ELBOW

## Clinical Summary

The elbow can be affected by a variety of inflammatory arthropathies, the most common of which is rheumatoid arthritis (RA) (**Table 6.1**). RA has been described as causing isolated elbow monoarthropathy in 5% of cases and as part of a polyarticular pattern in up to 65% of cases. Historically, patients presented with significant articular destruction through inflammatory erosive changes, and the only treatment option was elbow arthroplasty.

The advancement of disease-modifying anti-rheumatic drugs (DMARDs) has altered the natural history of the disease and reduced the number of patients presenting with advanced joint destruction.

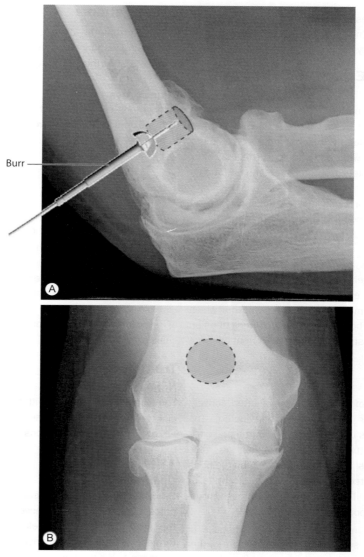

Fig. 6.11 OK Procedure: A) Lateral X-ray demonstrating reamer used to remove osteophyte and drill through the base of the olecranon fossa. The tip of the olecranon can also be removed, if impinging. Through this hole, anterior osteophytes in the coronoid fossa and on the coronoid tip can be removed. B) AP X-ray demonstrating circular hole created. Care should be taken to avoid breaching the distal 'columns', which risks a supracondylar fracture.

Other causes of arthrosis should be considered, including seronegative arthropathy, gout and other crystal arthropathies.

## Clinical Examination

### Look

The whole patient should be evaluated to assess their overall pattern of joint involvement, particularly in other upper limb joints such as the wrist and shoulder. This may alter the subsequent treatment recommendation.

Extra-articular signs may be noticed, such as rheumatoid nodules and olecranon bursitis.

### Feel

The joint is palpated to evaluate any heat, swelling or tenderness. Joint swelling may arise from either effusion or synovitis. An effusion tends to be more fluctuant than synovitis, which tends to be boggy in nature. A pointing effusion may be associated with the formation of a sinus.

### Move

The range of movement is evaluated actively, and further passive correction noted. The flexion arc is assessed along with the presence of contracture. Forearm rotation is also recorded as the proximal radioulnar joint is often affected as well as the radiocapitellar articulation. The pattern of pain through movement is important:

- Is there impingement pain in extension or flexion, suggesting pathology in either fossa?
- Is there pain when the patient is asked to grip and rotate their forearm, suggesting pathology in the radiocapitellar articulation?
- Is there pain in the midrange of flexion, suggesting humeroulnar pathology?

The ulnar nerve should be evaluated for any sensory or motor deficit.

## Investigation

It is likely that the diagnosis will have been made using immunological tests by the time of referral to an orthopaedic surgeon.

### Plain X-rays

Radiographs can assist with the classification of the extent of disease (**Table 6.1**) and help to plan treatment (**Fig. 6.9**).

- Loss of joint space
- Erosive changes
- Periarticular osteopaenia
- Cyst formation
- Hypertrophy of the radial head
- Thinning of the olecranon

Ultrasound or magnetic resonance imaging (MRI) with contrast may be useful in early disease to evaluate for the ongoing presence of synovitis and early bone and cartilage changes.

## Treatment

### Nonoperative

The surgeon should liaise with the rheumatologist to determine whether the patient has tried all available DMARD options and biological therapy.

### Operative

Synovectomy +/- radial head excision: This procedure attempts to remove the inflammatory synovium. A capsular release can be performed to attempt to increase range of movement. When there is significant involvement of the radial head with pain on rotation, this can usually be excised. Caution should be exercised if there is evidence of instability through attrition of the MCL. The procedure can be performed either arthroscopically or using the limited open approach. The approach will depend on the available surgical skill and need to excise the radial head.

**Total elbow arthroplasty:** The worn joint surfaces are excised and replaced with stemmed implants. The long-term survival of total elbow arthroplasty in patients with rheumatoid arthritis is 92% at 10 years, 83% at 15 years and 68% at 20 years. This operation is good at relieving pain. If there is limitation of the range of movement prior to surgery, the aim is to return it a functional range of 30 to 130 degrees. It is unrealistic to expect return of a full range of motion. The risks of surgery include infection, aseptic loosening, bearing wear and periprosthetic fracture. The risk of loosening and future revision is greatest in younger male patients who have an expectation of returning to heavier tasks. Traditionally, patients were advised to limit lifting following arthroplasty (e.g., carry less than 5 kg in their hand). Although such advice is often still given, compliance in younger patients is poor. Consideration should be given to the present or future need for shoulder surgery. Historically, soft tissue interposition arthroplasty has been described for patients who were unsuitable for total elbow replacement by virtue of age.

## Surgical Technique: Total Elbow Replacement

*Total elbow replacement (arthroplasty) involves replacing both the humeral and ulnar side of the elbow articulation. It can be undertaken for inflammatory arthritis, osteoarthritis or post-traumatic arthritis. Patient selection is crucial. Dissatisfaction and early failure are high in younger age groups with higher daily and occupational demands.*

*In most cases the radial head is excised, although some implant systems include the option to replace the radial head.*

*Traditionally, exposure was gained with a triceps-off approach, whereas more recent attempts have been made to preserve the triceps to improve postoperative extension control and strength. This approach most commonly utilizes the paraolecranon interval.*

*The ulnar nerve is either decompressed and left in situ or transposed.*

*The worn joint surfaces are removed, and stemmed implants are cemented into the humerus and ulna. Many systems are linked to provide a degree of constraint (semicon-strained) and stability. This allows for full release of collateral ligaments and anterior capsule. If an implant is over-constrained, the forces transmitted to the implant–cement–bone interfaces would be too great and result in early loosening.*

## NEUROPATHY AROUND THE ELBOW

### Background

The ulnar, radial and median nerves cross the elbow. Neuropathy can develop as a result of extrinsic compression from fascial or other anatomical structures. It may also develop with no obvious cause. It can result in paraesthesia, dysaesthesia, pain and weakness in the distribution of the affected nerve.

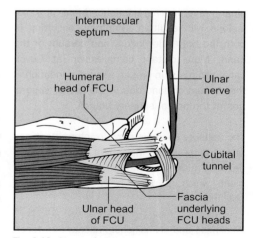

Fig. 6.12 Sites of ulnar nerve compression (FCU flexor carpi ulnaris).

## Ulnar Neuropathy

The ulnar nerve provides sensory innervation to the ulnar border of the hand, little finger and ulnar half of the ring finger. The dorsal branch arises proximal to the wrist. It provides motor innervation to the flexor carpi ulnaris (FCU) muscle and the deep flexors (flexor digitorum profundus [FDP]) to the little and ring fingers. Within the hand, it provides motor innervation to the intrinsic muscles, with the exception of the thenar muscles and lateral two lumbricals (which are supplied by the median nerve).

The ulnar nerve can become compressed at several locations (**Figs 6.13–6.15**): the medial intermuscular septum, cubital tunnel retinaculum and the fascia beneath the heads of the FCU. The ulnar nerve can also be compressed more distally at Guyon's canal, where the ulnar nerve passes into the hand.

Ulnar neuropathy may occur in the acute phase following injury or surgery. It can also occur as a later complication (tardy ulnar nerve palsy).

## Symptoms

Altered sensation in the distribution of the ulnar nerve is characteristic. More proximal lesions will result in symptoms occurring in both the ring/little fingers and dorsum of the hand. More distant compression at Guyon canal can result in preservation of sensation in the dorsum of hand due to the earlier separation of the dorsal sensory branch.

The sensory changes may be intermittent and provoked by certain movements such as elbow flexion. Patients commonly report symptoms at night, which is probably linked to sleeping position.

Weakness and clumsiness: Patients may report a weaker hand grip. They may also notice difficulty with fine manipulation such as fastening buttons.

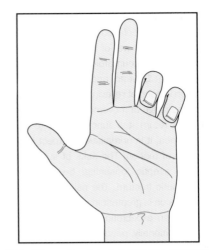

Fig. 6.13 Ulnar claw hand deformity. Hyperextension of the ring and little finger MCPJs is caused by weakness of the ulnar innervated lumbricals.

## Signs

The whole upper limb should be observed to determine whether there is any deformity around the elbow, such as the cubitus valgus. The presence of any scars at the elbow or wrist and restriction of movement should be assessed.

Intrinsic muscle wasting may be noted in the hand. It is most obvious in the first dorsal interosseous space (between the thumb and index finger). The patient may have difficulty in crossing their fingers as this involves interossei muscles to abduct and adduct the neighbouring fingers.

Ulnar clawing can occur in more advanced cases (**Fig. 6.13**), affecting the ring and little finger. There is extension at the metacarpophalangeal joint (MCPJ) and flexion at the proximal interphalangeal joint and distal interphalangeal joint. This results from select loss of the ulnar two lumbricals and their flexion action at the MCPJ. The ulnar claw deformity is more pronounced in more distal lesions, such as compression at Guyon canal. This is due to the more unbalanced deformity as the deep

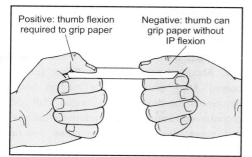

Fig. 6.14 Froment's Sign: The patient is asked to grasp a piece of paper flat between the thumb and index metacarpal. Ulnar neuropathy can lead to loss of first dorsal webspace adduction. A patient can therefore only grip by recruiting FPL, leading to interphalangeal joint flexion.

flexors are relatively preserved in this situation. This phenomenon is called the 'ulnar paradox'.

The Wartenberg sign is relative abduction ("escape") of the little finger during finger extension due to the loss of the adducting interosseous nerve.

The Froment sign (**Fig. 6.14**) can be elicited by asking the patient to grasp a piece of paper between their thumb and the side of the index finger without flexing the thumb interphalangeal joint. With loss of intrinsic hand muscles, this movement is not possible, and the thumb flexes (median nerve) to maintain the paper in position.

The Tinel sign is sensory alteration or tingling elicited by tapping on a nerve at the point of compression or damage. The ulnar nerve may be tapped over the cubital tunnel or Guyon canal.

The ulnar nerve should be also palpated during elbow flexion to detect other pathology such as ulnar nerve subluxation or an accessory snapping triceps.

## Investigation

A patient with minor, intermittent sensory symptoms and no muscle involvement does not require investigation. Such symptoms can be transient and are common in the population. Nonoperative management should be instituted. This includes advice to avoid leaning on the elbow, nocturnal splintage and performing nerve gliding exercises.

Where symptoms are more prolonged and affecting day-to-day life, or where there is evidence of motor involvement, nerve conduction studies should be performed. These tests can be used to pinpoint the location of compression. The degree of neuropathy can be estimated. Other causes of neuropathy can be excluded, such as more widespread polyneuropathy.

## Treatment

Nonoperative management consists initially of lifestyle advice. Pressure on the cubital tunnel should be avoided. The patient should be counselled to avoid leaning the elbow on surfaces such as chair arms or tables. Patients can also try the use of a night splint to prevent excessive nocturnal flexion. This can often simply be achieved by wrapping a towel around the arm before going to bed. Nerve gliding exercises may be provided by physiotherapy.

Operative management can be used where nonoperative methods fail, and when there is significant limitation or motor involvement. Surgery normally consists of *in-situ* decompression. When the nerve is unstable or a revision is being undertaken, the nerve can be transposed anteriorly and placed in the subcutaneous plane.

## Other Nerve Entrapment
### Radial Nerve Entrapment

The radial nerve can be injured in association with a humeral shaft fracture, leading to acute radial nerve palsy. Its terminal branch, the posterior interosseous nerve, can be compressed in the radial tunnel or within the supinator

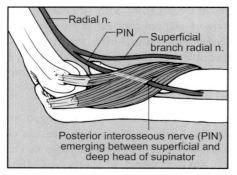

Fig. 6.15 The posterior interosseous nerve (PIN) is the terminal motor branch of the radial nerve. It runs through a deep tunnel through the supinator muscle, where it can be compressed.

(**Fig. 6.15**). There are several potential locations of compression, with the leash of Henry, fibrous edge of the extensor carpi radialis brevis, arcade of Frohse and the distal edge of the radial tunnel all being implicated. Weakness is less commonly described. The patient usually reports lateral elbow pain distal to the epicondyle (distinguishing it from lateral epicondylitis). They may report fatigue of the arm, rather than weakness. Pain can be reproduced by pressure over the path of the radial nerve in the between brachioradialis and the flexor/pronator compartment. Diagnosis is difficult as nerve conduction studies are usually normal and imaging findings are not specific. Care must be taken to exclude other causes of lateral elbow pain. Treatment is conservative initially, with splintage of the wrist to rest the extensor musculature. In cases that are refractory to rest and do not settle over time, surgical decompression may be offered, with care to decompress the nerve along the whole radial tunnel.

### Median Nerve Entrapment

While the most common form of median neuropathy is carpal tunnel syndrome, more proximal compression of the median nerve around the elbow can also lead to similar symptoms. The median nerve innervates the palmar sensory aspect of the thumb to the radial border of the ring finger, along with the muscles of the thenar eminence and lateral two lumbricals (mnemonic 'LOAF' = **L**umbricals, **O**pponens, **A**bductor pollicis brevis, **F**lexor pollicis brevis). More proximally, the median nerve innervates the flexor pollicis longus, FDP and pronator quadratus via the anterior interosseous nerve (AIN). The median nerve can be trapped proximally around the elbow. This can occur at several distinct locations (**Fig. 6.16**). When it occurs due to entrapment between the two heads of the pronator teres, it is called 'pronator syndrome'. The clinical presentation is similar to carpal tunnel syndrome but with the added proximal dysfunction. This is most commonly seen in the muscles innervated by the AIN (**Fig. 6.16**).

Nerve conduction studies can be useful to pinpoint the site of compression and exclude alternate or simultaneous, compression at the carpal tunnel.

Treatment initially consists of conservative measures, with rest. Splintage, particularly at night, may be useful. If symptoms persist beyond 6 months, consideration can be given to decompression. This procedure is performed through an anterior incision, ensuring decompression of all the potential sites of constriction.

## TENDINOPATHY AROUND THE ELBOW

### Background

Tendinopathy (or more strictly, enthesopathy) is common around the elbow. It most commonly affects the common extensor origin at the lateral epicondyle (**Fig. 6.17**), followed by the common flexor origin at the medial epicondyle. These conditions have traditionally been called lateral epicondylitis (tennis elbow) and medial epicondylitis (golfer's elbow). These terms are still

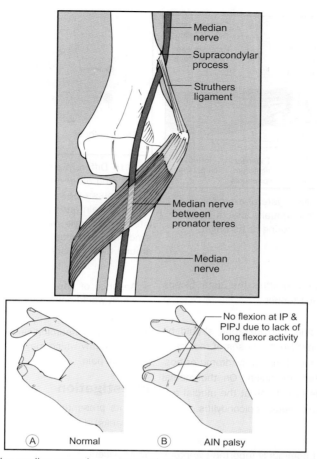

Fig. 6.16 Where the median nerve is compressed at the level of pronator teres, it can result in anterior interosseous nerve palsy and the "Okay Sign". When asked to form an "okay" sign A), a patient with an anterior interosseous nerve (AIN) palsy is unable due to an inability to move FPL and FDP tendons, resulting in the attempt seen in B).

commonly used, although the nomenclature has changed to reflect the fact that these processes are more complex chronic inflammatory and degenerative conditions rather than simple acute inflammation. These conditions are commonly associated with overuse through sports, recreation or work. They normally occur slowly, with an insidious onset, but may also occur after an acute injury. An acute injury may lead to a full or partial thickness tear at the tendon insertion site and thereafter develop into a chronic inflammatory picture.

These conditions are very common in the population, with the majority of people suffering symptoms at some point in their lives. The majority of cases are self-limiting and respond to rest and activity modification. A small proportion prove refractory and may require consideration of intervention.

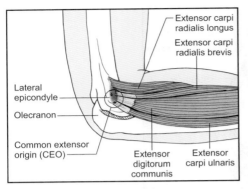

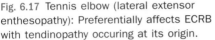

Fig. 6.17 Tennis elbow (lateral extensor enthesopathy): Preferentially affects ECRB with tendinopathy occuring at its origin.

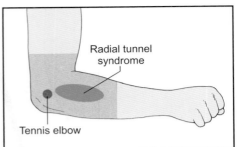

Fig. 6.18 Differentiating between "tennis elbow" and other causes of lateral elbow pain. Tennis elbow usually produces well localised pain and tenderness around the lateral epicondyle, whereas radial tunnel syndrome produces more diffuse symptoms around the extensor wad.

Tendinopathy can also affect the distal biceps tendon and triceps tendon.

On the lateral side, consideration should be given to the alternative diagnoses of radiocapitellar arthrosis, radial tunnel syndrome or posterolateral rotatory instability. On the medial side, ulnar nerve symptoms at the medial epicondyle can mimic medial epicondylitis.

## Symptoms

Pain is the most commonly reported symptom. It is described in a localised area of the enthesis, at, and just distal to, affected epicondyle. It is aggravated by activities that require contraction of the affected muscle group (extensor or flexor). The pain can come on suddenly during a gripping or moving manoeuvre.

## Signs

- Localised tenderness over the lateral or medial epicondyle (rare to be distributed more widely). **Fig. 6.18** outlines the difference between lateral epicondylitis and radial tunnel tenderness.
- Reproduction of pain on resisted extension (lateral elbow tendinopathy) or flexion (medial tendinopathy)

- Absence of grip and grind pain (**Fig. 6.19**), which would point to underlying radiocapitellar arthritis
- Absence of neurological signs such as ulnar neuropathy which may also result in medial elbow pain

## Investigation

Patients presenting with short-lived symptoms (<6 weeks) do not need routine investigation.

When patients have symptoms that persist beyond 6 to 8 weeks and do not respond to first-line treatment, it is reasonable to investigate further.

- Plain X-rays may reveal another cause for pain, such as arthrosis or tumour. They may also reveal other signs of tendinopathy, such as calcification at the tendon insertion.
- Ultrasound scanning or MRI can examine the area in greater detail and demonstrate irregularity in tendon structure, along with partial and full thickness tears.

## Treatment

### Nonoperative Management

Nonoperative management consists initially of lifestyle advice. Where possible, the aggravating sport or occupational activity should be

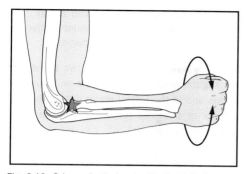

Fig. 6.19 Grip and grind pain: Radiocapitellar arthrosis causes pain when the patient is asked to rotate their forearm with a clenched fist.

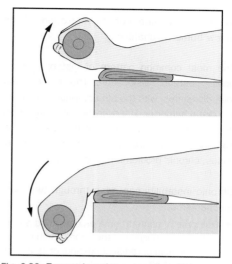

Fig. 6.20 Eccentric wrist extension. This exercise for lateral elbow tendinopathy should be performed for three sets of 15 repetitions, four times a day. A light weight is held in the hand, and the wrist is supported by the other hand or on a rolled up towel. The wrist is raised with support then slowly lowered. It is the lowering phase that is effectively "eccentric" as the extensor muscles are contacting and lengthening simultaneously.

reduced and modified. In most cases, the key factor is time, and healing can take up to a year.

Physiotherapy should include eccentric exercises (**Fig. 6.20**). These lead to reorganization of disordered tendon fibres into a more normal pattern during the tendon healing and remodelling.

Corticosteroid injections are not recommended for the treatment of tendinopathy at the elbow. They are associated with short-lived symptom improvement and the likelihood of worsening of symptoms in the longer term. They can also lead to tendon thinning, degenerative tears and, in rare cases, entities such as posterolateral rotatory instability through attrition of the lateral ligament complex.

Although occasionally offered, there is no significant evidence to demonstrate the superiority of other biological injections (such as platelet rich plasma hyaluronic acid) in the management of elbow tendinopathy.

In refractory cases, where physiotherapy and time have failed, surgical management can be considered. These treatments aim to cause acute damage at the site of the tendon insertion and thereafter provoke a healing reaction that results in more normal scar tissue. This can be accomplished through open or arthroscopic techniques.

## ELBOW INSTABILITY

### Background

The elbow is a congruent hinge joint, with rotation movement arising from the proximal radioulnar articulation. It derives its inherent stability from static and dynamic stabilizers (**Table 6.2**). In full extension the olecranon locks into its fossa, providing sagittal stability. As the elbow moves into flexion, it increasingly relies on other static and dynamic stabilizers for support. The elbow is also less stable in forearm supination due to relaxation of the screw home mechanism.

The most common pattern of instability is an acute posterior dislocation. The humeroulnar joint dislocates, with the ulna moving posterior to the distal humerus. The overwhelming majority of acute dislocations without fracture resolve with no long-term instability. In a small number of cases, chronic problems may develop.

Chronic instability can arise through two main mechanisms:

- Outcome of acute trauma as described above, through damage to the bony architecture (i.e., coronoid or radial head) and/or ligaments (MCL or LUCL).
- Accumulation of microtrauma and stretching of collateral ligaments through repetitive motion, most commonly seen in throwing athletes who participate sports such as baseball, cricket and javelin throwing (**Fig. 6.21**).

It can sometimes be observed as an iatrogenic complication of corticosteroid injection or surgery for lateral epicondylitis.

Instability can be described in two planes. In the sagittal plane it is described as varus and valgus and in the lateral plane it described as anterior or posterior (depending on the direction of displacement of the ulna on the humerus). It is usually a more complicated pattern, involving rotation instability, due to the combination of structures that are weakened or absent. Two main patterns are described.

**Posterolateral rotatory instability (PLRI)** is most common and can occur following injuries to the LUCL and/or radial head (**Fig. 6.22**). When a valgus load is applied to an extended and supinated elbow, the radial head can slip posteriorly, rotating under the lateral column of the humerus. It is then spontaneously reduced on bringing the elbow into flexion, sometimes with an audible and visible clunk.

| Table 6.1 | Mayo Classification of the Rheumatoid Elbow |
|---|---|
| I | Osteopaenia, subchondral cysts and synovitis without marked joint line space narrowing |
| II | Joint line space narrowing with preservation of overall bony architecture |
| IIIA or B | Moderate bone loss affecting one (IIIA) or both (IIIB) humeral columns |
| IV | Complete disintegration of the elbow joint with dysfunctional instability (mutilans rheumatoid arthritis) |
| V | Ankylosis secondary to juvenile rheumatoid arthritis |

| Table 6.2 | Static and dynamic stabilizers of the elbow | |
|---|---|---|
| | **Static** | **Dynamic** |
| **Valgus** | Radiocapitellar articulation<br>Anterior band of medial collateral ligament | Forearm flexors |
| **Varus** | Coronoid<br>Lateral ulnar collateral ligament (LUCL) | Forearm extensors |
| **Posterolateral rotation** | Lateral ulnar collateral ligament (LUCL) | Anconeus |
| **Posteromedial rotation** | Medial collateral ligament | |

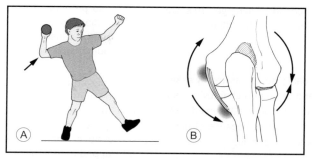

Fig. 6.21 Chronic instability though repeated microtrauma from throwing. A) 'At-risk' throwing motion. B) Valgus overload on radiocapitellar joint and repetitive tension microtrauma to the MCL.

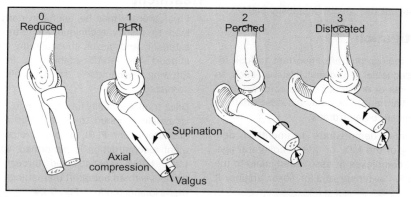

Fig. 6.22 Posterolateral rotator instability: Supination of the forearm through the elbow, with deficiency of the LUCL and other lateral restraint, can result in a 'rotatory' subluxation of the radiocapitellar joint.

**Posteromedial rotatory instability (PMRI)** is less common and is associated with medial coronoid deficiency, along with obligate LUCL injury.

## Symptoms

- Mechanical symptoms such as clunking. They occur predominantly during axial load on the extended arm, with the forearm supinated. PLRI will result from valgus load and postero-medial rotatory instability from varus load, which can be disabling and prevent the patient from lifting or pushing. This can be commonly seen when pushing up from a chair.

- Pain is more commonly seen in overload types, with inflammation forming at the site of the stretched MCL and also at the lateral joint. It is aggravated by throwing and can lead to restriction in recreation and sporting performance.

- Ulnar nerve: In some cases, particularly with longer histories, there can be traction on the ulnar nerve with valgus overload. This can lead to tardy ulnar nerve palsy, with related sensory and motor symptoms in the ulnar nerve distribution.

- Arthritis: In the late stages, osteoarthritis can develop due to the consequences of instability and chondral damage. This can lead to pain and ultimately stiffness.

## Signs

Instability can be easily demonstrated by asking the patient to stand up from a chair by pushing themselves up from the arms. Observed instability or the inability to do so because of apprehension supports the diagnosis.

PLRI can be formally detected by performing the pivot–shift test (**Fig. 6.23**). This can be challenging to perform in an awake patient and an examination under anaesthesia can be useful to investigate the specific instability pattern.

## Investigation

- Plain radiographs are important to look for the sequelae of previous trauma, such as fractures or deficiency of the coronoid and/or radial head. They may also demonstrate secondary osteoarthritis.
- MRI may demonstrate ligamentous deficiency of the MCL or lateral collateral ligament complexes or associated injury to the common extensor and/or flexor origins. It

can also be useful to exclude other differential diagnoses such as loose bodies (alternative cause of clicking and locking) or tendinopathy on the lateral or medial side.

- Dynamic studies are useful to characterize the nature of instability. Fluoroscopy can be used while taking the elbow through a range of motion and then under provocative manoeuvres such as the lateral and medial pivot shifts, where joint subluxation is caused and then reduction is detected through inspection and audible clunks.

## Treatment

- Physiotherapy may be useful in early overload to modify technique and strengthen extensor and flexor musculature and to support the static stabilizers. Improper throwing technique should also be corrected.
- Once frank instability has developed, surgery is usually required to correct the deficient stabilizers. For PLRI, a lateral elbow ligament reconstruction is performed, with the LUCL being reconstructed through bone tunnels with an autograft (hamstrings or palmaris longus tendon) (**Fig. 6.24**). In a similar manner, the MCL can be reconstructed through bone tunnels with an autograft when conservative measures have failed.

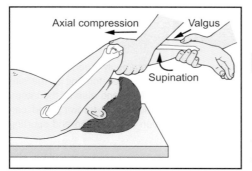

Fig. 6.23 The lateral pivot–shift test for PLRI. An axial and valgus force is applied to an extended and hypersupinated arm. This can cause the radial head to sublux posteriorly. The elbow is them flexed, leading to reduction of the radial head with a clunk. The test is most easily performed under GA.

## EXAMINATION OF THE ELBOW

### Look

Examination of the elbow commences with inspection. The patient should be asked to stand with their arms straight by their sides. The palms should point forwards. The most common deformity seen is a varus deformity (**Fig. 6.25**). The hand and forearm are closer to the body. The carrying angle is reduced. This deformity most commonly arises as a consequence of previous childhood trauma. In a similar way, valgus deformity may arise from trauma to the lateral column and growth arrest.

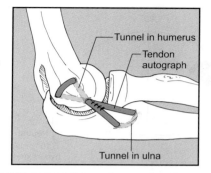

Fig. 6.24 Lateral ligament reconstruction: Autograft or allograft tendon is passed through tunnels in the humerus and ulna to recreate the stability normally provided by the LUCL and other lateral structures.

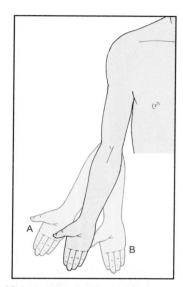

Fig. 6.25 Inspection in the coronal plane can reveal valgus (A) or varus (B) deformity.

Scars are noted, along with overlying phenomena such as rashes, nodules and other skin conditions. Swelling may be noted over the olecranon bursa with an underlying bursitis. Swelling arising from the joint may manifest in the triangle between the lateral epicondyle, radial head and olecranon. It may result from effusion or synovitis in this area.

### Feel

Palpate the lateral and medial condyles, which may be tender in tendinopathy.

### Move

The elbow joint movements are described from a position of full extension (**Fig. 6.26**). This denotes zero degrees. The arc of flexion is defined by the range that the forearm can flex, relative to this fully extended position. Loss of active and passive flexion is common after trauma and is described as a flexion contracture.

While the full arc of flexion is zero degrees to 140 degrees, the functional flexion arc is accepted as being 30 to 130 degrees. With this range the arm can be flexed to bring the hand to the face and extended far enough for most situations of reach.

Forearm rotation is assessed with the elbow held against the side (**Fig. 6.27**). Neutral is with the thumb pointing up. Supination brings the palm face up (imagine carrying a bowl of soup). Pronation brings the palm face down.

## Extended Tests

Impingement can be noted through pain at the furthest extent of extension and flexion. It is likely to correlate with pathology in the posterior or anterior aspects of the elbow, respectively. Impingement pain on rotating the forearm with the forearm clenched is termed 'grip and grind' pain (**Fig. 6.20**).

The elbow joint can be examined for varus/valgus instability in the coronal plane. This may reveal gross insufficiency of the medial or lateral collateral structures. The elbow should be slightly flexed to unlock the olecranon from its fossa during the manoeuvre.

More subtle rotatory instability can sometimes be elicited by pivot–shift testing (**Fig. 6.23**).

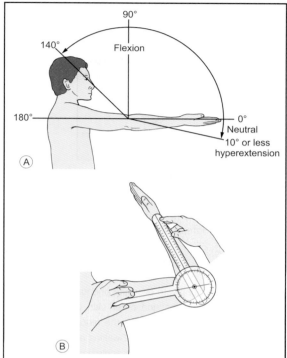

Fig. 6.26 Assessment of flexion: A) The range of motion is described as an arc of a circle. With the arm straight, there are 0 degrees of extension. B) A goniometer should be used to ensure accuracy as esti-mated visual determination is inherently inaccurate.

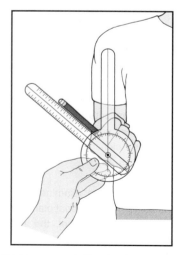

Fig. 6.27 Forearm rotation is also measured with a goniometer. A pencil can be grasped to aid measurement. Neutral is considered when the pencil is pointing directly up and down. Supination and pronation are measured from this reference.

To assess for PLRI, a supination/external rota-tion force is applied distally at the hand/wrist, along with a valgus stress across the elbow. In PLRI, this may cause the radial head to rotate 'under' the inferior edge of the capitel-lum. As the joint is then flexed, it is palpated to determine relocation of a subluxed radial head.

Tendinopathy around the elbow can be deter-mined using provocative tests that stress the respective muscle common origins (**Fig. 6.28**).

## Neurovascular Examination

Neurovascular examination is essential. In the case of the elbow, pulses should be palpated distally at the wrist. The ulnar nerve in particular should be assessed as ulnar neuropathy is most commonly associated with elbow conditions. This

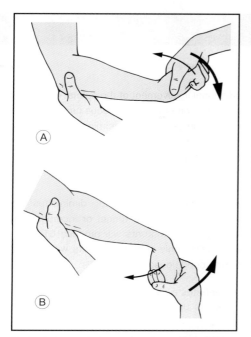

Fig. 6.28 Provocative testing for lateral and medial elbow tendinopathy. Resisted motion is applied through the wrist. Resisted dorsiflexion produces pain at the lateral epicondyle in tennis elbow A) and at the medial epicondyle in "golfer's elbow" B).

leads to muscle wasting in the intrinsic muscles of the hand along with altered sensation in the ulnar border of the hand. An ulnar claw deformity is sometimes present due to imbalance between the long flexor muscles of the fingers and the local hand intrinsic muscles (**Fig. 6.14**).

The ulnar paradox describes a situation where a more proximal ulnar lesion results in less ulnar clawing. This is due to the muscle loss being balanced, as the more proximal long flexors are also affected.

The Froment test can be used to demonstrate intrinsic weakness in the hand (**Fig. 6.15**). The ulnar nerve can be assessed for sensitivity in the cubital tunnel by tapping over the nerve, behind the medial epicondyle. This is the generic Tinel sign. If positive, shooting discomfort and paraesthesia are experienced in the ulnar nerve distribution.

# The Hand

## INTRODUCTION

The hand and wrist are composed of 27 bones. There is motor innervation from the median and ulnar nerves. The sensory innervation comes from both nerves, with additional innervation from the radial nerve over the dorsum of the radial side of the hand. The hand's main function is to provide power and precision grip to manipulate and manoeuvre objects. Hand function is vital for self-care, personal hygiene, activities of daily living, education, employment and recreation. Therefore, disorders of the hand can lead to significant impairment and disability.

## Clinical Summary

The carpal tunnel is bound on the palmar side by the transverse carpal ligament. On the radial side it is limited by the scaphoid. The hamate bounds the ulnar border. The carpal tunnel contains the median nerve, along with the fingers' superficial and deep flexors (flexor digitorum superficialis [FDS] and flexor digitorum profundus (FDP)) and the thumb's flexor pollicis longus (FPL) (**Fig. 7.1A–B**).

The median nerve carries sensory information from the palmar aspect of the thumb, index and middle fingers and the radial border of the ring finger. It provides motor innervation to the muscles of the thenar eminence.

Dysfunction of the median nerve produces a pattern of sensory and motor symptoms in the hand. The most common cause of this condition is carpal tunnel syndrome (CTS), where the median nerve is compressed within the carpal tunnel. When compression of the median nerve occurs at elbow level or more proximally, a different pattern of symptoms is seen, with additional involvement of the palmar cutaneous nerve and anterior interosseous nerve. Cervical root compression can mimic median nerve compression in some aspects, but the sensory and motor patterns are very different (**Fig. 7.2**) (Cross Reference Elbow Chapter).

Any condition which either diminishes the volume of the carpal tunnel or increases the volume of its contents will produce CTS. It is more commonly seen in patients with the following conditions:

- Diabetes mellitus: associated with a greater risk of underlying neuropathy
- Pregnancy: probably due to a more oedematous state, leading to compression of the contents of the carpal tunnel
- Osteoarthritis: associated joint swelling
- Trauma: CTS can occur in the acute or chronic phase following trauma to the wrist, such as a fracture of the distal radius.

CTS has also been reported to be associated with certain occupational activities that require repetitive movements or use of certain vibrating tools. Epidemiological studies of such effects are difficult to perform and interpret. CTS also commonly occurs spontaneously in the population. Occupational association should not be made lightly.

## Symptoms

- Numbness, more symptomatic at night. The classic description is of waking at night and shaking the hand to bring the feeling back.
- Pins and needles (paraesthesia)
- Pain (dysaesthesia)
- Weakness, particularly of the thumb

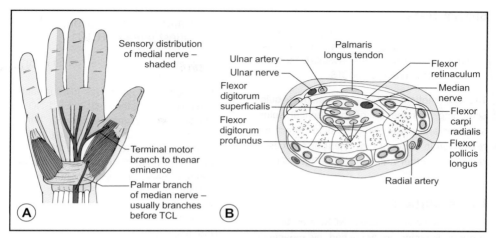

Fig. 7.1 A) Carpal tunnel on volar aspect of wrist. The palmar branch usually divides proximal to the transverse carpal ligament (TCL). Care should be taken not to damage it during approaches around the wrist. B) Cross-section through carpal tunnel. This demonstrates the arrangement of the flexor tendons in relation to the median nerve. Flexor carpi radialis (FCR) is outside the tunnel, in a separate sheath. The radial artery has traversed dorsally by this point.

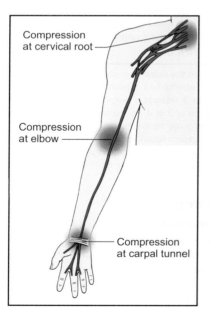

Fig. 7.2 Although the most common point of compression of the median nerve is at the carpal tunnel, it can also be compressed at the cervical roots or around the elbow. More proximal compression tends to lead to wider extent of signs, such as anterior interosseous nerve (AIN) palsy.

## Clinical Examination

### Look
- Muscle wasting, particularly of the thenar eminence

### Feel
- Tinel sign: percussion over the carpal tunnel aggravates symptoms
- Check sensation, in particular assess for reduced sensation over the thenar eminence, as this may signify a more proximal lesion (as the palmar cutaneous branch usually arises before the carpal tunnel).

### Move
- Assess abductor pollicis brevis (APB) strength (grade 1–5 on the Medical Research Council (MRC)] scale) to examine motor function.
- Assess for ability to make the 'OK' sign, with flexion of the index distal interphalangeal joint (DIPJ) and thumb interphalangeal joint (IPJ). If there a deficit, this may point to a more proximal lesion, affecting the motor anterior interosseous nerve branch of the median nerve (**Fig. 6.17.**)

## Special Tests

- The Phalen test involves resting the elbow on a surface, allowing the wrist to flex under gravity. Onset of paraesthesia within 60 seconds indicates the presence of CTS.

The examination should also include a quick screening examination of the cervical spine, shoulder and elbow, which should detect any restriction in range of movement or sources of radicular or other radiating pain (**Fig. 7.2**).

## Investigation

Nerve conduction studies (NCS) may be performed. Function is assessed by measuring how long stimulation takes to travel along motor and sensory fibres. This is measured as latency. The size of the nerve's action potential (amplitude) can also be measured. The combination of these results, along with comparison to the contralateral limb and ulnar nerve, can indicate the presence and degree of median nerve compression.

NCS may not be needed in all cases. When symptoms and examination findings indicate classical CTS, NTS may not add to the diagnosis. The studies may therefore lead to delays in diagnosis and treatment, along with additional treatment cost.

NCS are useful where there is doubt regarding symptoms and diagnosis. Patients may have sensory deficits that do not fully fit with CTS, or they may have other comorbidities, such as a cervical disc disease, other upper limb pathology or chronic pain syndromes. NCS may be useful in such cases to help counsel the patient as to the likely success of surgery.

Specially designed questionnaires may be useful in determining which patients should undergo NCS and which may proceed directly to treatment.

## Kamath and Stothard Carpal Tunnel Questionnaire (CTQ)

- Has pain in the wrist woken you at night? YES 1 NO 0
- Has tingling and numbness in your hand woken you during the night? YES 1 NO 0
- Has tingling or numbness in your hand been more pronounced first thing in the morning? YES 1 NO 0
- Do you have/perform any trick movements to make the tingling or numbness go from your hands? YES 1 NO 0
- Do you have tingling and numbness in your little finger at any time? YES 1 NO 3
- Has tingling and numbness presented when you were reading a newspaper, steering a car or knitting? YES 1 NO 0
- Do you have any neck pain? YES -1 NO 0
- Has the tingling and numbness in your hand been severe during pregnancy? YES 1 NO -1 N/A 0
- Has wearing a splint on your wrist helped the tingling and numbness? YES 2 NO 0 N/A 0

When the score is greater than or equal to 5, 90% of patients had a positive NCS. A score of less than 3 predicts a negative NCS. Patients with a score of 3 or 4 are equivocal and NCS can therefore guide treatment.

Need permission from: *Kamath V, Stothard J. A clinical questionnaire for the diagnosis of carpal tunnel syndrome. J Hand Surg Br. 2003 Oct;28(5):455-9*

## Treatment

**Resting splint:** A wrist splint should be offered, particularly for use at night, if symptoms are problematic at this point. Care should be taken to avoid splints that hold the wrist in extension. Splints can often be shaped to reduce such positioning.

**Corticosteroid injection:** An injection may be useful in certain cases where avoiding surgery is desirable, such as in patients with diagnostic uncertainty, mild symptoms and other health issues such as pregnancy and those who work in very manual occupations, where pillar pain and scar sensitivity may be limiting.

**Surgery:** Open carpal tunnel decompression is the standard of care, with an anticipated success rate of approximately 95%. Keyhole techniques have been described and are hypothesised to lead to fewer complications and faster return to work. There are, however, greater risks of median nerve injury.

## Surgical Technique: Carpal Tunnel Decompression

*The palmar skin overlying the carpal tunnel is anaesthetised using a fine gauge needle and a mixture of local anaesthetic and adrenaline (1:100,000). A tourniquet can be used to provide a clearer bloodless field. Some surgeons advocate a tourniquet-free technique, and evidence supports equivalent outcomes and less tourniquet-related discomfort. If a tourniquet is used, it should be inflated after preparation of the skin to minimise the application time and discomfort. The arm is elevated, and pressure is applied over both the radial and ulnar arteries (similar to an Allan test). The tourniquet is inflated. A longitudinal incision is made at the lowest point between the thenar and hypothenar eminences, midway between the scaphoid tubercle and hamate. This is usually in line with the radial border of the ring finger. The proximal extent of the wound is the wrist crease, and the distal extent must not cross a transverse line from the medial border of the thumb to the hamate (Kaplan line) (**Fig. 7.3**). This prevents damage distally to the recurrent motor branch and palmar arterial arch. The subcutaneous tissue is dissected, taking care to avoid damage to rare anatomical variants of the palmar cutaneous sensory branch. A self-retainer is used sequentially until the transverse carpal ligament (TCL) is reached. It is incised carefully in line with the skin incision. Once the median nerve is visible, it is protected, and the division of the TCL is completed distally until palmar fat is seen. Care*

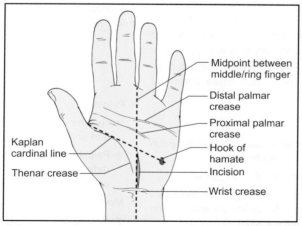

Fig. 7.3 Carpal tunnel decompression – surface anatomy. The distal extent of the incision is bordered by Kaplan's cardinal Line. This is an imaginary line drawn from the hook of hamate to the base of the ulnar border of the thumb. The proximal extent is the wrist crease. It is in line with an imaginary line drawn proximally from the intersection of the middle and ring finger, in the lowest point between the thenar and hypothenar eminences. Observing these rules will protect the superficial palmar arch distally and the recurrent motor branch of the median nerve.

*must be taken to ensure full release of any thickened forearm fascia proximal to the wrist crease. Incomplete release is the most common reason for failure to improve following surgery. Haemostasis is secured, and the wound is closed with interrupted sutures. The patient should be advised to maintain finger and wrist movements. Sutures should be removed at 10–14 days.*

## TRIGGER FINGER

### Clinical Summary

The flexor tendons to the fingers and thumb run through a pulley system (**Fig. 7.4**). This prevents 'bow-stringing' of the tendons and enables compound finger flexion at the metacarpophalangeal joints (MCPJs), proximal interphalangeal joints (PIPJs) and distal interphalangeal joints (DIPJs). The pulley is a fixed, inelastic fibrous structure. As the flexor tendon runs through the pulleys, it can accumulate damage and inflammation, which leads to localised swelling of the tendon, which in turn can cause painful clicking or jamming. It is sometimes called 'stenosing flexor tenosynovitis'. The A1 pulley is the most common site (**Fig. 7.4**). There is an increased incidence in patients with diabetes mellitus or other connective tissue disorders such as rheumatoid arthritis, but in most cases the cause cannot be identified.

### Symptoms

- Clicking (sometimes audible) during flexion and extension of the finger
- Pain can accompany the 'triggering'.
- A tender lump in the region of the flexor tendon over the A1 pulley (at level of the MCPJ on the palmar side)
- Inability to extend the finger

### Clinical Examination

- Inspect
  - Deformity/finger held in flexion

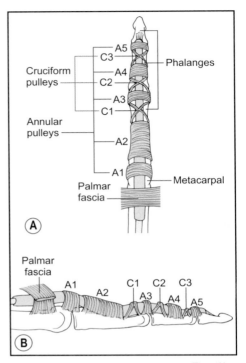

Fig. 7.4 Flexor tendon pulley system. The 'A' pulleys are annular, while the 'C' pulleys are cruciform. The 'C' pulleys can crimple during flexion. A) coronal view; B) lateral view.

- Palpate
  - Feel for a tender lump in the A1 pulley and snapping on movement of the finger.
  - Palpate for other causes of finger flexion deformity, such as palmar nodules associated with Dupuytren disease.
- Move
  - Palpate the flexor tendon during passive finger flexion. A mobile lump around the A1 pulley can sometimes be detected.
  - Check range of movement in the MCPJ, PIPJ and DIPJ to ascertain if there are any secondary flexion contractures.

## Investigation

- No investigation is required when the diagnosis is clear from the history and clinical examination.
- Ultrasound scanning may be useful if the diagnosis is not clear to assess for flexor tendon damage, swelling and synovitis, along with dynamic assessment of tendon movement through the pulley.

## Treatment

- **Extension splintage**, particularly at night, may result in resolution of the underlying tendinopathy and prevention of flexion to the point of triggering.
- **Corticosteroid injection (Fig. 7.5)** may provide permanent relief in up to 90% of cases.
- **Trigger finger release (Fig. 7.6)**: This is most commonly performed with a local anaesthetic procedure to release the A1 pulley.

## DUPUYTREN'S DISEASE

## Clinical Summary

Dupuytren's disease is a disorder that affects the palmar fascia of the hand. It leads to progressive thickening that results in contracture of one or more fingers. It tends to affect the ring and little fingers more often (**Fig. 7.7**).

At a histological level, there is overactivity of myofibroblasts. The disease starts with the development of firm nodules in the palm. It can then progress with the development of thick cords that lead to tethering of the fingers. It is important to note that these cords are not thickened tendons, as is sometimes thought.

Once contractures have developed, secondary changes occur to the capsule of the MCPJ and PIPJ.

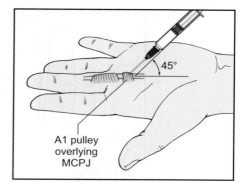

Fig. 7.5 Corticosteroid injection for trigger finger release. A narrow gauge needle (insulin syringe or orange – 25G) is used. The surface anatomy is noted. The injection is in the midline of the finger (to avoid the neurovascular bundles which lie laterally), 1 cm proximal to the MCPJ joint crease. The needle is aimed at 45 degrees to the skin heading distally. Resistance is felt as the needle passes through the pulley. Care should be taken to avoid injection into the tendon. If resistance to injection is felt, withdraw the needle slightly. Usually only a small amount of volume can be injected due to the small space. The patient should be warned of the risks of infection, neurovascular damage, recurrence, failure to improve and skin thinning/pigmentation.

Dupuytren's disease has been reported to be more common in older men and people of northern European descent. There is also a strong genetic component. It has also more prevalent among people with diabetes and higher tobacco and/or alcohol usage.

## Symptoms

- Palmar nodules: initially painful during formation and then painless
- Development of cords in palm and fingers

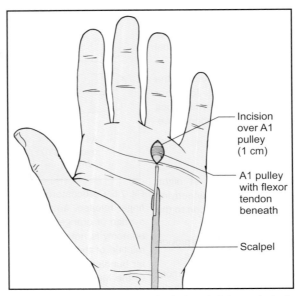

Fig. 7.6 Open trigger finger release. Local anaesthetic is administered. An incision is made longitudinally over the A1 pulley. Blunt dissection is used to clearly visualise the pully, which is incised in line with the skin incision. The underlying flexor tendons are inspected to ensure that they move freely. The patient is asked to make a fist several times to ensure that triggering has been abolished.

- Deformity with flexion contractures affecting the MCPJs and PIPJs
- Functional impairment with the inability to open the hand to initiate grasp. This can also cause trouble when putting a hand into a pocket or washing the face.
- Skin hygiene problems in tight flexion creases

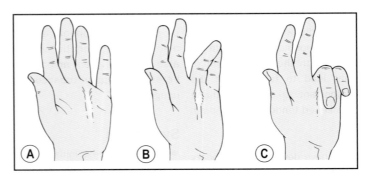

Fig. 7.7 Stages of Dupuytren's Disease. A) Palmar nodules without deformity. B) Palmar cords leading to flexion at the MCPJ. C) Cord progression causing deformity at PIPJs.

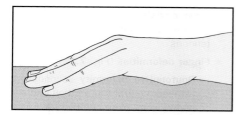

Fig. 7.8 Tabletop test. The patient cannot place their hand flat on a table, palm down.

## Clinical Examination

- Observe and palpate to determine the location and extent of cord(s). The table-top test is positive if the patient is unable to place their hand palm down on the table (**Fig. 7.8**).

- Measure maximal extension possible at the MCPJ, PIPJ and DIPJ.

- Ensure it is not another pathology such as trigger finger (cross reference).

- Assess distal sensation and perfusion (important when considering operative intervention).

## Investigation

- No specific investigation is required. Diagnosis and management are based on levels of symptoms, functional impairment and clinical examination findings.

## Treatment

Where there is no deformity no active treatment is required. The patient should be counselled to watch for the development of any contracture.

Intervention may be offered if there is functional impairment and the flexion contracture at the MCPJ is >30 degrees or the contracture at the PIPJ is >15 degrees. Intervention options include the following:

- Fasciotomy: This approach is suitable for simple cords with mild to moderate contracture affecting the MCPJ. It can be achieved via the percutaneous needle technique (needle fasciotomy (NF)) or more traditional open techniques. NF has a higher rate of recurrence but can be undertaken in an out-patient setting. Fasciotomy can also be achieved with injection of collagenase around the cord. At the time of writing the availability of collagenase for the treatment of Dupuytren's disease has been affected by licensing and supply issues.

- Fasciectomy: The cord is dissected free and traced into the digit. Care is taken to avoid damage to the neurovascular bundles, particularly around the spiral bands. The overlying skin can also be contracted and released with a Z-plasty during closure (**Fig. 7.9**).

- Dermofasciectomy: In complex cases, such as those with recurrence or severe deformity and contracture of skin, a skin graft can be placed following release of the contracture. This can also act as a 'firebreak' for the disease.

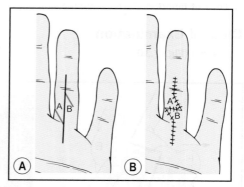

Fig. 7.9 After dissection of the cord and correction of deformity, there can be an associated overlying skin contracture. The resulting scar can be lengthened using a z-plasty. Use of 45 degree flaps results in an overall 50% increase in scar length. A) planning additional incisions (red). B) The apex of each flap is then rearranged (angles A and B). An alternative is to plan zig-zag incisions, a so called "Bruner" incision.

## THE RHEUMATOID HAND AND WRIST

### Clinical Summary

Rheumatoid arthritis (RA) is a common inflammatory polyarthropathy (Chapter 1, Principles of Elective Orthopaedics). It may affect the small joints of the hand along with the wrist. It is associated with a diffuse synovitis that leads to articular cartilage loss and periarticular joint erosions. There can also be extraarticular damage to tendons leading to rupture and loss of function. The introduction of disease-modifying antirheumatic drugs and biological treatments for rheumatoid arthritis has reduced the occurrence of severe hand manifestations of RA.

### Symptoms

- **Pain.**
- **Joint swelling.** Principally in more proximal joints (i.e., wrist and MCPJs)
- **Stiffness.** Particularly for extended periods on waking
- **Loss of function.** Power and precision grip

### Clinical Examination

- Inspect (**Fig. 7.10**)

- **Ulnar deviation** of fingers due to joint erosion and subluxation of extensor tendons
- **Finger deformities** (**Fig. 7.11**)
  - **Boutonnière deformity** secondary to extensor central slip attrition and secondary volar plate contracture
  - **Swan neck deformity** secondary to volar plate rupture and secondary compensatory changes

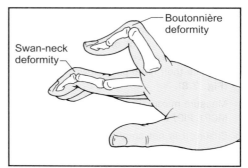

Fig. 7.11 Finger deformities. **Boutonnière Deformity** arising from attrition and deficiency of the central slip of the extensor tendon at the PIPJ, with compensatory hyperextension of the DIPJ. **Swan-neck Deformity** arising from attrition and deficiency of the volar plate of the PIPJ.

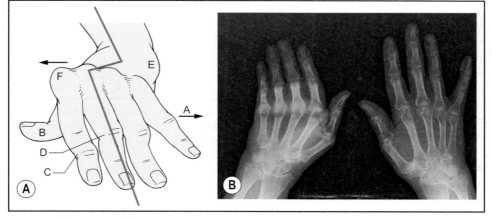

Fig. 7.10A Observation of the rheumatoid hand. A) ulnar deviation of the fingers; B) Z-shaped thumb; C) swan-neck deformity; D) boutonnière deformity; E) subluxation of the ulnar head; F) swelling of the MCPJs.

Fig. 7.10B Corresponding radiological findings in the rheumatoid hand.

- **Z-shaped thumb**
- **Dropped fingers** due to extensor tendon rupture
- **Muscle wasting**
- **Palpate**
  - Gently examine sequentially for pain, swelling and synovitis of individual MCPJs, PIPJs and DIPJs along with the wrist.
- **Move**
  - Examine active and passive range of movement of individual small joints and wrist.
  - Examine extensor and flexor tendon function for each finger individually.

## Investigation

- Plain radiographs of the whole hand are useful to look for loss of joint space, periarticular erosions, osteopaenia and deformity such as joint subluxation (**Fig. 7.10B**).

## Treatment

Treatment should be targeted at the particular joint, tendon or deformity causing pain and loss of function. In many cases deformity will be asymptomatic and not require treatment. Care should be taken to ensure that the patient is receiving maximal medical therapy under the care of a rheumatology department.

- Corticosteroid injections may be useful to treat particular small joints that are painful and synovitic.
- Significant tenosynovitis that is not responsive to antirheumatological therapy may be considered for synovectomy to reduce the risk of subsequent tendon rupture.
- Joint replacement
- Joint fusion
- Tendon reconstruction

## OSTEOARTHRITIS OF THE HAND AND WRIST

### Clinical Summary

Osteoarthritis (Chapter 1, Principles of Elective Orthopaedics) of the hand and wrist is a heterogeneous group of degenerative disorders. There are several distinct patterns (**Fig. 7.12**):

### Generalised Hand Osteoarthritis

This condition tends to affect older patients and the more distal small joints (PIPJ and DIPJ). It is characterised by the onset of bony swelling, pain and stiffness (Heberden [distal] & Bourchard [proximal]). Over time the pain usually resolves, leaving residual stiffness.

### Base-of-Thumb Osteoarthritis

The carpometacarpal joint at the base of the thumb is commonly affected by degeneration. Patients complain of pain just distal to the anatomical snuffbox. As the disease progresses, stiffness and contracture of the adductor muscle can occur, leading to compensatory hyperextension at the MTPJ.

### Wrist Osteoarthritis

The majority of wrist osteoarthritis occurs as a late complication of injury around the scaphoid (scaphoid nonunion advanced collapse (SNAC)) and scapholunate ligamentous complex (scapholunate advanced collapse (SLAC)). The end result of both processes is widespread osteoarthritis of the wrist.

A separate form of osteoarthritis can affect the lateral side of the wrist, with abutment of distal ulna on the capitate. This initially leads to attrition of the triangular fibrocartilage complex and finally full-thickness cartilage loss and frank osteoarthritis. This tends to arise as a result of trauma to the distal radius or forearm, leading to a secondary ulnar positive deformity of the wrist.

## Avascular Necrosis

The wrist can be affected by avascular necrosis. The lunate is affected, and it has been given the eponymous name 'Keinbock disease' (**Fig. 7.12E**). It is most common in men between the ages of 20 and 40 and leads to pain and stiffness of the wrist. It is thought to arise from a disruption to the blood supply to the lunate. This can result from congenital abnormalities such as an ulnar minus deformity of the wrist, a systemic illness such as autoimmune disorders or sickle cell disease or trauma.

## Symptoms

- Pain
- Joint swelling
- Stiffness

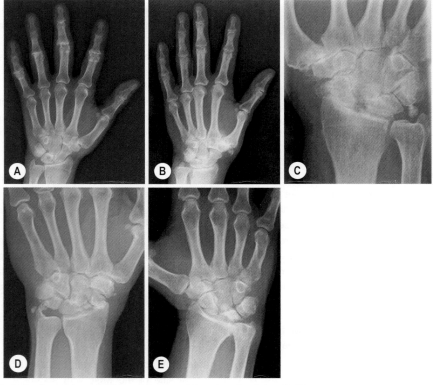

Fig. 7.12 Radiographs of different forms of hand and wrist arthritis:

A: Generalised osteoarthritis

B: First carpometacarpal (CMC) joint osteoarthritis (base of thumb OA)

C: Scapholunate dissociation advanced collapse (SLAC)

D: Scaphoid nonunion advanced collapse (SNAC)

E: Keinbock's (avascular necrosis of the lunate)

## Clinical Examination

- Inspect for joint swelling and muscle wasting.
- Palpate the joints of the hand and wrist for swelling and pain.
- Observe movement of wrist dorsiflexion, palmar flexion, radial and ulnar deviation and forearm rotation. Assess movement of the fingers and look for compound movements.
- Assess for any secondary problems such as CTS of tendon dysfunction.

## Investigation

- Radiographs targeted to area of symptoms: whole hand, wrist and/or base of thumb

## Treatment

Patients suffering from early osteoarthritis of the fingers or thumb base do not require treatment. Since the development of osteoarthritis is frequently part of the ageing process, simple reassurance and advice on modification of activity are sufficient to alleviate anxiety regarding the diagnosis.

Treatment, when necessary, should be targeted at the particular joint, tendon or deformity causing pain and loss of function. In many cases the deformity will be asymptomatic and not require treatment.

### Nonoperative

- Systemic therapy with the occasional use of analgesia and antiinflammatory medication may be useful. Surgical intervention should only be considered after a prolonged period of nonoperative management. This is because the natural history of these conditions is generally one where symptoms are most troublesome during their initial period of onset and then reduce or disappear over time.
- Splintage may be of benefit for base-of-thumb or wrist osteoarthritis, particular during activities that may provoke discomfort.
- Activity modification should be considered where possible and appropriate.

### Surgical

- **Joint arthroplasty** may be considered for small joints that have not responded to conservative management. There is a risk of infection, component wear, loosening and reoperation.
- **Joint fusion (arthrodesis)** may be considered for symptomatic small joints, particularly the DIPJs.
- **Trapeziectomy.** Excision of the trapezium can be considered for symptomatic base-of-thumb osteoarthritis. This procedure has been associated with thumb shortening and weakness, therefore a ligament reconstruction and tendon interposition (LRTI) with half of the flexor carpi radialis (FCR) can be considered to reduce the change in thumb shortening. Alternatively, in younger patients, arthrodesis can be performed to improve grip strength at the cost of motion.
- **Other Carpal Procedures.** Several procedures have been described to manage wrist osteoarthritis. These need to be tailored to the pattern of disease. In SNAC and SLAC wrists, there are options of proximal row carpectomy, scaphoidectomy and four-corner fusion, along with total wrist fusion in the most severe cases. When disease has resulted from ulnar abutment, ulnar shortening can be offered.

## EXAMINATION OF THE HAND

## Look

The hands should be observed for the following:

- Deformity
- Joint swelling
- Cords
- Nail changes
- Rashes, nodules or other skin changes

## Feel

The joints of the hand and wrist should be sequentially palpated to assess for the following:

- Swelling
- Tenderness

## Move

The following movements are examined:

- **Deficit in range of motion and power due to joint/soft tissue pathology**
  - Assessment of power and precision grip
  - Assessment of deficit in finger flexion (tip to palm distance)
  - Assessment of deficits in finger extension (i.e., joint contracture or Dupuytren disease)
- **Deficit in movement of wrist +/− fingers due to tendon pathology or injury**
  - Flexion to each finger should be assessed by isolating the deep and superficial flexors sequentially.
- **Deficit in movement due to nerve injury**
  - Gross examination of median, radial and ulnar motor function can be carried out using the 'rock–paper–scissors' test (**Fig. 7.13**).

## Neurovascular Examination

### Perfusion

- The radial pulse is commonly palpated to assess distal limb perfusion. It also provides a readily accessible method to assess the patient's pulse.
- Capillary refill is assessed by pressing on the nail bed to make it turn white. When pressure is released, blood should return. Blood normally takes less than 2 seconds to return. Delay in capillary refill can signal impaired central perfusion (cardiovascular) or a distal structural deficit (i.e. damaged digital artery).

### Examination of the Median Nerve

When there is greater suspicion of a peripheral nerve deficit, the patient should be examined in greater detail. More proximal compression in the neck or brachial plexus should be considered in the differential diagnosis, along with possible central nervous system causes.

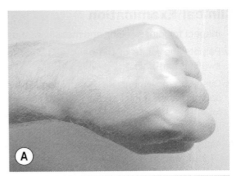

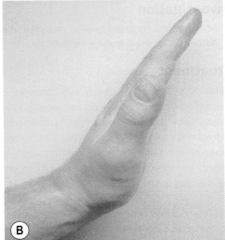

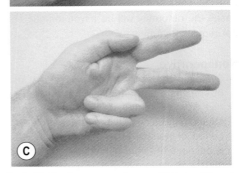

Fig. 7.13 Rock–paper–scissors: This traditional 'game' can be used to assess all nerve function in the hand. A) Rock – pronated fist – median nerve. B) Paper – wrist and finger extension – radial nerve. C) Scissors – finger abduction – ulnar nerve.

- **Sensory**

  - The median nerve supplies sensation to the palmar aspect of the thumb, index and middle fingers. The palm itself is supplied by the palmar cutaneous branch. It usually leaves the main nerve before the carpal tunnel, and therefore palmar sensation is usually preserved in CTS.

  - Phalen's test is performed by asking the patient to flex both wrists and hold the position for 30–60 seconds. The test is positive if symptoms of paraesthesia are reproduced (**Fig. 7.14**)

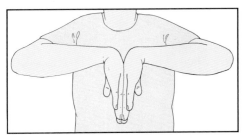

Fig. 7.14 Phalen's Test-can be performed as demonstrated, or by resting the elbow on a surface and letting the hand hand in flexion.

- **Motor**

  - Muscle loss and weakness of the muscles of the thenar eminence are assessed (**Fig. 7.15**).

## Examination of the Ulnar Nerve

- **Sensory**

  - The ulnar nerve supplies sensation to the little finger and the ulnar half of the ring finger.

- **Motor**

  - More distal lesions of the ulnar nerve (i.e., at the level of the Guyon Canal) can lead to a more pronounced ulnar claw hand deformity (**Fig. 7.16**).

  - The ulnar nerve supplies the intrinsic muscles of the hand, excluding those of the thenar eminence. Muscle wasting in the first dorsal interosseous is assessed.

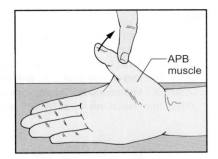

Fig. 7.15 Abductor pollicis brevis (APB) strength is tested by asking the patient to abduct their thumb against resistance. The strength of abduction is felt and assessed, along with observation of the contraction of the APB muscle in the thenar eminence.

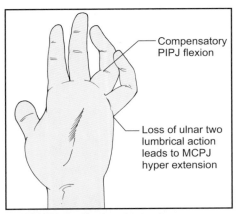

Fig. 7.16 Ulnar claw hand: sign is more pronounced in a distal nerve lesion (ulnar paradox) as action of long flexors is unopposed.

- Loss of the ability to cross the fingers can arise from ulnar neuropathy.

- More proximal lesions can lead to weakness of the long deep flexors (FDP) of the little and ring finger.

## Examination of the Radial Nerve

- **Sensory**

  - The radial nerve supplies a diffuse and variable area on the dorsum of the radial side of the hand, thumb and fingers. This is from the terminal superficial radial nerve.

- **Motor**
  - The radial nerve does not supply any intrinsic musculature of the hand. Motor deficit can result from compression of the either the radial nerve or the terminal posterior interosseous nerve branch (PIN). True radial nerve palsy will also include weakness of the extensor carpi radialis brevis and extensor carpi radialis longus, resulting in loss of wrist extension. Isolated PIN palsy may include preservation of some wrist extension and sensation in the superficial radial nerve territory.

Odhràn Murray, Eoghan Donnelly, Ignatius Liew

## BACK PAIN

Patients presenting with back pain should be assessed according to Waddell's diagnostic triage:

1. **Mechanical low back pain:** This type of back pain is not related to any specific disease, although it is often occurs with degeneration. Presentation may follow an incident where the patient has fallen or attempted to lift something. The precipitating incident may be surprisingly innocuous. Pain is usually worse with movement and relieved by rest.

2. **Radiculopathy**. Radiculopathy (nerve root pain) is characterised by pain, paraesthesia and numbness in a dermatomal distribution. The pain is often described as electric, shooting or burning in nature. Sensory symptoms may be accompanied by motor weakness. The term sciatica implies symptoms in the distribution of the sciatic nerve, below the knee, but is frequently used imprecisely and is best avoided.

3. **Major spinal pathology**. It is important to identify any "Red Flag" features potentially indicating fractures, infections, tumours or cauda equina syndrome, which require prompt assessment and treatment.

## MECHANICAL BACK PAIN

### Clinical Summary

Mechancial Low back pain is extremely common, representing the leading cause of activity limitation and work absence throughout most of the world. Eighty percent of the population will experience back pain at some point in their lifetime, with a 1-year prevalence of 22%–65%. In order to reach a sound diagnosis, an accurate history and physical examination are essential.

## Symptoms

It is important to identify the site and nature of the pain. Pain is often located in the lower back but may be referred from other sources such as the hip or sacroiliac (SI) joint. In some cases, it can be severe and may be associated with debilitating muscle spasms.

The diagnosis of mechanical low back pain ("non-specific low back pain") can only be reached after the exclusion of more sinister conditions, such as infection, inflammation, tumour, trauma or cauda equina syndrome (**Box 8.1** Red Flags of Back Pain). It is also important to consider factors that may adversely affect assessment and long-term outcome. These are often referred to as yellow flags. These include psychosocial and occupational components. Waddell's signs are useful in evaluating patients with non-organic causes of back pain and as possible indicators of a poor prognosis (**Box 8.2**).

## Clinical Examination

Clinical examination (Pages 230–234) includes spinal inspection of overall coronal and sagittal balance, areas of tenderness, range of motion (including Schober test) and lower limb neurological assessment. Examination of the hip, knee and/or SI joints is often useful in order to exclude other sources of pain.

## Investigation

Patients often request investigations such as radiographs and magnetic resonance imaging (MRI) scans. However, in the absence of red flags, these are of little value and are

## Box 8.1 Red Flags for Low Back Pain

- History of malignancy
- History of Trauma
- Constitutional symptoms (fever, night sweats, unexplained weight loss)
- Thoracic pain
- Age <20 years or >55 years
- History of infection, foreign travel, steroid use, intravenous drug use or being immunocompromised
- Autonomic dysfunction (bowel or bladder dysfunction)
- Saddle anaesthesia
- Bilateral radiculopathy
- History of trauma
- Severe/progressive neurological deficit

## Treatment

Acute back pain is often self-limiting, with 90% of patients reporting recovery within 6 weeks. In 2% to 7% of patients, chronic low back pain can develop. Management of these patients includes education, symptom control and active mobilization with return to activities of daily living and work.

Patients should be advised to avoid bed rest and can be referred to exercise programmes or physiotherapy with the aim of maintaining an active lifestyle. A short course of oral analgesia such as nonsteroid anti-inflammatory drugs (NSAIDs), paracetamol and weak opioid medication can be recommended in conjunction with the above lifestyle and mobilization advice. Strong opioids, muscle relaxants and anti-neuropathic pain medications should not be routinely prescribed. Orthoses, traction therapy, acupuncture and electrotherapies such as transcutaneous electrical nerve stimulation have not been proven to be beneficial. Psychological therapy such as cognitive behavioural therapy may be of benefit, especially when combined with physical rehabilitation.

Invasive procedures such as injections and surgery should only be considered in patients

not recommended. Radiographs have low sensitivity and specificity for spinal pathology. With increasing age, the prevalence of incidental spinal pathology increases on MRI, even in the absence of symptoms. For example, all people over 80 years of age have one or more positive MRI findings but are asymptomatic.

## Box 8.2 Factors Which Negatively Affect Assessment and Long-term Outcome

**Waddell's Signs**

- Superficial tenderness
- Nonanatomical tenderness
- Exaggerated response to superficial palpation
- Pain on spinal axial loading (i.e., downwards pressure on head)
- Pain on acetabular rotation
- Distracted straight leg raise discrepancy (sitting patient up on couch)
- Regional sensory disturbance
- Regional weakness

**Yellow Flags**

- A negative attitude that back pain is harmful or potentially severely disabling
- Fear avoidance behaviour and reduced activity levels
- An expectation that passive, rather than active, treatment will be beneficial
- A tendency towards depression, low morale and social withdrawal
- Social or financial problems

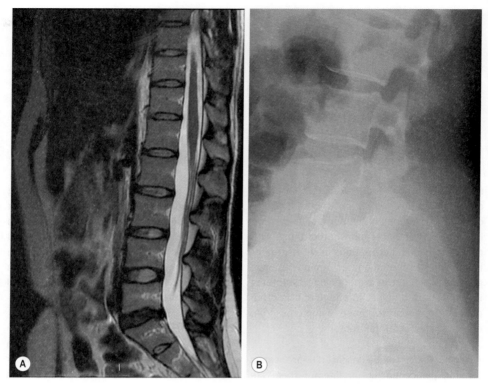

Fig. 8.1 Anterior lumbar intervertebral body fusion (ALIF) in a 30-year-old nurse with recalcitrant severe back pain who failed 18 months of conservative management. A) Sagittal T2 MRI demonstrating isolated degenerative disc disease at L5–S1 and loss of lumbar lordosis due to painful muscle spasms. B) Lateral radiograph at 15 months demonstrating fusion (patient back at work and pain-free, with and significant improvement in all PROMs).

with severe/and debilitating low back pain, in the absence of yellow flags and when at least 3 months of conservative measures have been exhausted. Surgical procedures such as anterior or lateral lumbar intervertebral fusion have shown good results in correctly selected patients (**Fig. 8.1**). However, patient selection remains difficult as it is challenging to predict who will improve and who will suffer chronic pain following surgery.

## RADICULOPATHY

Radiculopathy is pain, paraesthesia (pins and needles) and/or numbness in the distribution of a nerve root (Latin: radix), and may be accompanied by motor weakness. The nerve root is commonly irritated as a result of compression by a lumbar disc herniation, or spinal stenosis (narrowing)

## LUMBAR DISC HERNIATION

### Clinical Summary

**Lumbar disc herniation** is defined as 'a localised displacement of disc material beyond the limit of the disc space'. It affects men more than women (57% versus 43%, respectively), with an average age of onset at 41 years. Smoking, raised body mass index and family

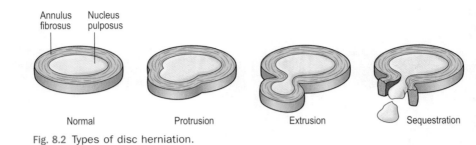

Fig. 8.2 Types of disc herniation.

history are independent risk factors for developing lumbar disc herniation. The association of work with the risk of lumbar disc herniation is complex. It is uncertain whether those with more strenuous occupations have a greater incidence of herniation, or simply a have greater likelihood of experiencing symptoms in a degenerate spine. In addition, it is often difficult to separate these symptoms from other psychosocial risk factors.

A disc herniation can be described by its location (central, paracentral or far lateral). There are several stages of disc herniation (**Fig. 8.2**). The degenerative spine develops with age and is often multifactorial. The disc dehydrates with

decreasing levels of proteoglycans, increasing the stress and abnormal load on the disc. Other contributing factors include loss of disc nutrition and abnormal collagen, which can eventually lead to loss of disc height and tearing of the annulus. Inflammatory cytokines are often released, which can contribute to the patient's symptoms, as well as resorption of the herniated disc.

## Symptoms

Patients present with radiculopathy with which results from the mechanical compression or chemical irritation of one or more nerve roots causing pain numbness, paresthaesia and/or weakness in the distribution of the affected nerve roots Note that pain radiating into the buttocks

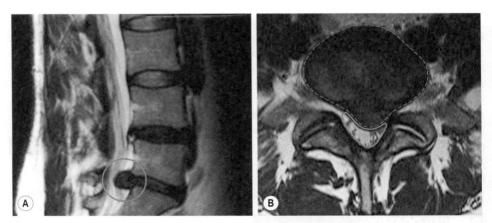

Fig. 8.3 Lumbar disc herniation. A) Sagittal and B) axial image demonstrating a moderate central/left paracentral disc protrusion at L5–S1. Clinical correlation would include left S1 radiculopathy, potential left S1 sensory and motor deficit, reduced ankle reflex, a positive SLR and likely positive cross-over sign.

and posterior thighs (ie not below the knee) is not usually radicular, and is considered to be simply part of mechanical back pain. The lay term 'sciatica' is imprecise and is best avoided.

## Clinical Examination

Examine the lumbar spine and lower limb neurological function, following the sequence look-feel-move (pages 230–234). are A suggests.

## Investigation

MRI is the investigation of choice and should be correlated with the clinical findings (**Fig. 8.3**). It is noninvasive, does not expose the patient to radiation and provides high-definition images of the spinal soft tissues and neural structures. Computed tomography (CT) myelogram can be utilized when MRI is contraindicated. Plain radiographs are generally not useful. Gadolinium-enhanced (contrast) MRI is useful to differentiate recurrent disc herniation from scar tissue in patients with previous spinal surgery.

## Treatment

Management of lumbar disc herniation is similar to that of back pain. Initially, conservative treatment with physiotherapy, simple analgesia and self-management advice is recommended. Radiculopathic pain improves within 6 to 12 weeks in approximately 90% of patients. Paraesthesia and motor deficit may take longer to improve, and if they are still present at 18 months following onset, they are usually permanent. Anti-neuropathic medication such as gabapentin may be considered in persistent neuropathic pain. However, most anti-neuropathic pain medications require careful titration, taking several weeks to become efficacious. They are often associated with significant side effects such as drowsiness.

Surgery is indicated in patients who fail initial non-operative management or in the presence of a progressive neurological deficit. In cases of cauda equina syndrome, investigation and management are indicated on an emergency basis (**Box 8.3**. Single-level disc disease can be managed with discectomy. Surgery leads to improvement in radiculopathic pain in over 85% of correctly selected patients. Paraesthesia and numbness take longer to settle, and improvement in motor function is less likely, although it can occur, especially with early intervention. Importantly, the pain felt in the back is often not significantly improved by decompression surgery. Complications of microdiscectomy are uncommon but include infection, haemorrhage (rarely damage to the great or iliac vessels which can result in loss of life or local bleeding that can cause cauda equina syndrome postoperatively), scar tissue formation, disc recurrence, dural tear, nerve injury, blindness, deep vein thrombosis and pulmonary embolism.

---

### Box 8.3 Clinical Emergency – Cauda Equina Syndrome

Cauda equina syndrome is a surgical emergency.

- The cauda equina nerve roots are compressed within the spinal canal, typically by a large disc herniation (but may also be due to tumour, infection, spinal stenosis or haematoma).

- Diagnosis is difficult. Clinical signs are not sensitive or specific, and MRI is indicated.

–Suspicions should be raised in any patient presenting with red flags: bilateral radiculopathy, severe or progressive bilateral neurological deficit of the legs, difficulty initiating micturition or impaired sensation of urinary flow, loss of sensation of rectal fullness, saddle anaesthesia and/or laxity of the anal sphincter.

–Bladder scanning is useful, with a postvoid residual volume >200 mL as an important indicator for emergency MRI.

–Emergency decompression is required to alleviate pressure as soon as possible and to reduce the chance of permanent neurological dysfunction.

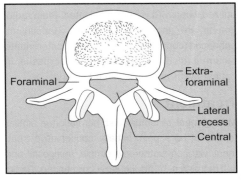

Fig. 8.4 Anatomical classification of spinal stenosis.

## LUMBAR SPINE STENOSIS

### Clinical Summary

Spinal stenosis in the lumbar spine is the most common indication for spinal surgery. It most commonly affects the L4/5 level and L5 nerve root. Lumbar spinal stenosis is defined as a clinically significant reduction in space for traversing neural and vascular structures. It affects almost 50% of patients over the age of 60 with significant impact on quality of life due to pain. It is most commonly classified based on the site of narrowing or defined by the cause of the narrowing.

### Classification

Spinal stenosis can be classified as either acquired (e.g., degenerative, iatrogenic or traumatic) or congenital (short pedicles or medially placed facets). The anatomical classification system is more commonly used and clinically useful (**Fig. 8.4**).

**Central stenosis:** Typical presentation includes leg weakness, heaviness and/or the 'feeling of walking on cotton wool' up on walking or standing.

**Lateral recess:** Radiculopathy of the traversing nerve root (e.g., L5 at the L4–5 level). A paracentral disc will cause compression in the lateral recess.

**Foraminal stenosis:** Radiculopathy of the exiting nerve root (e.g., L4 at the L4–5 level).

### Symptoms

Patients often present with spinal claudication, with symptoms worsening when the spine is in extension due to the narrowing of the spinal canal as well as axial loading. In contrast, the symptoms are relieved with flexion, typically upon sitting (leaning forwards) and cycling. Neurogenic claudication can be differentiated from vascular claudication, as outlined in **Box 8.4**.

### Investigation

MRI scanning should be performed if surgery is clinically indicated. Neural compression from facet

### Box 8.4 Differentiating Vascular and Neurogenic Claudication

|  | Vascular Claudication | Neurogenic Claudication |
|---|---|---|
| Concomitant vascular disease and absence of peripheral pulses | Yes | No |
| Cycling | Aggravates symptoms | Relieves symptoms (lumbar flexion) |
| Stairs/hills | Aggravated on ascent | Aggravated on descent (lumbar extension) |
| Standing | Relieves symptoms | Aggravates symptoms |
| Sitting | Relieves symptoms | Relieves symptoms |

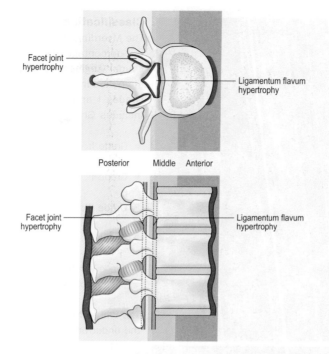

Posterior | Middle | Anterior

Facet joint hypertrophy

Ligamentum flavum hypertrophy

Facet joint hypertrophy

Ligamentum flavum hypertrophy

Columns

Fig. 8.5 Facet joint hypertrophy and osteophyte leading to nerve root and spinal cord compression.

hypertrophy and ligamentum flavum thickening +/− disc protrusion is pathognomonic (**Figs 8.5** and **8.6**). Reduction or absence of fat and obliteration of cerebrospinal fluid surrounding neural structures indicate severe compression. CT myelogram is useful when MRI is contraindicated.

## Treatment

Nonoperative measures in spinal stenosis are similar to those for mechanical low back pain. Simple analgesia, physiotherapy and active mobilization are advocated. Nerve root injections can be offered in patients with multiple comorbidities who are not fit for surgery to provide symptomatic relief. They are also useful to help identify the location of painful stenosis in patients with multilevel lateral recess or exit foraminal stenosis but not central stenosis.

The absolute indications for surgery include cauda equina syndrome, progressive neurological deficit, failure of conservative measures and disabling claudication. Surgical management has been shown to relieve leg pain and may improve back-related functional status of patients.

The surgical strategy should be based on the patient's clinical presentation and comorbidities, along with MRI correlation. Depending on the level and type of spinal stenosis, surgical management may include discectomy, laminotomy, laminectomy, foraminotomy and/or (partial) facetectomy. These can be done simultaneously in order to achieve the desired decompression. Spinal fusion can be considered in patients who exhibit signs of instability intraoperatively or when radical decompressive strategies require removal of >50% of the facet joints.

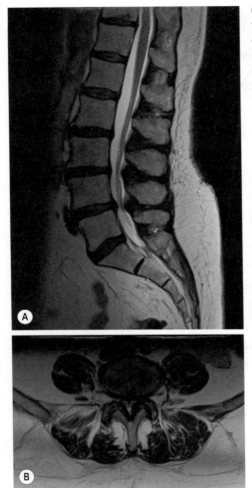

Fig. 8.6 Features of spinal stenosis. The cord and nerve roots are compressed by osteo-phytes and hypertrophy of the facet joint capsule and ligamentum flavum. There is effacement of the cerebrospinal fluid (CSF). A) Sagittal slice B) Axial slice.

## SPONDYLOLISTHESIS

### Clinical Summary

Spondylolisthesis is the displacement of adjacent vertebrae. It most commonly involves anterior displacement of the cranial (upper) segment in relation to the caudal (lower) vertebrae.

### Classification

The Myerding classification is used to define the percentage of slippage in relation to the caudal segment (**Fig. 8.7**). It can also be simplified into stable (<50%), which includes Grades I and II, or unstable (>50%), which includes Grade III, IV and IV.

● Grade I: <25%

● Grade II: 25%–50%

● Grade III: 50%–75%

● Grade IV: 75%–100%

● Grade V: >100% (also known as spondyloptosis)

The Wiltse–Newman classification is based on the underlying case.

● Dysplastic

● Isthmic (pars defect, ~6%)

● Degenerative

● Traumatic

● Pathological

● Iatrogenic

Both classifications are commonly use together, for example, a Grade II isthmic L5–S1 anterolis-thesis (**Fig. 8.8A**).

### Symptoms

Patients can present with low back pain and/or radiculopathy or neurogenic claudication. The presentation can be similar to lumbar spinal stenosis, depending on whether the neurological impingement is central, in the lateral recess, or (more commonly) foraminal.

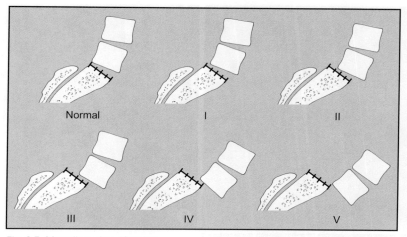

Fig. 8.7 Myerding classification

## Clinical Examination

### Investigation

MRI is the imaging modality of choice and clearly delineates the presence and location of neurological compression. CT scanning is much better at demonstrating bony patho-anatomy, such as pars defects. Weight-bearing plain radiographs are useful to identify patients with dynamic instability, an increase in the degree of slippage compared to the (supine) MRI scan (**Fig. 8.8**). Radiation exposure has largely confined the oblique 'Scottie Dog' lateral plain radiographic view to history, and CT should only be used when necessary (if diagnosis cannot be reached on MRI/plain radiograph or if MRI is contraindicated).

### Treatment

The management of spondylolisthesis depends on the clinical features, as well as the underlying cause and severity of the slip. Conservative measures as described in the section on mechanical low back pain, spinal stenosis and lumbar disc herniation apply. Simple analgesia and physiotherapy should be first-line management. Surgical strategies primarily involve decompression of the neurological structures, usually with direct posterior decompression and fusion +/− of the intervertebral body cage (**Fig. 8.8C**). Anterior approaches can also be considered and are particularly useful when restoration of foraminal height is important. Spondylolysis and back pain are both common findings in the spinal clinic, but the relationship is not necessarily causative. Therefore pars injections are recommended to confirm pathology prior to fusion.

## NECK PAIN

## Clinical Summary

Most patients presenting with neck pain have simple machanical neck pain. In most cases there is no specific pathoanatomical or radiological abnormality. Approximately two-thirds of the population will describe experiencing neck pain at some point in their life, with the majority presenting in middle age. It is the second-most common musculoskeletal presentation to general practitioners in the UK, after back pain. It also accounts for a considerable socioeconomic burden in the form of time off work. Most acute episodes should resolve with expectant and conservative management within 6–12

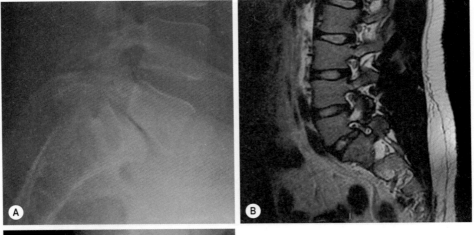

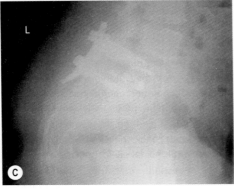

Fig. 8.8 Spondylolisthesis. A) Standing radiograph demonstrating Grade II Isthmic Spondylolisthesis, B) parasagittal T2 MRI with compression of exiting L5 nerve root (note slip partially reduced on supine MRI compared to standing radiograph) and C) lateral radiograph demonstrating insitu transforaminal intervertebral fusion (TLIF).

weeks. The list of differential diagnoses is broad and detailed in **Box 8.5**.

## Symptoms

A diagnosis of simple mechanical neck pain can usually be reached with clinical history and examination alone, supplemented with simple investigations. Mechanical neck pain can be defined as neck pain without featurs of radiculopathy radiation and normal neurological examination in the absence of red flags.

Pain is in the neck region, and description is usually vague, with radiation up towards the base of the skull/occipital region or down towards the trapezius muscles and over the posterior aspect of the shoulder girdle. It may sometimes reach down into the arms. Patients may describe numbness or tingling as well as weakness in the upper limbs, but this should not follow a segmental distribution. Red flags for neck pain are highlighted in **Box 8.6** and should be ruled out in every patient.

## Clinical Examination

Examination of the neck should be carried out carefully to assess for pain, movement, symmetry and stiffness. This should be accompanied by full lower and upper limb neurological examination to assess for focal neurological abnormalities as these may point to a secondary diagnosis.

## Box 8.5 Differential Diagnoses in Patients Presenting With Neck Pain

- Acute disc prolapse
- Acute trauma – including whiplash injury
- Acute torticollis
- Degenerative disease of the cervical spine
- Cervical myelopathy
- Cervical radiculopathy
- Cervical spinal stenosis
- Infection
- Meningitis
- Malignancy

## Box 8.6 Red Flags Associated with Neck Pain That Warrant Further Investigation

Suggestive of cancer/infection/inflammatory disease
- Malaise fever or weight loss
- Night pain/sleep disturbance
- Progressive increasing pain
- Exquisite bony tenderness
- Previous history of cancer/inflammatory arthropathy/chronic infection/immunosuppression
- Lymphadenopathy

Suggestive of myelopathy and spinal cord compression
- Insidious onset
- Gait disturbance/loss of balance
- Feeling of clumsiness/weak hands
- Loss of bowel/bladder/sexual function
- Lhermitte's sign*

History of major trauma

Age <20 years and >55 years

Weakness, especially progressive

Severe progressive pain that is not treatable with standard analgesics

*Lhermitte's sign is an electric shock sensation produced on flexion of the neck that may radiate down into the spine and upper or lower limbs.

## Investigation

If clinical history or examination suggests a cause for symptoms other than simple neck pain, further investigation should be initiated. Initial investigation should include laboratory tests to look for evidence of inflammation, infection and malignancy. These should include full blood count, C-reactive protein (CRP), erythrocyte sedimentation rate (ESR), bone profile, serum electrophoresis and urinary Bence Jones protein. In non-traumatic neck pain, radiographs are of limited value, as they tend to demonstrate degenerative changes only. Such changes can be misleading as they are commonly present without symptoms. MRI provides the most useful diagnostic detail, and CT scanning is useful when bony pathology is suspected.

## Treatment

In patients with neck pain lasting less than 12 weeks, the mainstay of treatment is nonoperative. These patients should be reassured that most neck pain settles over time, resolving within a few weeks. Treatment with simple analgesics, such as paracetamol, NSAIDs or weak opiates, is appropriate based on the level of pain or discomfort. Muscle relaxants such as benzodiazepines are generally not recommended. Return to activities of daily living and work, where possible, should be encouraged. The use of neck braces should be avoided as this may prolong pain and stiffness. Referral to a physiotherapist for strengthening and range of motion exercises should be considered. Neck pain related to work activities may benefit from assessment by an occupational therapist, in terms of treatment and avoiding further episodes of pain. Individuals with persistent pain lasting more than 12 weeks should be reassessed for red flags or the evolution of symptoms that may point to another diagnosis. When a patient has chronic severe symptoms with no treatable cause, referral to a chronic pain service may be appropriate.

## CERVICAL RADICULOPATHY

### Clinical Summary

Cervical radiculopathy is the presence of symptoms related to the cervical nerve roots and has a peak onset in the sixth decade of life. The incidence in the general population is approximately 84 per 100,000 people, with the incidence in men slightly higher than women. The natural history of the disease in most cases in reassuring, with 80%–90% of patients showing improvement in symptoms with nonoperative management alone.

Radiculopathy occurs when conduction of a spinal nerve is slowed or blocked at its exiting root. The symptoms are variable and include sensory and motor disturbances as well as pain. Radiculopathy is not the same as radicular pain.

The pathological process usually develops as a result of compression or inflammation around a nerve root. This typically relates to an ongoing degenerative process and can be caused by the following:

- Intervertebral disc herniation secondary to degeneration of the annulus fibrosis (**Fig. 8.2**)

- Osteophyte formation secondary to cervical spondylosis and degeneration

- Facet joint hypertrophy

- Loss of disc height causing distortion of the surrounding ligaments

- Inflammatory arthropathy

Important secondary causes such as malignancy or infection should also be considered.

Red flags should be looked for in the history and examination (**Box 8.6**).

### Symptoms

Symptoms are variable, and are usually unilateral with pain starting at the neck and radiating into the upper extremity. The patient may report burning or shooting pain in a dermatomal distribution as well as concurrent weakness of the limb. Patients often also complain of pain in the trapezius +/− intrascapular region.

There are eight cervical nerve roots (C1–C8), with the root exiting above the pedicle of the corresponding vertebra except for C8, which exits below C7 and above T1 (**Fig. 8.9**). The nerve roots most commonly affected are C6 and C7. Sensory and motor examination should be performed to identify the affected nerve root, remembering that patterns of dysfunction sometimes do to fully conform to "textbook" dermatomes and myotomes.

### Clinical Examination

Active spine movements are assessed. The Spurling test is performed by fully extending the

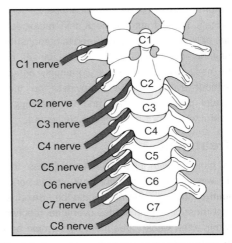

C1
C1 nerve
C2
C2 nerve
C3
C3 nerve
C4
C4 nerve
C5
C5 nerve
C6
C6 nerve
C7
C7 nerve
C8 nerve

Fig. 8.9 Arrangement of cervical nerve roots in relation to their corresponding vertebra. C1 to C7 roots emerge above the pedicle of the same vertebrae where as C8 emerges below.

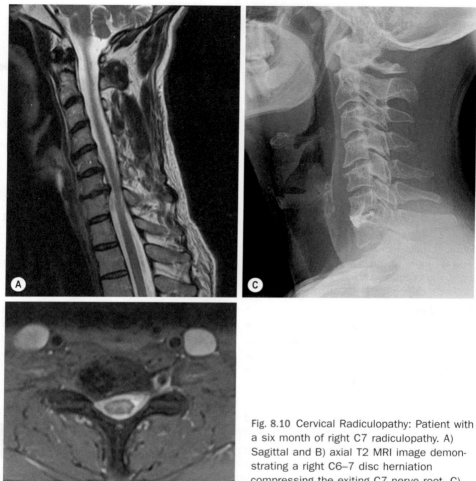

Fig. 8.10 Cervical Radiculopathy: Patient with a six month of right C7 radiculopathy. A) Sagittal and B) axial T2 MRI image demonstrating a right C6–7 disc herniation compressing the exiting C7 nerve root. C) Postoperative Anterior Cervical Discectomy and Fusion (ACDF) radiographs.

patient's head and turning towards the affected side. This is particularly useful when positive to help differentiate from pathology arising in the shoulder. Upper motor neuron signs such as the Hoffman sign (see examination section) should be identified. A neurological examination is performed to assess tone, power, sensation and reflexes in both upper limbs. Finally, examination of the peripheral nerves is necessary when peripheral nerve compression is suspected, such as in carpel or cubital tunnel syndrome.

## Investigation

For cervical radiculopathy, MRI of the cervical spine is the investigation of choice. It allows good visualization of soft tissues such as the intervertebral discs and is noninvasive (**Fig. 8.10**). CT myelography can be used for patients when MRI in contraindicated. A preoperative plain CT is useful for planning when compression by osteophytes, ossification of the posterior longitudinal ligament or disc calcification is suspected.

## Treatment

In most cases, cervical radiculopathy is self-limiting. Around 90% of patients will have mild or no symptoms 1 year after onset. Therefore, the first-line treatment in most cases is non-operative.

### Medications

The recommended first-line therapy is paracetamol, NSAIDs and weak opioid analgesia. Muscle relaxants such as benzodiazepines may provide some symptomatic relief but should generally be avoided. Anti-neuropathic pain medication may be useful when troublesome chronic neuropathic pain is a predominant feature. The role of medication is to help with symptom control and help patients mobilize and engage with physical activity.

### Physiotherapy

A combination of manual and exercise therapies may be superior to either therapy alone. Exercises focused on opening the intervertebral foramina yield the best results in terms of symptom relief. These are active range-of-movement exercises such as contralateral rotation and side flexion and can be combined with stretching exercises to increase range of movement and stability after symptoms have settled. Input from an occupational therapist may also be beneficial in developing strategies to avoid further episodes or exacerbation of symptoms.

### Epidural Corticosteroid Injections

Injection of local anaesthetic and steroids around the affected nerve root may provide some symptomatic relief and can be useful diagnostically in trying to determine the contribution of a specific nerve root to a patient's symptoms. These interventions are carried out with the aid of CT or an image intensifier in theatres. Care should be taken as there is an associated morbidity with these procedures, especially around the cervical spine. Risks include nerve injury, vertebral artery injury/vascular injection, stroke, haematoma and paralysis.

### Operative Management

Surgery is indicated in two situations:

- Failed conservative management or progressive unrelenting pain in which conservative management has failed.

- Severe/progressive neurological deficit.

Outcomes in this patient group are generally favourable, with a 80%–90% of patients showing improvement in their radicular symptoms.

Surgery can be performed through an anterior or posterior approach according to surgical preference/experience and the location of the compressive pathology. Common approaches include anterior cervical decompression and fusion (**Fig. 8.10**) for anterior pathology and posterior laminoforaminotomy for posterior compression.

## DEGENERATIVE CERVICAL MYELOPATHY

### Clinical Summary

Degenerative cervical myelopathy (DCM) is the most common cause of spinal cord impairment in adults worldwide. The incidence and prevalence are estimated at between 4.1 and 60.5 per 100,000 people, respectively. DCM occurs when a narrow spinal canal results in compression on the spinal cord leading to neurological injury, usually secondary to degenerative (spondylosis) disease of the cervical spine. Consequently, DCM tends to present more frequently in the elderly population. Men are affected more than women at a ratio of 2.7 to 1, and the average age of diagnosis is 64 years. Multilevel disease is not uncommon, with the most commonly affected

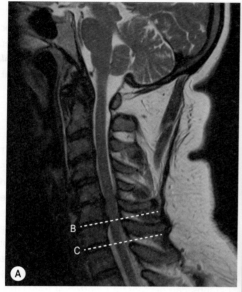

Fig. 8.11 MRI scan of degenerative myelopathy. A) Sagittal view showing posterior disc bulge at c5/6 and c6/7 and myelomalacia at c6/7 – dotted lines demonstrate axial slices. B) Axial view at c6/7. C) Comparison view at c7/T1 showing no compression and capacious CSF surrounding cord.

levels being C5/6. The risk of hospitalization for DCM is 4 per 1,000 patient years.

The pathophysiology of cervical myelopathy is a multifactorial process resulting in the narrowing of the central spinal canal due to changes in adjacent anatomical structures including intervertebral discs, vertebral bodies, facet joints, uncovertebral joints, the posterior longitudinal ligament and ligamentum flavum (Fig. 8.11). Ossification of the posterior longitudinal ligament (OPLL) is a potential cause of cervical myelopathy, especially in the Asian population. OPLL is thought to be influenced by genetic, hormonal (e.g., diabetes) and environmental (e.g., high-salt, low-meat diet) factors. The resulting local compression on the cord leads to microvascular disruption, causing persistent hypoxia with a resulting neuroinflammatory response leading to cell death and disability.

Some congenital disorders do not cause DCM on their own but can indirectly influence the disease's natural history through various gross/microstructural abnormalities. This can occur in patients with Down syndrome, Klippel–Feil syndrome and congenital cervical stenosis or in

**Box 8.7** Signs and Symptoms Associated With Cervical Myelopathy

| Symptoms | Neurological Signs |
|---|---|
| • Clumsy/numb hands | • Ataxic gait |
| • Paraesthesia | • Lhermitte's sign |
| • Abnormal gait/ balance | • Hyperreflexia |
| • Weakness in upper and lower limbs | • Positive Hoffman's sign |
| • Neck pain/radicular symptoms | • Positive Babinski sign |
| | • Clonus |

patients with generalized hypermobility syndrome, for example, Ehrler–Danlos.

## Symptoms

Disease presentation in DCM is often insidious due to the slow progressive nature of the disease. Patients can present with signs and symptoms in both upper and lower limbs. Any established neurological deficit is prone to deterioration over time without intervention.

The progression can be in a stepwise decline, or patients can experience long periods of quiescence. Some identified risk factors for deterioration over time include the following:

• Female sex

• Increased cervical mobility

• Intervertebral disc herniation

• Increased kyphosis at the level of greatest compression

Patients can present initially with loss of fine motor control in the upper extremities and gait imbalance, which may be due to the corticospinal and spinocerebellar tracts being affected first.

## Clinical Examination

There is a mixture of upper and lower motor neuron signs up on examination, with upper motor neuron signs present below the level of compression and lower motor neuron signs at the level of compression (**Box 8.7**).

## Investigation

Investigation is best performed using cross-sectional imaging in the form of MRI and CT scanning. MRI scanning will confirm the diagnosis of myelopathy showing cord changes and allows for an assessment of the cause, degree of compression and canal stenosis (**Fig. 8.11**). CT scanning may be useful in surgical planning as it provides high resolution and is excellent for defining the bony pathoanatomy of the spinal canal. Flexion and extension lateral radiographs can demonstrate vertebral translation at the site of cervical instability.

## Treatment

In most instances of degenerative myelopathy, surgical management is the treatment of choice and can be approached through an anterior or posterior approach. The decision is based on relevant pathoanatomy, number of levels involved, spinal instability and sagittal alignment. A combined anterior and posterior approach may be used, although this increases the risk of complication. The aim is to reduce the acquired stenosis by removal of diseased tissue, relieving compression on the spinal cord. Anteriorly, the surgeon can perform anterior cervical discectomy and/or corpectomy with fusion (**Fig. 8.12**). Posteriorly, the options available are cervical laminectomy +/− fusion or laminoplasty.

## INFLAMMATORY ARTHRITIS OF THE SPINE

## Clinical Summary

An important subset of patients presenting with back pain to any spinal service are those with an inflammatory arthropathy (IA). Recently, the

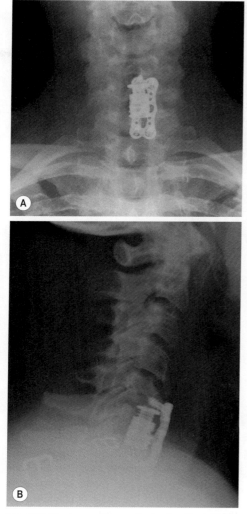

Fig. 8.12 Postoperative radiographs (A – AP, B – lateral) following anterior corpectomy and fusion.

use of disease-modifying antirheumatic drugs (DMARDs) for conditions such as ankylosing spondylitis (AS) has demonstrated the potential to slow and halt disease progression, but only if identified in a timely fashion. Therefore, IA should form part of the differential diagnosis in an attempt to avoid end-stage disease, which is extremely debilitating for this group of patients.

## Rheumatoid Arthritis

Rheumatoid arthritis is a chronic inflammatory disease characterized by progressive damage of synovial joints. It is characteristically symmetrical, although any synovial joint may be affected, including the SI joints and the synovial joints of the spine.

Spinal disease tends to present later in the disease process and is generally more common with a higher number of peripheral joints involved. The cervical spine is the most common region to be affected, but other regions may be involved. It is important to enquire about pain at the base of the skull and in the neck in rheumatoid patients.

## Psoriatic Arthritis

Up to 50% of patients with psoriatic arthritis may have disease involving the axial skeleton. Plain X-ray or MRI scans may show erosive disease. Risk factors associated with developing spinal disease include increased number of joints involved, psoriatic nail changes and longer disease duration.

## Reactive Arthritis

Reactive arthritis occurs secondary to an infection usually involving the gastrointestinal or urogenital tract. Men under the age of 40 are most commonly affected, and the symptoms of arthritis typically begin 2–4 weeks after infection. It is commonly associated with cystitis and arthritis. Sexually transmitted infections (e.g., chlamydia) are associated with larger joints of the lower limb most commonly being symptomatic, but the pelvic girdle and SI joints may be involved. The goal of treatment is eradication of infection and symptomatic management.

## Enteropathic Arthritis

Inflammatory arthritis is associated with a form of inflammatory bowel disease (IBD)–most commonly Crohn's disease or ulcerative colitis. Around 20% of patients with IBD will go on to

**Box 8.8** Features of Diffuse Idiopathic Skeletal Hyperostosis (DISH) versus Ankylosing Spondylitis (AS)

| | Diffuse Idiopathic Skeletal Hyperostosis | Ankylosing Spondylitis |
|---|---|---|
| HLA B27 Association | None | Associated |
| Abnormal Bone Formation | Nonmarginal: flowing ossification along the anterior or right anterolateral aspects of at least four contiguous vertebrae | Marginal: syndesmophytes are thinner, form over the annulus and are vertically oriented (bamboo spine) |
| Spinal Involvement | Cervical and Thoracic | SI joint, symphysis pubis, facets, costovertebral joints, and throughout whole spine |
| Disc Space | Preserved | Can become ossified |
| Bony Erosions | Absent | Frequent |
| Enthesopathies | Infrequent | Frequent |

develop enteropathic arthritis, with one in six of these showing spinal symptoms. Activity of arthritic disease is independent of bowel symptoms, and in many people only the SI joints are involved. In 5% of those with spinal disease the entire spine is involved. Arthritis may precede bowel symptoms.

## Ankylosing Spondylitis

AS is a seronegative chronic inflammatory disease mainly affecting the spine, SI joints and pelvis. The pathological hallmark is enthesitis and the formation of syndesmophytes around these joints due to ossification of soft tissues and eventually fusion. This accounts for much of the pain and stiffness seen in this patient group. Advanced disease results in a fused spine within these patients. Classic clinical features include reduced chest expansion and positive Schober test. Treatment has traditionally been with NSAIDs and symptomatic management, and attempts to treat with DMARDs have been met with varying success. Recent advances in understanding of the disease process have highlighted various cytokines such as interleukin-17 as potential mediators of the inflammatory process.

## Diffuse Idiopathic Skeletal Hyperostosis

Diffuse idiopathic skeletal hyperostosis (DISH) is characterized by abnormal ossification/bone formation of soft tissues surrounding the joints of the spine different from AS (**Box 8.8**). Ossification along the anterior longitudinal ligament and OPLL may lead to partial or complete fusion of adjacent spinal segments. The SI joints tend to be spared.

The majority of people are asymptomatic, and diagnosis tends to be made by incidental finding on imaging. The cause is unknown, and there is no association with HLA B27 haplotype. Treatment is generally conservative. Surgical intervention may be sought in patients with dysphagia or nerve impingement.

## Clinical Features

Clinical features which should alert the surgeon to the possibility of inflammatory arthritis include the following:

● Early morning stiffness which eases after 30–60 minutes of activity

- Swollen joints

- Uveitis

- History of IBD

- Swelling in peripheral joints that follows a palindromic pattern

- Skin rashes (psoriasis)

- Reduced lumbar flexion (Schober test)

- Reduced chest wall expansion

## Investigation

Often, plain radiographs will show evidence of joint disease in late presentations. Biomarkers such as CRP and ESR are useful in active disease and as a monitor of activity.

## Treatment

Surgical intervention in the spine is usually undesirable. It may be required in a small number of cases to correct deformity, manage instability or relieve neural compromise. Extreme caution should be exercised in treating patients with AS or DISH in the trauma scenario. Firstly, spinal immobilization should take preexisting deformities into consideration (standard triple immobilization may result in paralysis). In addition, even minor fractures should be considered as unstable until proven otherwise.

## SPINAL INFECTION: SPONDYLODISCITIS

## Clinical Summary

The incidence of pyogenic spinal infection of the vertebra and adjacent discs is approximately 1 in 250,000 people per year. These infections comprise approximately 2% to 7% of all musculoskeletal infections. It can affect the vertebrae, adjacent disc, spinal canal and local soft tissues. When it affects the canal, it can result in epidural abscess and empyema. It affects men more than women at a ratio of 3 to 1. Risk factors for infection include the following:

- Multimorbidity

- Diabetes

- Obesity/malnutrition

- Renal failure

- Chronic hepatitis

- Immunosuppression

- Long-term steroids

- Intravenous drug abuse

It is likely to be the result of three main mechanisms:

- Inoculation from direct trauma (or surgery)

- Spread from adjacent local source of infection, e.g., soft tissue infection

- Haematogenous or lymphatic in nature, spread from a distant site (genitourinary tract, cellulitic area of skin, gastrointestinal tract or distant abscess)

At presentation there is usually infection present in both the intervertebral disc and vertebral body. It is therefore often difficult to determine which was affected first, hence the name spondylodiscitis. The most prevalent infective organism worldwide is *Mycobacterium tuberculosis*, while in Europe *Staphylococcus aureus* is most common. Rarely, infection can also be caused by fungus or parasites. In most cases infection is with a single organism, but in more difficult-to-treat cases, there can be several different infective organisms. Prognosis is also dependent on the host status, with the best result in patients with normal function and low comorbidity. Patients with local or systemic disease and functional impairment have poorer outcomes.

## Symptoms

Pain is the most common physical finding. Normally, it is reported to have been present for an extended period due to the nonspecific nature in early disease. Often it is made worse by movement and up on sitting and standing, and it can be felt intensely during heel strike while walking.

Patients may also report fever-related symptoms such as sweating. It is an important diagnostic indicator as it can point to infection, but it not always present, and its absence does not exclude spinal infection.

Spinal canal and nerve root compression may also occur. It most commonly appears in a radicular pattern and can be associated with weakness/paralysis and cauda equina dysfunction.

The presence of neurological involvement should raise suspicion for formation of an epidural abscess and subsequent mass effect causing neurological impairment.

## Clinical Examination

Examination findings are usually nonspecific. Pyrexia, sweating and tachycardia may occur in advanced infection. Local tenderness and reduced range of movement of affected segments may occur. Lower motor neuron signs indicate compression of exiting nerve(s). Upper motor neuron signs suggest spinal cord compression from an epidural abscess, mandating emergency investigation and treatment.

## Investigation

Laboratory investigations are useful in diagnosing and managing infection and should include full blood count, ESR, CRP and blood cultures, especially in the presence of pyrexia as this suggests systemic infection. White cell count can be raised or may be normal. The most sensitive marker for aiding in diagnosis and response to treatment is CRP, as this is normally raised in spondylodiscitis, and a down-trending CRP suggests response to treatment.

Plain radiographs are not diagnostic in early stages of the disease process. However, radiographs are useful later if bone loss occurs and help monitor spinal deformity/stability. CT scanning is useful in the presence of bone loss and to guide biopsy in order to identify the causative organism. MRI is the diagnostic gold standard. It can help differentiate infection from malignancy. MRI shows hyper intense signal in vertebral bodies and soft tissues on T2 imaging. MRI will identify neural compression from an epidural abscess and may show myelomalacia if the scan is not performed in a timely fashion. Gadolinium contrast enhancement is often helpful in making the diagnosis, for example, by demonstrating epidural abscess ring enhancement.

## Treatment

The aim of treatment is to eliminate the focus of infection, restore stability, protect neurological function and reduce pain symptoms. The majority of patients with discitis are managed conservatively with analgesia, supportive bracing and targeted antibiotic therapy (after biopsy when possible) for at least 6 weeks, but the duration is tailored to the patient's response to treatment and can be monitored with weekly measurement of serum inflammatory markers. Non-operative treatment can be supplemented with percutaneous CT or ultrasound-guided drainage of paraspinal abscesses if present.

The indications for surgical management include the following:

- Treatment of sepsis or infection refractory to antibiotic therapy. This can involve obtaining tissue samples for histology and culture to guide future management.

- Neurological compromise

- Instability with progressive spinal deformity

- Refractory pain

- Drainage of epidural abscess (clinical emergency in presence of neurological deficit)

- Drainage of paravertebral abscesses not amenable to percutaneous drainage

## SPINAL MALIGNANCY

### Clinical Summary

Malignancy of the spine can be divided into primary tumours and metastatic disease. Primary neoplastic disease of the spine is rare, and secondary metastatic cancer comprises 95% of spinal malignancy. Approximately 70% of all osseous metastases occur in the spine. The spine is the third most common site where cancer cells metastasize, after the lung and liver. Breast, prostate, lung, renal and thyroid primary cancers are responsible for the majority of metastasis to the spine. In addition, haematological malignancies, such as myeloma and lymphoma, frequently involve the spine. Primary spinal malignancy is uncommon but accounts for approximately 10% of all bone and soft tissue sarcomas.

Primary central nervous system (CNS) tumours of the spine account for 2%–4% of all CNS tumours. Intradural tumours of the spine are separated into extramedullary (located outside the spinal cord but within the dural sheath) and intramedullary neoplasms (within the spinal parenchyma). Intradural extramedullary are the more common of these rare tumours and account for 70%–80% of cases.

### Symptoms

As with malignant disease in general, the clinical history is often vague and insidious. Almost all patients eventually present with pain; localised back pain may result from bony/soft tissue infiltration or pathological fractures, whereas direct compression of neurological elements tends to produce radicular symptoms. The red flags of back pain (**Box 8.1**) are an excellent tool to help differentiate serious pathology such as malignancy from (common) mechanical back pain. The most predictive red flag is a past medical history of cancer.

Metastatic spinal cord compression is a neurological emergency resulting from compression on the spinal cord from the tumour mass or from pathological loss of spinal column structural integrity. Patients present with sensorimotor deficits and/or autonomic dysfunction (bowel and bladder problems).

### Investigation

MRI is the gold standard in initial diagnosis due to its high sensitivity and specificity in detecting malignancy. When malignancy is suspected, a whole-spine MRI should be requested due to the possibility of noncontiguous lesions (>10% of patients). MRI allows qualification of the relationship between lesion and neurovascular structures and can help distinguish between infection and malignancy. CT scans are useful in defining the bony pathoanatomy, especially in quantifying the degree of lytic destruction, in order to help decide if operative stabilization is required. CT of the thorax, abdomen and pelvis is often requested as part of the general patient workup to help identify the primary tumour +/− metastases. Plain radiographs are useful as part of the preoperative planning but should not be relied upon to exclude spinal tumour due to their poor negative (and positive) predictive value. X-ray can demonstrate both sclerotic and lytic lesions (only identifiable after >50% of trabecular bone loss) as well as identify pathognomonic signs such as the 'winking owl' sign (**Fig. 8.13**).

### Treatment

Treatment should be tailored to each patient according to their prognosis and personal preferences, where appropriate. The patient's thoughts, concerns and expectations should be explored in detail. Broadly speaking, management will

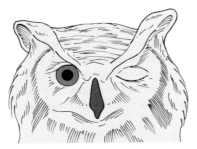

Fig. 8.13 The 'Winking Owl' Sign. AP radiograph of the lumbar spine demonstrating the 'winking owl' sign at L1 and L2, due to destructions of the pedicles by tumour. Note the adjacent levels with intact pedicles bilaterally (owl's eyes) and spinous process (owl's beak).

either be palliative (most common) or curative. Both aim to control pain, provide spinal column stability and protect the neurological structures, such as the cauda equina and spinal cord. Surgery, radiotherapy and/or chemotherapy constitute the main treatment modalities, although other modalities such as immunotherapy, bone marrow transplant and specialized radiotherapy such as proton beam therapy and stereotactic ablative radiotherapy may be utilized. The benefits of any surgical intervention should outweigh the associated morbidity, and in the case of palliative surgery, the recovery period should not significantly impair the patients remaining life. For example, surgery with a recovery time of 6 weeks in a patient with a similar life expectancy would be inappropriate.

## CLINICAL EXAMINATION OF THE SPINE

## Musculoskeletal Spine Examination

As with other examinations of the musculoskeletal system, examination of the spine is carried out in a systematic fashion starting with inspection of the patient, followed by palpation and finishing with assessment of the various movements (Look–Feel–Move). Each region of the spine is considered separately at each point in the examination. This is then followed by a series of special tests designed to assess for specific pathology.

### Look

Patients should be adequately exposed (with a chaperone). From behind, examine for evidence of asymmetrical shape/posture (**Fig. 8.14**), scars, muscle wasting, swelling and skin change associated with spinal dysraphism (e.g., cutaneous haemangioma, hypertrichosis or pathological sacral dimple). Next, inspection should be carried out looking from the side, noting the presence or absence of normal cervical lordosis, thoracic kyphosis and lumbar lordosis as well as overall sagittal balance.

### Feel

Start centrally and proximally at the base of the skull. The spinous processes should be palpated sequentially in a distal fashion, finishing with the SI joints. The patient should be observed for pain throughout this part of the examination. Then, the paraspinal muscles can be examined looking for evidence of pain or discomfort. Palpation rarely imparts significant information to the examiner, except in certain situations such as trauma, where contusion, boggy swelling and spinous process tenderness/increased interspinous distance should alert the examiner to the disruption of the posterior spinal column and instability.

### Move

Continue with the patient standing and start with lumbar flexion and extension. Place two to three fingers on the lumbar spine and ask the patient to bend over and touch their toes. The examiner's fingers should move apart during flexion and come back together during extension. If not, this suggests that most, if not all, of the movement is coming from the hips and pelvis. Pain during extension may indicate a lytic spondylolisthesis.

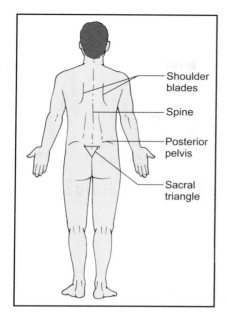

Fig. 8.14 Observation of the spine. It is important to observe the spine from the back and side to detect the presence of any curves (scoliosis in the coronal plan and/or kyphosis in the sagittal plane)

Lumbar lateral flexion is assessed by asking the patient to run each hand down the outside of their ipsilateral thigh as far as they can to the knee alternatively. It is worth bearing in mind that some of the movements may be complicated for patients; therefore, a useful technique is to demonstrate first and then ask them to copy.

Thoracic rotation is assessed by asking the patient to sit on the edge of the bed to stabilize the pelvis and cross their arms over their chest; their shoulders can then be rotated to the right and the left. The movement may be guided by the surgeon at this point.

Cervical spine movements can be carried out last with the patient sitting.

- In flexion, the patient is asked to put their chin to their chest.

- In extension, they tilt their head backwards as far as possible.

- Lateral flexion is carried out by trying to place each ear on the ipsilateral shoulder.

- With rotation, the patient looks over each shoulder alternatively by turning their neck.

## Neurological Examination

The neurological system should also be examined to determine if there is any associated upper or lower motor neuron lesion and/or sensory impairment. The ASIA chart is a useful aide-mémoire of dermatomes, myotomes and Medical Research Council power grading (**Fig. 8.15**).

### Sensation

Light touch assesses the integrity of the dorsal (posterior) column pathway and pinpricks the spinothalamic (anterolateral) pathway in the spinal cord. The area of least dermatomal crossover should be tested and compared to the contralateral side.

### Motor Function (Power and Tone)

The myotomes of each limb should be assessed individually. The examiner should stabilize the joint being tested with one hand and provide resistance with the other. The stablizing hand should also be used to palpate the muscle belly/tendon for contraction. The presence of increased tone indicates an upper motor lesion.

### Reflexes

The deep tendon reflexes should be sequentially tested with the patient's limbs relaxed. Using a tendon hammer, strike the tendon being examined either directly or via the examiners finger or thumb (reduce patient discomfort and palpate involuntary contraction) (**Fig. 8.16**). If a reflex cannot be evoked, a reinforcement manoeuvre may help, such as asking the patient to clench their jaw. Reduced reflexes may be due to abnormalities in sensory neurons, lower motor neurons,

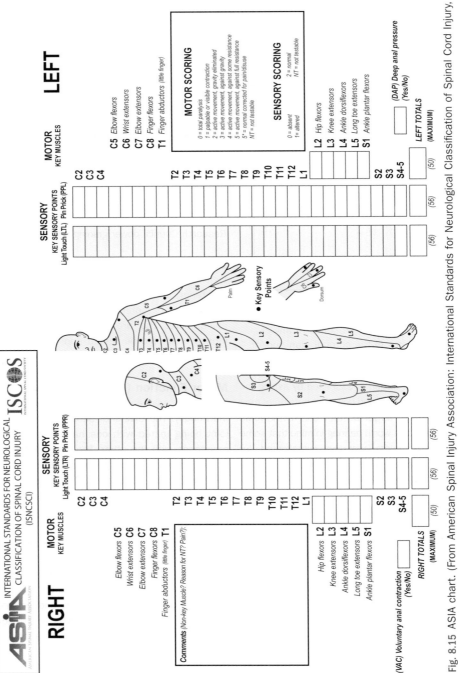

Fig. 8.15 ASIA chart. (From American Spinal Injury Association: International Standards for Neurological Classification of Spinal Cord Injury, revised 2013; Atlanta, GA. Reprinted 2013. With permission.)

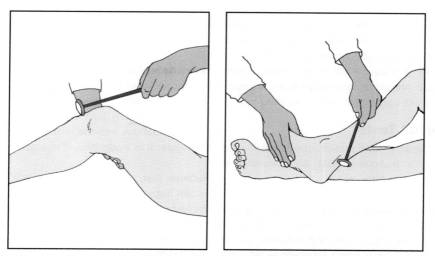

Fig. 8.16 Testing of reflexes. Spinal reflexes are useful to determine the level of pathology and differentiate between upper and lower motor neuron lesions. The knee jerk represents the L4 level and ankle jerk the S1 level. Brisk reflexes may represent upper lesions while sluggish or absent may represent lower lesions.

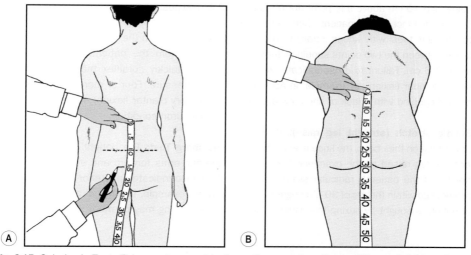

Fig. 8.17 Schober's Test. This can be used to formally assess and record forward flexion. The dimples of Venus are identified and marks are made in the midline 10 cm above and 5 cm below. The patient is instructed to bend forwards to the maximum limit. The length is remeasured. An increase of less than 5cm denotes the presence of objective stiffness.

muscles and the neuromuscular junction; acute upper motor neuron lesions, such as spinal shock; endocrine abnormalities, such as hypothyroidism; and mechanical factors, such as joint disease. Abnormally increased reflexes are associated with upper motor neuron lesions.

## Special Tests

The following special tests may be performed during a musculoskeletal and neurological examination of the spine.

**Adam's forward bend test:** If scoliosis is suspected, observe from behind and ask the patient to bend forwards. Chest wall deformity will be exacerbated due to increased rotational deformity of the thoracic vertebra (with attached ribs). The deformity is often referred to as a rib hump.

**Schober's Test (Fig. 8.17):** While the patient is standing, the examiner marks a line between the dimples of Venus. Two points are made 5 cm below and 10 cm above this point (for a total of 15 cm distance). The patient then bends to touch their toes with knees straight. The distance between the two points should increase by at least 5 cm. Failure to do so indicates restriction in lumbar flexion, for example, in AS, especially if coupled with a lack of chest expansion.

**Sciatic stretch (straight leg raise):** With the patient flat on their back, the knee is kept straight and the leg raised by the examiner. The test is positive if the patient's radicular symptoms are reproduced within the arc of 30–70 degrees. Confirmation is sought by flexing the patient's knee to ease the symptoms, not by seeking to exacerbate pain via dorsiflexing the foot.

**Lhermitte's Sign:** The patient is asked to flex his/her neck, resting their chin on their chest. This test is positive if they experience radicular symptoms into any limb or describe electric shock sensations into the arms legs or down their back. It is suggestive of myelopathy.

**Hoffman Test:** Hold the middle phalanx of the middle finger and then flick the distal phalanx. Involuntary flexion of the interphalangeal joint of the thumb indicates the presence of an upper motor neuron condition, such as cervical myelopathy.

**Plantar Reflex:** The lateral border of the foot is stroked from the heel towards the toes with the back of a tendon hammer. Toe flexion is normal. Extension in patients older than 1 year of age indicates an upper motor neuron lesion (Babinski-positive).

**Clonus:** Establish the absence of ankle pathology/pain from the patient. With the patient relaxed, quickly dorsiflex the ankle with sustained pressure. Four or more beats of clonus (involuntary plantar flexion) suggests an upper motor neuron condition.

**Rhomberg Test:** The patient stands with feet together, arms forward and eyes closed. Loss of balance indicates posterior column dysfunction, for example, in cervical myelopathy. Heel-to-toe walking may be more sensitive.

## INTRODUCTION

Orthopaedic oncology is a specialty which encompasses benign and malignant tumours of soft tissue or bone. Depending on the nature of the tumour (and the patient), the treatment may range from surgery to radiation, chemotherapy or palliative care. Decisions are often made as part of a multidisciplinary team (MDT) due to the complexity of certain management plans.

The treatment of tumours involves applying skills learned from the breadth of trauma and elective orthopaedics. There is a large spectrum of bone lesions that may require resection followed by reconstruction with an arthroplasty procedure or stabilization with a plate or an intramedullary nail. Equally, soft tissue lumps may require a wide local excision and flap reconstruction or a marginal resection if proven benign. A thorough knowledge of anatomy is essential for what is a truly general and varied practice.

There are many different types of musculoskeletal tumours. Due to this wide range and a conscience effort to avoid endless lists, attention in this chapter focusses on the general principles of managing tumours, as well as the most common and clinically relevant pathologies.

## ASSESSMENT

### Clinical History

The symptoms described by patients with a tumour are as diverse as the range of potential pathologies. Recognition is therefore challenging; consideration of the possibility of a tumour by the receiving clinician is crucial.

A tumour may be picked up in a previously asymptomatic individual having an X-ray performed in the emergency department after a sporting injury. In other cases a patient may present complaining of swelling or persistent pain which clearly requires further assessment and investigation.

Children frequently have a diagnosis of growing pains or muscle sprains that can lead to delayed presentation. Nerve-based tumours can be exquisitely tender and may have associated motor or sensory disturbance, while vascular tumours are often painful following exercise. There may be a history of trauma, but this is usually non-contributory to the aetiology.

Obtaining a past medical history is vital, particularly in the older patient with a history of prior malignancy. Details of previous treatments including radiotherapy or any ongoing chemotherapy aid in decision-making. Smoking and alcohol history may point toward a primary tumour. Family history is occasionally relevant with conditions such as Li–Fraumeni syndrome, retinoblastoma and neurofibromatosis associated with an increased risk of a bone or soft tissue malignancy.

**Patients with a sarcoma often lack classic systemic symptoms of malignancy** such as sweats, malaise and weight loss. Swelling in otherwise healthy patients must still be viewed with suspicion.

### Examination

The swelling should be palpated. Those that have **grown rapidly** and are **larger than 5cm** and are **painful** and **deep** have a higher risk of malignancy (**Fig. 9.1**). The depth of the tumour is

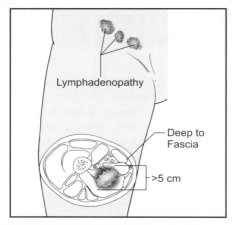

Fig. 9.1 Soft tissue lesion signs of malignancy: >5 cm, deep to fascia, painful, growing, infrequently lymphadenopathy.

| Table 9.1 Modified Glasgow Prognostic Score | |
| --- | --- |
| **Biochemical Characteristics** | **Score** |
| CRP ≤10 mg/l + any albumin | 0 |
| CRP >10 mg/l + albumin ≥3.5 g/dL | 1 |
| CRP >10 mg/l + albumin <3.5 g/dL | 2 |

evaluated by tensing potentially involved muscles. Superficial tumours remain mobile after muscle contraction, but deep tumours become fixed. The relationship to surrounding structures must be assessed with a neurovascular assessment. Regional lymph nodes should be felt. In the setting of a potential metastatic tumour, common sites of origin (breast, prostate, lung, renal, thyroid) should also be examined and investigated appropriately.

## Investigations

The tests one orders should be considered and pertinent to the likely pathology.

**Laboratory** investigations include the following:

- Full blood count: check for anaemia
- Urea and electrolytes: baseline function prior to chemotherapy
- Liver function tests: baseline function prior to chemotherapy. Albumin levels
- Inflammatory markers: C-reactive protein (CRP) in conjunction with albumin makes up the modified Glasgow prognostic score (**Table 9.1**), which is a prognostic indicator in soft tissue sarcoma for metastatic spread and overall survival.

- Coagulation screen: safe to proceed to biopsy
- Bone profile: calcium level can be raised in metastatic disease. Alkaline phosphatase is a prognostic indicator in osteosarcoma.
- Lactic dehydrogenase: prognostic indicator in Ewing sarcoma
- Serum electrophoresis/urinary Bence Jones protein: assess for myeloproliferative disorder
- Tumour markers (PSA, CEA, CA-125): dependent on the likely primary tumour in the setting of metastatic bone disease

**Imaging options** (**Fig. 9.2**):

- Radiograph: Interpretation is covered in 'seven questions'
- Computer tomography (CT) scanning: useful to assess bone stock in reconstructions for metastatic disease, finding the nidus of an osteoid osteoma and in patients who cannot undergo magnetic resonance imaging (MRI). Used for systemic staging of a sarcoma
- MRI: characterizes the lesion and helps with local staging to identify any tumour. Crucial to examine surrounding neurovascular structures and their relationship to the tumour for surgical planning
- Bone scan: assess the rest of the skeleton in bone sarcomas
- Positron emission tomography scan: a staging adjunct usually combined with CT scanning that gives an idea of possible systemic disease. The exact indications for the use in sarcoma staging are yet to be established

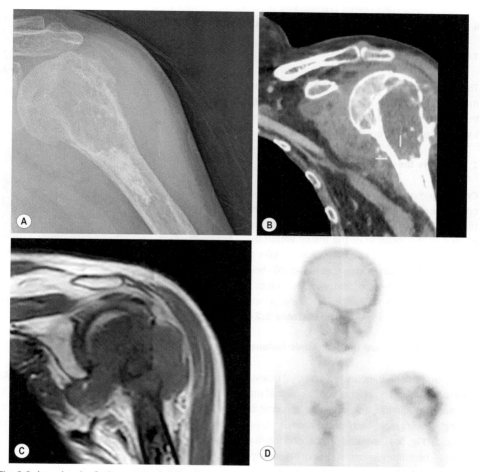

Fig. 9.2 Imaging in Orthopaedic Oncology. Lesions are evaluated by several modalities to fully understand their nature and extent. A) A proximal humeral lesion is seen with areas of lysis, B) this is confirmed by CT scanning, C) chondroid matrix formation and soft tissue extension. D) It is 'hot' on a bone scan.

## BONE TUMOURS – GENERAL PRINCIPLES

### Seven Questions

A bone tumour is most commonly picked up on a plain X-ray. When reviewing the plain radiograph, the following questions must be asked:

1. **Where is the abnormality?**

2. **Is it solitary, or are there multiple lesions?**

3. **What is the lesion doing to the bone?**

4. **What is the bone doing in return?**

5. **Is there any erosion of the bone cortex?**

**6. Is there any associated soft tissue mass?**

**7. What is the matrix?**

The answers to these questions allow placement of the lesion on a spectrum (harmless through to concerning) and narrows down the list of potential differential diagnoses.

**1. Where is the abnormality?**

Certain tumours have a predilection for specific bones (such as an adamantinoma of the tibia). However, the crux of this question relates to the location of the lesion within the bone, i.e., is it in the epiphysis, metaphysis or diaphysis (**Fig. 9.3**)? Once this is established, the lesion will either be central or eccentric. If the abnormality is not within the bone, it may be surface-based or periarticular (**Table 9.2**).

**2. Is it solitary, or are there multiple lesions?**

Most primary bone tumours are solitary. However, there are a limited number of conditions that may present with multiple abnormalities apparent on a single radiograph; enchondromatosis (Ollier) Maffucci) (**Fig. 9.4**), exostosis/osteochondromas (multiple hereditary exostosis) and fibrous dysplasia (polyostotic). Metastatic disease and haematological malignancies (myeloma, lymphoma)

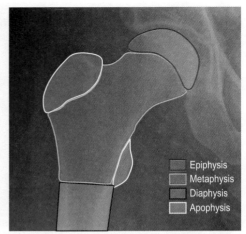

Epiphysis
Metaphysis
Diaphysis
Apophysis

Fig. 9.3 Zones within a bone in which lesions can occur.

are, however, the most common cause for multiple lesions in bone.

**3. What is the lesion doing to the bone?**

The lesion can either be eroding (lytic) (**Fig. 9.5A**) or forming additional bone (**Fig. 9.5B**) on a radiograph. Bone has a limited repertoire of tricks that involve the regulation of osteoblast and osteoclast cell response.

Lesions may be well demarcated, commonly referred to as a narrow zone of transition and

| Location | Differential Diagnosis |
|---|---|
| Epiphysis/ Apophysis | Infection, chondroblastoma, clear cell chondrosarcoma |
| Epi-metaphyseal | Giant cell tumour, aneurysmal bone cyst, osteoblastoma |
| Metaphyseal | Enchondroma, unicameral or simple bone cyst, nonossifying fibroma, chondrosarcoma, osteosarcoma |
| Diaphyseal | Osteoid osteoma, fibrous dysplasia, adamantinoma, Ewing sarcoma |
| Surface | Osteochondroma, periosteal chondroma, parosteal osteosarcoma |
| Periarticular | Synovial chondromatosis, pigmented villonodular synovitis |

**Table 9.2  Differential Diagnosis of Lesion by Location**

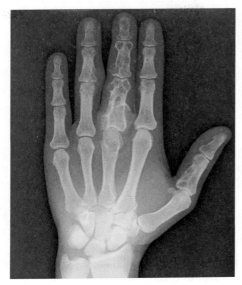

Fig. 9.4 Multiple lesions (enchondromas) evident in Ollier's Disease.

associated with low biological activity slow growing lesions. Equally, they may be permeative and poorly defined, described as having a wide zone of transition and associated with a more aggressive pathology.

4. **What is the bone doing in return?**

This is primarily an assessment of whether there is a periosteal reaction. The classic lifting of periosteum associated with primary malignant tumours of bone creates a Codman triangle (**Fig. 9.6**). The periosteum typically attempts to lay down bone. If there is time for a full layer to form, it can have an 'onion skin' appearance. With rapidly growing bone tumours, there may be streaks/patches of ossification along Sharpey fibres leading to a 'hair on end' or 'sunray spiculation' appearance (**Fig. 9.7**).

5. **Is there any erosion of the bone cortex?**

For there to be erosion or lysis visible on a radiograph, around 50% or more of the cortical

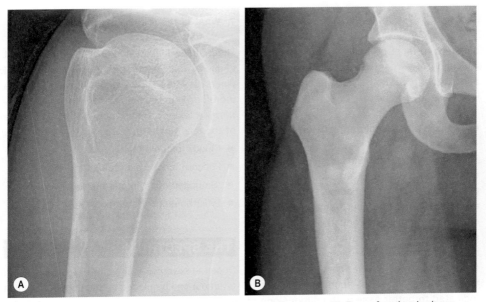

Fig. 9.5 Plain radiographic analysis A) Lytic lesions eroding bone. B) Bone forming lesions.

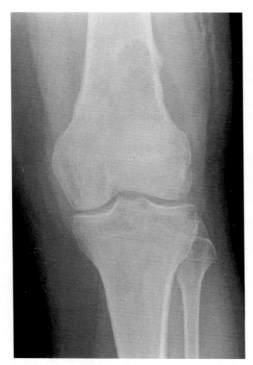

Fig. 9.6 Periosteal reaction: 'Bone in Return' – Codman's triangle on the lateral border of the femur.

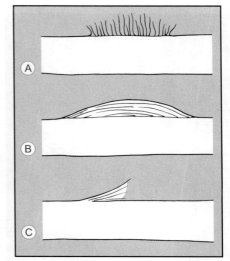

Fig. 9.7 Periosteal Reactions. A) Sunray spicule. B) Onion skin. C) Codman's Triangle.

architecture must be destroyed. This gives an indication of a more biologically active lesion and, furthermore, that a fracture is impending, if not already complete.

### 6. Is there any associated soft tissue mass?

There may be a soft tissue shadow associated with the abnormal area of bone on the plain radiograph. This may be the periosteal reaction or a true tumour outgrowth. If cortical destruction is present, there must be a soft tissue mass. The mass may have elements of calcification or simply be displacing the surrounding muscles and visible as a bulge. If present, cross-sectional imaging is indicated to better assess the dimensions of the soft tissue mass and assess any association it has with surrounding neurovascular structures.

### 7. What is the matrix?

The matrix will give an idea of the predominant tissue of origin and in turn the likely differential diagnosis. This can be difficult to judge and is therefore kept as the last of the seven questions. A lesion's matrix may described as one of the following (**Fig. 9.8**):

- Cloudy: osteoid matrix
- Popcorn: chondroid matrix
- 'Smudged out': fibrous matrix
- Lytic: absence of matrix

## THE SPECTRUM

Once the seven questions have been answered, a tumour can be placed on the spectrum, which is a method of categorizing the behaviour of a

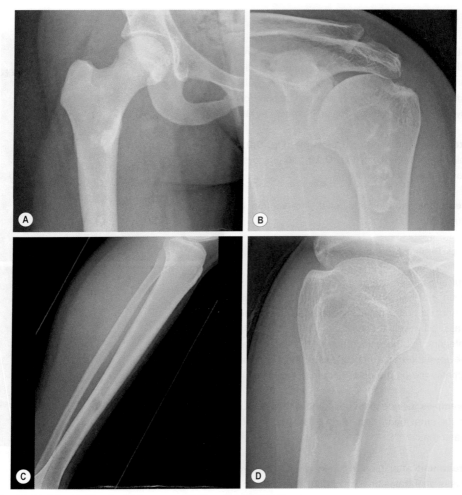

Fig. 9.8 Matrix. A) Cloudy. B) Popcorn. C) Smudged. D) Lytic.

lesion. Not all tumours behave typically, but this process helps to assess whether a tumour is harmless and can be left alone or if it is sinister and requires urgent investigation.

### 1. Benign bone tumours

#### a) Benign Latent

Benign latent lesions are classically asymptomatic and are found incidentally on a radiograph following trauma to the area. There is no periosteal reaction, cortical destruction or soft tissue mass, and the tumour will be well demarcated or have a 'geographic' appearance. A matrix may be present.

**Examples** include enchondroma and nonossifying fibroma.

**Treatment** is not routinely indicated. Alternative causes for symptoms should be sought.

### b) Benign Active

Patients with benign active tumours often present with local symptoms. The radiographs usually demonstrate a geographic lesion with a well-ordered periosteal reaction and an absence of any significant soft tissue mass, if present at all.

**Examples** include osteoid osteoma (**Fig. 9.9**), unicameral bone cyst (**Fig. 9.10**), fibrous dysplasia and osteochondroma.

**Treatment** Symptomatic relief, intervention if refractory.

### c) Benign Aggressive

Typically, benign aggressive lesions are symptomatic with lytic areas and cortical destruction. In turn, they often have an associated soft tissue mass. However, the hallmark features of this category are the epi-metaphyseal location and the formation of a neocortex, an eggshell-type appearance on the outer border of the lesion.

**Examples** include giant cell tumour (**Fig. 9.11**), aneurysmal bone cyst (**Fig. 9.12**) and osteoblastoma.

**Treatment** after biopsy confirmation. Typically, this is an intralesional procedure, but resection may be required if the joint is not thought to be salvageable.

### 2. Malignant bone tumours

Patients typically present with a localised persistent pain or swelling. They may present with a pathological fracture and systemic symptoms such as malaise or weight loss however these frequently may be absent.

### a) Low grade

Radiologically, these low-grade primary malignant bone tumours are permeative. These

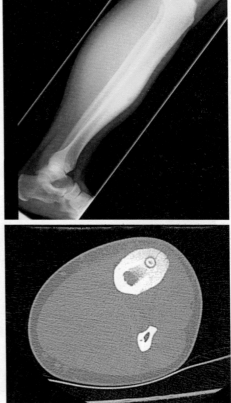

Fig. 9.9 X-ray and CT slice with osteoid osteoma in left tibia.

include entities such as adamantinomas, parosteal osteosarcomas and chordomas (**Fig. 9.13**). However, their appearance may otherwise be relatively nonspecific, with variable cortical erosion, soft tissue mass and matrix. However, the specific types have a predilection for certain specific locations (**Table 9.3**).

**Treatment** begins after biopsy confirmation and staging. Adjuvant treatments are not typically recommended, and surgical-wide local excision is the mainstay of treatment (except chordoma where proton beam therapy may be utilised).

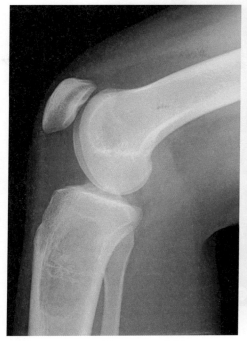

Fig. 9.10 Unicameral bone cyst (UBC).

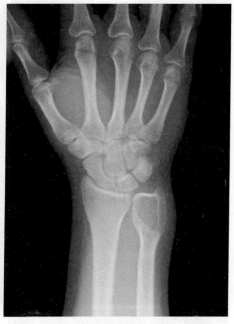

Fig. 9.11 Giant cell tumour located in distal ulna. Typically arises in the epiphysis and frequently extends into the metaphysis.

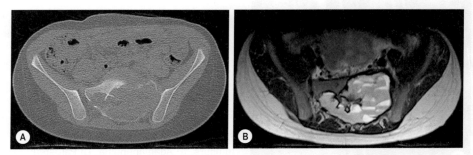

Fig. 9.12 Cross-sectional imaging A) CT images of an Aneurysmal bone cyst (ABC). The sacrum is involved, showing an expansile lesion. B) The MRI (Figure 9.12 B) (T1 weighted) demonstrates the fluid levels typically observed.

### b) High grade

High-grade primary malignant bone tumours are usually poorly demarcated and have a permeative appearance on X-ray. There is typically a soft tissue mass with a malignant periosteal reaction but no cortical destruction. The matrix is variable and dependent on the tissue of origin affected.

**Examples** include osteosarcoma, chondrosarcoma and Ewing sarcoma (**Fig. 9.14**).

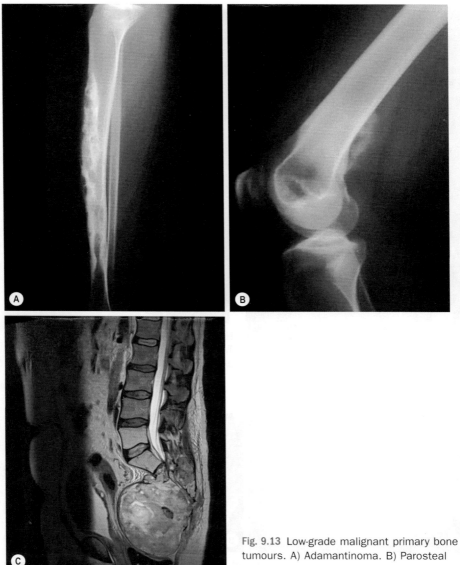

Fig. 9.13 Low-grade malignant primary bone tumours. A) Adamantinoma. B) Parosteal osteosarcoma. C) Chordoma.

**Treatment** occurs after biopsy confirmation and staging. Neoadjuvant chemotherapy followed by wide local excision and adjuvant chemotherapy is the routine management. Ewing's sarcoma may benefit from radiotherapy, especially in the axial skeleton/pelvis. Chondrosarcoma is typically tresated with surgery only.

## SOFT TISSUE TUMOURS – GENERAL PRINCIPLES

### Assessment of Soft Tissue Tumours

Lumps and bumps are extremely common presentations to both the general practitioner and

| Table 9.3   Low-grade Primary Malignant Bone Tumour by Classic Location | |
|---|---|
| **Low-grade Primary Malignant Bone Tumour** | **Classic Location** |
| Adamantinoma | Diaphysis of tibia |
| Parosteal osteosarcoma | Posterior cortex surface of distal femur |
| Chordoma | Sacrum, base of skull |

the orthopaedic surgeon. It is vital that clinicians have a system of triaging to facilitate timely investigation.

The four key history and examination features include the following:

1. Size >5 cm

2. Increasing size

3. Pain

4. Deep to fascia

If a patient has a lump with none of these features, it has been demonstrated that they have almost no chance of having a sarcoma. If, however, they have all four features, the risk of having a sarcoma approaches 90%.

Patients with a soft tissue sarcoma often have no systemic features of malignancy such as malaise or weight loss.

## Imaging

The modalities most often used to assess a soft tissue swelling are either ultrasound scan (USS) or MRI scan. The exact indications for each remain debatable between radiologists and surgeons.

USS is user-dependent but can give dynamic information about a lump, including how vascular the lesion is. A small (<2 cm) tumour may not be adequately characterized by an MRI scan and is dependent on slice thickness and

a relative indication for an USS. USS can be challenging to interpret, and MRI scans can usually better visualize the tumour and how it interplays with the surrounding anatomy. Cross-sectional imaging is therefore vital for surgical planning.

Unless a patient has a ganglion on the volar aspect of their wrist that transilluminates, both radiologists and orthopaedic oncologists agree that some imaging should be carried out to reduce the likelihood of missing an atypical sarcoma presentation.

### Benign soft tissue tumours

If the imaging has pathognomonic features of a benign tumour, treatment is usually symptom-based. There are broadly two options: conservative management or an intervention. Most conservatively managed patients will require no further follow-up, but if there is any concern, an interval scan may be appropriate to ensure no growth or change. If symptomatic, the treatment is usually a marginal excision. Vascular tumours may be amenable to minimally invasive treatment by interventional radiologists.

### Malignant soft tissue tumours

Soft tissue sarcomas are a very heterogenous group. They are usually diagnosed after an MRI scan and biopsy and must be staged. Assuming local disease, the treatment for most involves a combination of radiotherapy and surgery in the form of a wide local excision. Chemotherapy has a role in selected subtypes.

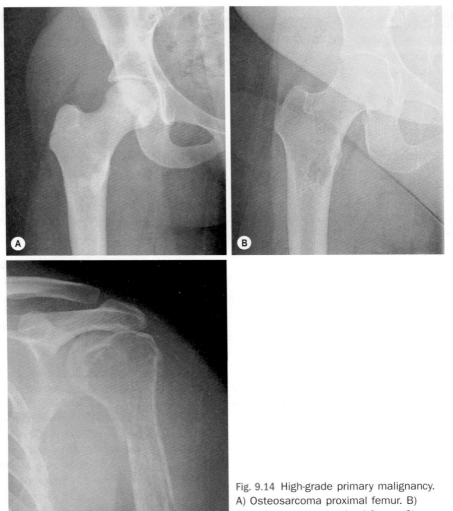

Fig. 9.14 High-grade primary malignancy. A) Osteosarcoma proximal femur. B) Chondrosarcoma proximal femur. C) Ewing's sarcoma – late progression with pathological fracture.

## STAGING

Staging is the method by which the extent of any cancer is defined. It involves local, regional and systemic assessment of the disease. For **bone sarcomas**, this involves getting a full-length MRI scan of the affected area, a bone scan and a CT scan of the chest, abdomen and pelvis. For **soft tissue sarcomas**, a bone scan is not required. The staging scans look for the most common sites of disease spread, i.e., locally within the limb or the lungs. For this reason, there is no international consensus as to whether the CT scan should include the abdomen/pelvis or not. Lymph nodes are typically assessed with clinical examination, but no formal imaging is standard. Staging is completed with a biopsy.

The key **aims of staging** are:

- Aid treatment planning
- Indicate prognosis
- Evaluate results
- Exchange information

The most common staging system used for both bone and soft tissue sarcomas was proposed by Enneking in 1986 and is also known as the Musculoskeletal Tumour Society system. The factors considered are the histological grade, local extent and distant metastasis (**Table 9.4**).

| Table 9.4 | Enneking Staging System | |
|-----------|-------|------|
| **Stage** | **Grade** | **Site** |
| IA | Low | Intracompartmental |
| IB | Low | Extracompartmental |
| IIA | High | Intracompartmental |
| IIB | High | Extracompartmental |
| III | Any | Metastasis |

## BIOPSY

Following a detailed history, examination and imaging investigations, the biopsy will ideally serve to confirm the diagnosis. Benign latent and active lesions do not routinely require a biopsy, and neither do benign soft tissue lesions with classical radiological appearances such as a lipoma. However, if there is any doubt, it is safer to perform a biopsy.

Prior to proceeding to a biopsy, a coagulation screen and cross-sectional imaging should be performed. This will permit a safe, targeted biopsy. The sampling technique is either **percutaneous, incisional** or **excisional.** Percutaneous sampling is most commonly a core-needle biopsy, such as a Tru-Cut for soft tissue tumours or a Jamshidi for a bone core.

Incisional or an open biopsy is something all orthopaedic surgeons are expected to be able to safely perform after discussion of the approach with the regional tumour unit. The principles include the following:

1. **Longitudinal incision**. The biopsy track can be easily excised as part of the definitive extensile approach.

2. **Through involved compartment/single muscle**. Internervous planes must be avoided, as they increase the zone of contamination that will require subsequent excision.

3. **Avoid neurovascular structures**. Otherwise, they will need to be resected as part of any definitive excision for a sarcoma.

4. **Generous sampling** with rongeur/curette/knife. Take care not to crush the specimen with forceps or burn it with cautery, making histopathological analysis more difficult.

5. **Meticulous haemostasis/watertight closure**. This decreases the area of contamination and bruising. A haemostatic foam or sponge placed into the biopsy site reduces ooze.

6. **Drains should not be routinely used**. If they are, they must be brought out in line with the incision, such that the track can be easily excised later.

A poorly performed biopsy can lead to diagnostic error at best, but at worst can adversely affect treatment and patient outcome.

## HAEMATOLOGICAL TUMOURS

Blood-based malignancies such as lymphoma, plasmacytoma and multiple myeloma may present to the orthopaedic surgeon as an incidental finding or the first presentation of the cancer due to pain/fracture or be referred by the haemoncologists with recognized bone disease that is no longer responding to medical therapies.

The patient should be worked up as per earlier described principles. As a rule, bone involvement is common with haematological malignancies. Though surgical stabilization of pathological fractures or replacement surgery is frequently performed, the first-line treatment for impending fractures, especially of the upper limb, tends to be nonsurgical (including but not limited to; chemotherapy, radiotherapy, bisphosphonates +/− stem cell transplantation) as there is reasonable potential for the fracture to heal.

## METASTATIC DISEASE

As a pathological process, metastatic disease is the most common cause of bone destruction in adults. As the population lives longer and treatments develop, there is an increased incidence of cancer accompanied by improved overall survivorship. Bone is the third most common site of metastasis, following the lung and liver.

While any malignancy has the potential to metastasize, the carcinomas which classically spread to bone are **breast, prostate, lung, renal, and thyroid**. Though not listed in the top 5, due to large incidences of malignancies of the gastrointestinal tract, deposits in bone are frequently seen. Much like haematological malignancies, the presentation to orthopaedics may be as an incidental lesion on a radiograph, the first presentation of the cancer as a fracture/impending fracture or as a referral by the oncologists with previously known disease that

has spread or is no longer responding to medical therapies. The patient will need to be worked up as discussed previously.

Contrary to haematological malignancies, and in particular multiple myeloma, metastatic lesions and fractures have **poor healing potential**. Breast, prostate and renal bone metastases are the most likely to heal, but in less than 50% of cases at best. The nonoperative treatment options include the following:

- Bisphosphonates/denosumab
- Radiotherapy
- Chemotherapy
- Hormone therapy

Predicting the risk of fracture in a metastatic lesion is challenging. Various scoring systems based on clinical and radiological parameters have been devised, but all have their limitations. The most widely quoted system by **Mirel (Table 9.5)** suggests a 6 month risk of fracture of 15% with a score of 8 increasing to 100% with a score of 12. A score of 8 has conventionally been used as the threshold at which to consider prophylactic stabilization. This is preferable to treating a completed fracture for technical ease, but more importantly because of the reduced blood loss and length of stay along with the improved mobility and overall survival. The implant selected should ideally exceed the patient's life expectancy. Potential options are covered in the surgical techniques section.

## INFECTION

Finding a benign osseous lesion that radiologically resembles a bone tumour is not uncommon. The list of potential lesions is extensive, but probably the most clinically relevant one is a Brodie abscess. This is an intraosseous abscess related to pyogenic osteomyelitis.

The infections associated with normal inflammatory markers may be normal. Plain radiographs

## Table 9.5    Mirel's Scoring System

| Score | 1 | 2 | 3 |
|---|---|---|---|
| Site | Upper limb | Lower limb | Peritrochanteric |
| Pain | Mild | Moderate | Functional |
| Lesion | Blastic | Mixed | Lytic |
| Size | <1/3 | 1/3–2/3 | >2/3 |

often show an oval lytic appearance surrounded by a sclerotic rim. MRI is the key investigation, classically demonstrating the 'penumbra sign', a rim lining of an abscess cavity with higher signal intensity than that of the main abscess which enhances after contrast.

## SURGICAL TECHNIQUES

Sarcoma treatment is carried out in specialist centres as part of a MDT due to the complexity of its management. The MDT comprises radiologists, pathologists, oncologists (both medical and radiation), specialist nurses and surgeons who have experience in dealing with rare cancers.

## Margins

The type of tumour excision can be categorized under four key headings (**Fig. 9.15**):

- **Intralesional**: The pseudocapsule or reactive zone of the tumour has been entered; the surgeon has gone into the tumour. An example of this is an open biopsy. For treatment, this is reserved for benign tumours or as palliation in the setting of metastasis.

- **Marginal**: The tumour is excised as one. However, the surgeon has dissected in the reactive zone of the tumour. An example would be a lipoma resection. This is generally reserved for benign tumours. In select cases, when carried out by experts, this strategy may be used focally to preserve neurovascular structures in the setting of sarcoma.

- **Wide local**: Intracompartmental tumour excision "en bloc". The surgeon has excised

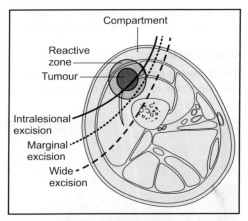

Fig. 9.15 Margins/types of excision.

the tumour in its entirety with a surrounding cuff of normal tissue. Examples include routine soft tissue and bone sarcoma resections. May be considered for solitary metastatic lesions with otherwise good prognosis.

- **Radical**: Extracompartmental tumour excision. The whole compartment is excised. Rarely performed for sarcoma unless there is a multifocal tumour.

**Amputation** is performed when it is not possible to achieve clear margins (i.e., neurovascular encasement by the tumour) or when the anticipated function of ablative surgery is superior to limb salvage. Techniques to improve mobility in amputees are evolving, and osseointegration (**Fig. 9.16**) is a method of reducing socket-related problems.

The remainder of this section will focus on some surgical and reconstructive strategies that may be employed for bone tumours.

## Radiofrequency Ablation

Radiofrequency ablation is a technique used to 'cook' the tumour. It is commonly used to treat osteoid osteomas, but some centres have expanded the indications to other tumours. Under CT guidance, a wire followed by drill is passed into the nidus of the tumour. A probe is then passed, heating up to approximately 90°C, causing a 1 cm area of necrosis (**Fig. 9.17**).

## Curettage

Benign lesions are often required to be 'scraped out'. After the tumour has been removed as

best possible to the naked eye, the base is burred and irrigated. Assuming the surrounding bone is healthy, the base is then filled with bone graft (**Fig. 9.18**). In the setting of diffuse pathology such as metastatic disease, cement is preferred as a larger volume defect can easily be filled (**Fig. 9.19**). The decision as to whether to augment this procedure with internal fixation is based on the intraoperative assessment of the risk of fracture.

## Geometric Osteotomies (with or without reconstruction)

Osteochondromas are one of the more common tumours encountered in orthopaedics. Though often managed conservatively, they may require excision. This procedure may be performed with an osteotomy flush to the bone, but if there is tumour overhang on a cylindrical bone, a section of cortex may need

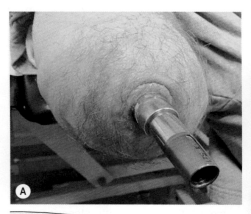

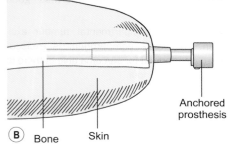

Fig. 9.16 Osseointegration prosthesis. A) Clinical picture. B) Diagram of intramedullary fixation.

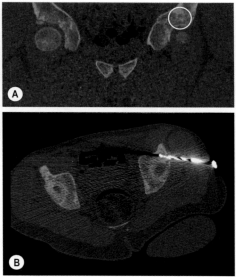

Fig. 9.17 Radiofrequency ablation of osteoid osteoma (OO). A) Sagittal CT reconstruction of lesion identified in left superior acetabulum. B) Axial CT slice demonstrating needle placed at site of OO to deliver radiofrequency ablation.

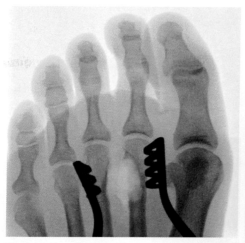

Fig. 9.18 Curettage and bone graft of chondroid lesion of left foot (intraoperative fluoroscopy).

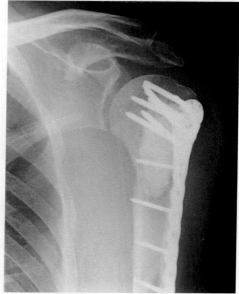

Fig. 9.19 Curettage with placement of bone cement and plate for renal metastasis.

to be excised to ensure that the tumour has not been entered.

Similarly, if such an osteotomy has been made and there is felt to be a fracture risk, then immediate or delayed stabilization should be considered using standard trauma principles. Locations such as the sacrum do not require bone reconstruction, but consideration must be given to spinopelvic stability and providing a muscle pad on which the patient can sit.

## Biological Reconstruction

Following wide local excision of a sarcoma there is often a large defect. Depending on the location, the defect may be filled using autograft or allograft. Taking the specimen, irradiating it and

reimplanting it is referred to as extracorporeal irradiation and can offer a satisfactory solution. Large allograft serves a similar purpose.

## Endoprosthesis

Enormous metal implants are probably what orthopaedic oncologists are most renowned for. They are used to fill sizeable voids and are often the adjacent joint. Custom implants are more commonly used in children. Endoprosthesis have a similar but more extensive list of potential complications than primary arthroplasty. The most common sites replaced are in the femur and humerus (**Fig. 9.20**).

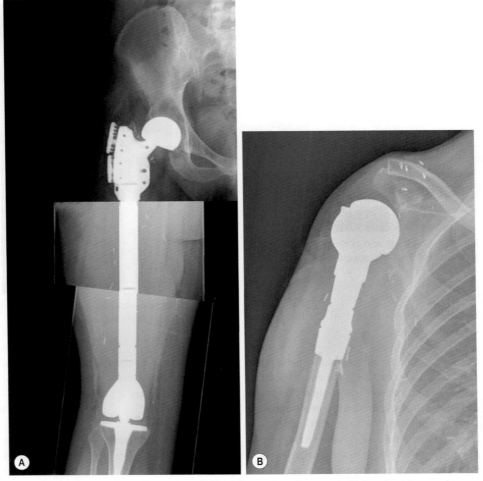

Fig. 9.20 Endoprosthetic replacement. A) Total femoral replacement. B) Proximal humeral replacement.

## HIP DISORDERS IN CHILDHOOD

### General Principles

A hip disorder should be considered in children who present with a painful or painless limp. Pain from a hip problem may be felt anywhere from the groin to knee, and it is a common pitfall to miss hip pathology in a child who presents with the complaint of knee pain.

## DEVELOPMENTAL DYSPLASIA OF THE HIP

### Clinical Summary

Developmental dysplasia of the hip (DDH) can range from mild misshaping (dysplasia) of the hip to complete dislocation of the joint. The incidence is 3–4 per 1000, with the majority affected at birth (congenital). A small proportion of children may develop the condition in early infancy despite having an apparently normally developed hip at birth.

It is not known what causes DDH, but the following are risk factors for the condition in infants:

- Breech position in the last one-third of pregnancy

- A first-degree relative had DDH

- Female infant

Other features that have an association with DDH

- High birth weight

- Gestation beyond due date

- Intrauterine crowding from twins or oligohydramnios

- Spina bifida

- Moulding features, e.g., torticollis, adducted position of leg, calcaneovalgus or metatarsus adductus of a foot

At birth, the hip is vulnerable to instability and displacement due to a combination of a relatively shallow acetabulum and increased joint ligament laxity caused by high levels of circulating maternal hormones (primarily relaxin). The mechanics of the foetal position in the final stages of pregnancy, together with passage down into the pelvis and through the birth canal, can position the foetus' leg into the at-risk position of adduction and/or hyperflexion. All of these factors contribute to, but are not the exclusive causes of, newborn hip decentring and being prone to subluxation or dislocation. For this reason, up to 6–8 per 1000 newborns in the UK are found to have some instability of the hip at birth, but most stabilize spontaneously in the joint within a few days or weeks. DDH is therefore a spectrum of disease from poorly formed hip joints to unstable hips, dislocated hips or irreducible hip joints.

As the hip decentres, the femoral head moulds the plastically deformable cartilaginous acetabular roof and labrum (comprising the limbus), which can then remodel medially, obstructing the femoral head from relocating in the true acetabulum (**Fig. 10.1**). In addition, as the femoral head migrates superiorly, it draws the inferior joint capsule via its attachment from

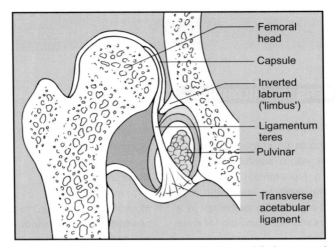

Fig. 10.1 Diagram showing dislocated femoral head with inverted limbus superiorly and elevated inferior capsule drawn up by ligamentum teres, resulting in narrowed introitus.

the ligamentum teres upwards to compound the narrowing of the inlet (introitus) into the true acetabulum. Over time, these changes become established and prevent spontaneous relocation of the femoral head. If the dislocation has occurred earlier in pregnancy, the hip may already be irreducible at birth, but in the more frequent situation of perinatal dislocation, the hip may well still be reducible with correct early intervention. If this can be achieved, then the limbus can remodel over the femoral head, creating a stable, well-centred joint with a good prognosis. If the dislocation is not identified within a few weeks of birth, a hip which may have been reducible will become irreducible and require surgical reduction +/− reconstruction.

## History

History taking should include a family history of hip problems, particularly those affecting a first-degree relative, details of the pregnancy including any history of breech positioning or oligohydramnios, whether this is the first-born child and the birth weight.

Parents should be asked about any history of hip problems in their or a sibling's past: Specific questions about the obstetric history should include the following:

● Was this a first pregnancy?

● Complications during pregnancy/abnormalities detected

● Breech presentation at birth

● Weight at birth

For delayed presentations, a developmental history should be detailed; however, note that the age of walking is not related to the presence/absence of DDH.

## Symptoms

DDH is asymptomatic in infancy; hence, careful examination of all newborn hips is essential in order to identify the condition before the hip becomes irreducible. A mild degree of acetabular dysplasia may remain asymptomatic for decades but is likely to predispose to early-onset osteoarthritis. A dislocated hip may also remain asymptomatic throughout childhood years, although patients can complain of abductor muscle pain (buttock and lateral pain) during adolescence and ultimately groin pain in early adulthood as degenerative osteoarthritis develops.

It is surprising how functional and symptom-free a dislocated hip can be during childhood. Typically, third-party concern about altered gait is what draws attention to the diagnosis in children.

## Clinical Examination

### Infant

The baby should be fully exposed; however, take care to avoid allowing overcooling. Begin with screening for associated conditions: torticollis, metatarsus adductus or other marked moulding.

Newborns should be placed on their back with their hips and knees flexed and abducted. An abnormal lie of the hip or knee should raise suspicion. Perform the Galeazzi test to inspect the relative leg lengths of the femur by comparing knee height with the hips flexed to 90 degrees (**Fig. 10.2**).

The thighs and groin are compared for symmetry of skin creases. In a relaxed infant it should be possible to abduct the flexed hip out to 70 or more degrees (females more than males), with asymmetry a warning sign of possible DDH.

Barlow Test: This test assesses the ability for the hip to be dislocated ('**B**arlow hips go out the **B**ack'). In this test, one hand is used to stabilize the pelvis, and the other hand flexes the hip to 90 degrees and then uses gentle pressure to attempt dislocation (**Fig. 10.3**). Note: if the hip is already dislocated, this will result in a negative result.

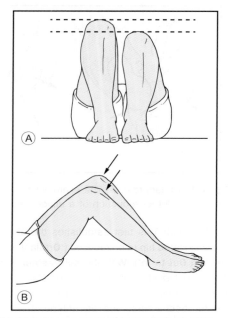

Fig. 10.2 Assessment of lower limb shortening. A) Difference in knee height shown with hips flexed (Galeazzi test) showing tibial shortening, compared with B) difference in knee height resulting from femoral shortening.

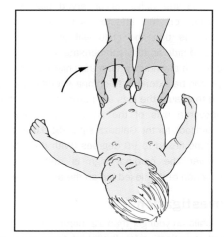

Fig. 10.3 Barlow test. Longitudinal force is applied along the femur, with the hip flexed at 90 degrees, to attempt posterior hip subluxation.

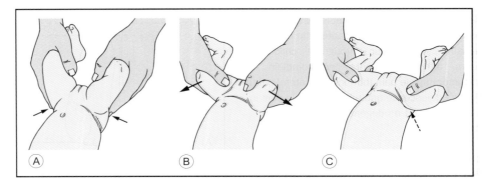

Fig. 10.4 Ortolani test. A) The examiner moves the hips into full flexion and B) abduction and aims to C) detect reduction of a dislocated head as abduction progresses.

Ortolani test: This test establishes the ability of a dislocated hip to be reduced ('**O**rtolani hips go from **O**ut to **I**n'). With the pelvis stabilized, the hip is flexed to 90 degrees and abducted. The examiner's fingers are placed over the greater trochanters, and an anterior translational force is applied to attempt reduction of the head back into the joint (**Fig. 10.4**).

Children of walking age may present due to concern about gait. Examination therefore includes assessment of walking with the shoulder, and the pelvis is observed closely for 'dipping' on the affected side. A common feature is that the child will tiptoe on the affected side as they compensate for the minor leg length asymmetry. With the child supine, the legs can be extended to compare length, taking care to ensure the legs are perpendicular to the transverse axis of the pelvis. The examiner should look for the Galeazzi sign (**Fig. 10.2**) with the hips flexed to 90 degrees. With the infant, however, the cardinal sign is restriction of abduction of the flexed hip on the affected side.

## Investigation

For children younger than 12 months of age, the best investigation is ultrasound scanning. This requires an experienced sonographer who can identify femoral head displacement. It can also assess the acetabulum for dysplasia and the

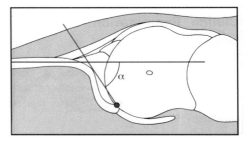

Fig. 10.5 Hip ultrasonography in DDH- the centre of the femoral head is appreciated in relation to the iliac wing (black line) and roof of the acetabulum (orange line). An 'alpha angle' greater than 60 degrees is considered normal.

position of the labrum (**Fig. 10.5**). It avoids ionizing radiation in this vulnerable age group. The Graf alpha angle is the key measurement indicating how steep the bony acetabular roof is, and an angle >60 degrees is considered normal.

In children from 4 to 6 months old, the hip ossification centres are visible on plain pelvic radiographs and can show hip displacement and acetabular morphology. Ultrasound screening beyond 1 year old is less useful as the view of the acetabulum is obstructed by the ossifying femoral head. Several key lines can be drawn on the plain anterior–posterior (AP) pelvis X-ray to help diagnose hip displacement and morphology (**Fig. 10.6**).

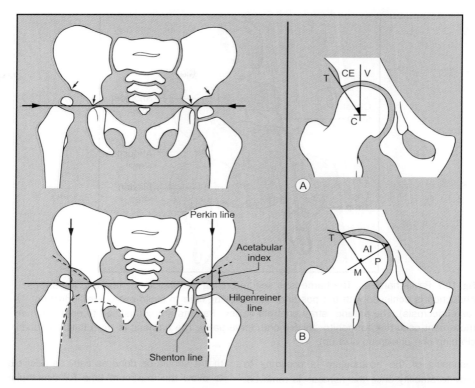

Fig. 10.6 Radiographic assessment of DDH. Interpretation of the hip radiograph in the older child is dependent on the presence of ossification in the epiphysis of the femoral head. This normally appears between 2 and 8 months but is often delayed in DDH. The position of the capital epiphysis in relation to the other pelvic elements must be determined. The Hilgenreimer (Horizontal) line is drawn across the pelvis, through the triradiate cartilage, touching the lowest point of the ilium (top left). The Perkins (Perpendicular, vertical) line is drawn from the lateral limit of the acetabulum (bottom left). These lines divide the hip into four areas. The epiphysis of the femoral head should normally lie within the lower and inner quadrant (epiphysis marked A), but in DDH the head moves upwards and outwards (B). Shenton's line (C) may be disturbed. Dysplasia of the acetabulum also alters it's slope. The "Centre-Edge Angle of Wiberg" (CE) is formed by the angle between the edge of the acetabulum (T – acetabular edge tangent), the centre of the femoral head (C) and a vertical line drawn upwards from the femoral head.

## Treatment

Abduction harness: For infants under the age of 3 months with unresolved instability or acetabular dysplasia, subluxation or dislocation of the hip most can be treated with an abduction harness. Several devices are available, with the most common being the Pavlik harness (**Fig. 10.7**). Use of the harness allows the infant's hips to be positioned in greater than 90 degrees of flexion while preventing adduction of the hips to less than 30 or 40 degrees. Care must be taken to avoid extreme flexion or abduction as this can lead to nerve palsy and avascular necrosis. The harness is worn 24 hours a day for 8 to 12 weeks. During this time, experienced practitioners will assess the position of the femoral head (clinically and using ultrasonography) and ensure it is reduced and that adequate

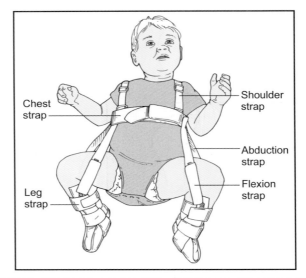

Fig. 10.7 Pavlik harness. The harness is secured using the shoulder, chest and leg straps. Abduction is achieved with the posterior strap, taking care to avoid excessive abduction (osteonecrosis). The anterior strap controls flexion. Parents are counselled to observe knee movement occurring to monitor for femoral nerve palsy. The harness is worn full-time (under clothing one age-group size up).

reshaping of the acetabulum is occurring to provide stability once the harness is removed. Weekly or fortnightly assessments are usually required during harness treatment to ensure that it remains well-fitted and to permit bathing and harness changes. In experienced hands, this treatment carries a 90% chance of the hip reducing and stabilizing, with an excellent long-term outcome. Where treatment is unsuccessful or where it is detected too late (typically beyond 3 months), surgical treatment is required. This is why it is imperative to attempt to identify DDH in infants in the first few weeks of life.

## Surgical Treatment for DDH

For hips which do not reduce and stabilize in an abduction harness, the next stage of treatment is surgical reduction. This approach is required for most affected hips which are diagnosed beyond 3 months of age as well as the few who have failed harness treatment. There is controversy about the optimal time for surgical intervention. Some advocate

that it should be done as early as possible to allow the maximum time for acetabular remodelling. Others argue that a delay until the appearance of the ossific nucleus of the femoral head is safer. It is proposed that this delay allows time for the collateral circulation to develop around the proximal femur, which reduces the chances of the serious complication of osteonecrosis.

The first surgical step is examination of the hip under general anaesthesia. The examiner assesses whether a palpable reduction of the hip can be achieved and whether the reduction is secure with the leg in the so-called safe position. If successful, this is termed a closed reduction. The typical position is with the hip flexed to 90 degrees and abducted sufficiently to secure it from posterior dislocation but not to the extent where osteonecrosis can be induced. This is usually somewhere between 40 and 60 degrees of abduction. The integrity of the reduction is usually aided with the use of an arthrogram (radio-opaque contrast injected into the hip joint) (**Fig. 10.8**).

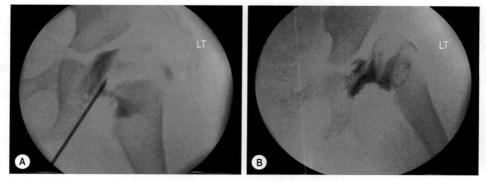

Fig. 10.8 Arthrogram demonstrating A) normal and B) dislocated hips.

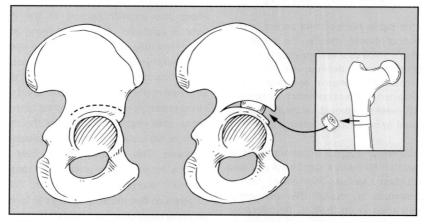

Fig. 10.9 Diagram showing Pemberton acetabuloplasty. The superior portion of the acetabulum hinges at the triradiate cartilage, improving anterior and lateral coverage of the femoral head. The osteotomy is held open by a bone graft usually obtained from the femur at the time of a femoral derotational osteotomy, or if no femoral osteotomy, then an a iliac crest graft is used. As the posterior column of the pelvis is not breeched, this reconstruction is intrinsically stable and does not require fixation.

If the hip will not reduce fully or is not sufficiently stable in a safe position, then open reduction is required. This is carried out via an anterior approach to the hip between the sartorius and tensor fascia lata. The rectus femoris is reflected inferiorly, and the hip capsule opened facilitating excision of the hypertrophic ligamentum teres and sufficient release of tight inferior and anterior capsular structures. This will usually allow reduction of the femoral head into the true acetabulum beneath the limbus. Historically, the limbus was excised or fenestrated, but it has been increasingly recognized that this structure is integral to subsequent superior and lateral stability and should be left intact.

Once reduced, the surgeon will assess the stability of the reduction in a manner similar to that used for a closed reduction. As a rule of thumb, if more than 30 degrees of internal rotation of the hip is needed to provide stability, many would advocate for an internal rotation osteotomy of the femur. Similarly, if the hip dislocates superiorly with less than 30 degrees of flexion an acetabular osteotomy is indicated (**Fig. 10.9**). However, this is not a practical proposition in children under 18 months old due to inadequate bone stock.

It is very important for the surgeon to assess the tension on the reduction as excessive pressure on the femoral head will increase the risk of osteonecrosis. This can be done by extending the knee once the hip is reduced. As the knee extends and hamstrings tighten, the femoral head may be seen or felt to push superiorly and redislocate. This is an indication for a femoral shortening osteotomy, which is increasingly commonly required as the patient approaches 2 years of age.

Once the hip is reduced and secure, either by open or closed means, the patient is placed in a spica cast immobilizing the pelvis and both hips in the desired, safe and stable position. Practice varies in how long casting is maintained, but it is commonly between 6 and 18 weeks, although a brace may be employed by some in the latter stages.

The outcome of surgical treatment is not as good as that for infants successfully treated in abduction harness. The risk of serious osteonecrosis is around 5%, with minor changes seen in up to 40%. Redislocation can occur (<5%), and subsequent inadequate development of the acetabulum with persisting dysplasia may require future femoral and/or acetabular surgery in childhood.

## PERTHES (LEGG–CALVÉ–PERTHES) DISEASE

### Clinical Summary

Arthurs Legg (USA), Jaques Calvé (France) and Georg Perthes (Germany) all described osteochondritis dessicans of the femoral head at roughly the same time. Approximately 1 per 1000 children are affected, typically between the ages of 3 and 8. It is more common in boys. The cause is unknown, but there is an increased frequency in some families, suggesting a weak genetic predisposition. Many environmental factors have been proposed and investigated, but none have been proven to be at fault. It is frequently observed that affected children are of short stature, which may implicate a systemic factor.

The current aetiological hypothesis is that the immature, proximal femoral epiphysis undergoes osteonecrosis followed by healing. The extent of femoral head involvement and adequacy of healing dictates the severity of the condition and prognosis.

Osteonecrosis follows a consistent pattern where the anterior portion of the proximal femoral epiphysis is most commonly involved. The infarct may extend from there to involve the entire epiphysis in the most severe cases. Following infarction and osteocyte death, the bony structure of the epiphysis is maintained until the blood supply is restored, delivering osteoclasts. These cells begin the removal of the damaged bone, which leads to progressive collapse of the epiphysis. This process evolves over several months before healing attempts to restore epiphyseal morphology. Long-term outcome depends on how much sphericity can be restored and how congruent the femoral head is with the acetabulum at the end of the process.

### Stages of Perthes Disease (Waldenström)

1. Initial: stage of infarction, shape preserved, but some increased sclerosis is seen on radiograph

2. Fragmentation: variable degree of collapse of the epiphyseal structure

3. Healing: gradual, attempted restoration of epiphyseal structure

4. Remodelling: a prolonged stage of slow reshaping of both the femoral head and acetabulum

Perthes usually affects only one hip, although approximately 15% of children may develop it in the contralateral hip in the following year or two. It is very unusual for Perthes to appear in both hips concurrently.

## Symptoms

Pain in the groin, thigh or knee may develop along with a limp. This may be intermittent at first, and children are often mildly symptomatic for weeks before presentation. The pain is aggravated by exercise, but rest pain and postsedentary stiffness become more common as the condition develops. The pain tends to improve slowly after 3–6 months but can flair up from minor injury for a much more prolonged period. Range of motion may never fully recover but gradually improves across approximately 6 to 18 months. Problematic symptoms from Perthes can exist for 1 to 3 years. In a small number of children with a poor outcome, pain and stiffness never fully resolve, but most children are able to return to normal activities after 18 months to 3 years.

Perthes increases the risk of premature osteoarthritis of the hip. The risk is increased if the hip has healed with poor sphericity or congruence. Predictors of a poor prognosis include the following:

- Age at onset of 8 years or more

- Herring Classification B or C (see below)

- Female

- Poor range of hip motion

## Clinical Examination

The child will be seen to limp. Examination when supine may reveal a slightly shorter leg (of 1 to 2 cm difference at most). The hip will be irritable on gentle rotation in extension, and abduction is usually restricted compared with the unaffected side. Frequently, the hip will move into external rotation as it is passively flexed, and internal rotation will be lost. Resistance to gentle adduction of the hip in flexion is an early sign of hip irritability and consistent in Perthes.

## Investigations

In early Perthes (before fragmentation), the radiograph may look unremarkable. As the condition progresses, features will become obvious on AP views (**Fig. 10.10**).

The best-known (and most prognostic) classification of Perthes is based on the appearance of the femoral epiphysis in the AP view (**Fig. 10.11**). This classification (lateral pillar or Herring) describes the morphology of the lateral one-third of the femoral head lateral to

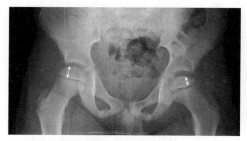

Fig. 10.10 AP Radiograph showing Perthes of the left hip with loss of height on the lateral aspect of the capital femoral epiphysis.

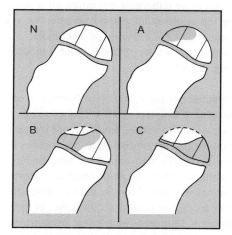

Fig. 10.11 Herring's lateral pillar classification (N=normal, with A, B and C representing increaseing severity of collapse).

the fovea. Notably, this classification system is only used at the end of the fragmentation phase, typically around 6 months from onset of symptoms. Group A has no loss in height, group B has <50% loss in height, and group C has >50% loss in height. A subsequent modification introduced the borderline B/C classification. When there is diagnostic uncertainty or a need to more fully establish the extent of the infarction, magnetic resonance imaging (MRI) is the best modality.

## Treatment

Mobility aids and analgesia are helpful, and early involvement of a physiotherapist to work on maintaining hip range of motion is thought to be beneficial. There is little evidence to support restriction of weight-bearing activity or the use of orthoses. Avoidance of aggravating activities is sensible for symptom control, but restrictions should not be too severe.

There is evidence that surgery to improve the containment of the hip can improve outcome for children older than 6 years with a Herring B classification. Containment can be achieved by reorientating the proximal femur into more varus or by enhancing the coverage provided by the acetabulum via reorientation or augmentation. An example of acetabular augmentation is the Staheli shelf procedure (**Fig. 10.12**)

Treatment of the sequelae of Perthes is challenging. A long-term loss of abduction can be helped with a valgus osteotomy of the proximal femur. This procedure also elongates the hip abductors and can allow adjustment of rotational deformity, all of which can improve patient function. There is little evidence that this procedure postpones the onset of osteoarthritis. Ultimately, early-onset osteoarthritis secondary to Perthes is best treated with total hip replacement after conservative

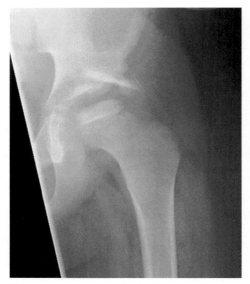

Fig. 10.12 AP radiograph showing acetabular augmentation using a shelf graft to improve containment of the femoral head affected by Perthes.

measures have been exhausted. The Stulberg classification (**Table 10.1**) is commonly used to describe the final hip morphology at the end of the disease process. It focusses on the morphology and congruency of the hip joint.

## THE LIMPING CHILD AND INFECTION

## Clinical Summary

A limp is one of the most common presentations in paediatric orthopaedics, and a wide variety of pathological locations and processes result in crossover in symptoms and signs. A thorough history followed by a focussed examination will usually localise the disease process. Supplemental information, such as blood results and imaging, can aid in diagnosis and monitor management.

**Table 10.1  Stulberg Classification**

| Class | Morphological Description | Radiological Appearance | Prognosis |
|---|---|---|---|
| I | Spherical congruency | Normal | Low risk of arthritis |
| II | Spherical congruency; loss of head shape <2 mm | Spherical head but at least one of the following:<br>• Coxa magna<br>• Steep acetabulum<br>• Short femoral neck | |
| III | Asymmetrical congruency; loss of head shape >2 mm | Nonspherical head but not flat | Mild to moderate risk of arthritis in mid-or late adulthood |
| IV | Aspherical congruency | Flat head and flat acetabulum | |
| V | Aspherical incongruency | Flat head, normal neck, normal acetabulum | Significant risk of early arthritis under 50 years old |

**Table 10.2  Essential Questions in the Evaluation of a Limp**

**Key Questions**

- Is there pain, and where is the maximal point of tenderness?
- Is the child generally unwell? Have they had a temperature?
- Was the onset gradual or sudden?
- Is the limp getting better, worse or staying the same?
- Can the child bear weight?

## History

Limping can be acute or chronic and be the manifestation of a large range of diagnoses. The diagnosis is often unclear from the initial presentation, but a detailed history narrows down the long list (**Table 10.2**). If infection is suspected, the history should also include details of recent infections, such as chicken pox, antibiotic courses and foreign travel, as this may shed light on the potential causative organism. Recent upper respiratory tract infection can be particularly relevant if reactive arthritis is suspected. Past medical history, including birth weight and gestation, alongside general health and well-being of the child, is essential in paediatric practice.

Developmental and past medial history are helpful in gauging walking age and functional abilities of the child, as well as evaluating risk of nonaccidental injury. A history of trauma (e.g., fracture) or activity-induced pain (slipped capital femoral epiphysis) should be elucidated. Symptoms such as insidious onset pain/swelling, night sweats, malaise, bruising or weight loss should raise suspicion of malignancy.

Drug history, including regular use of vitamin supplementation, should be noted. All children in the UK, particularly those with darke skin, should be taking vitamin D supplementation, which can prevents rickets and may lessen generalized bone pain.

| Table 10.3    Types of Gait | |
|---|---|
| **Gait Type** | **Examples of Associated Causes** |
| Normal | Wide-based gait of a toddler |
| Antalgic | Pain arising from the spine, SI joint, pelvis or lower limb |
| Toe walking (equinus) | Idiopathic |
| | Clubfoot |
| | Cerebral palsy (CP) |
| | Limb length discrepancy (LLD) |
| | Neurological disorder, e.g., Duchenne muscular dystrophy |
| Trendelenburg | Perthes |
| | DDH |
| | SCFE |
| | Hemiplegic CP |
| Circumduction | LLD |
| | CP |
| | Any cause of ankle or knee stiffness |
| Steppage | CP |
| | Spina bifida |
| | Charcot-Marie-Tooth disease |
| | Friedrich ataxia |

## Clinical Examination

If possible, the child should be observed walking and the type of gait observed (**Table 10.3**). Always examine the spine. A subtle loss of the normal lordotic curve and midline and spinal tenderness may indicate discitis.

Hip pain may be, in fact, arising from the abdomen, spine, sacroiliac (SI) joint, pelvis, or the psoas or iliacus muscles. A child may hold their hip in flexion due to a variety of conditions. If there is increased intracapsular pressure from septic arthritis, gentle rotation of the hip will produce pain. If there is no increase in pain with rotation, but pain with hip extension, then a diagnosis such as an iliopsoas abscess is more likely.

Knee pain may well be referred pain from the hip, and conditions such as slipped capital femoral epiphysis (SCFE) and Perthes should be actively excluded with a thorough hip examination.

## Investigation

The pace and intensity of the work-up for a limping child should be appropriate for the conditions on your differential diagnosis list (**Fig. 10.13**) but should generally involve a radiograph of the affected area. It is important to bear in mind that early infection may have few abnormalities on plain radiographs.

Subacute osteomyelitis may present with an intraosseous (Brodie) abscess (**Fig. 10.14**). Chronic osteomyelitis may display features such as a cloaca (sinus), sequestrum (devitalised bone), involucrum (new periosteal bone formation), avascular necrosis or bony defects (**Fig. 10.15**).

Blood tests should include full blood count, erythrocyte sedimentation rate, C-reactive protein and a blood film. If infection is suspected, blood cultures should be taken. In neonates and children with a diminished

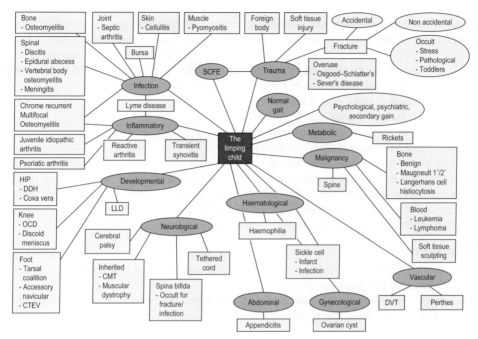

Fig. 10.13 Differential diagnosis of the limping child.

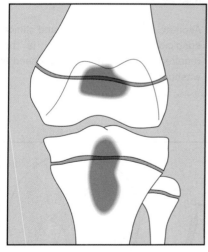

Fig. 10.14 Brodie's abscesses in the distal femur and proximal tibia.

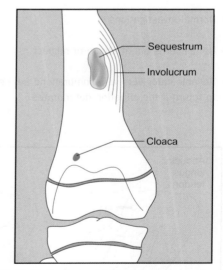

Fig. 10.15 Radiographic features of chronic osteomyelitis.

immune system, inflammatory markers may not be raised even in the setting of a severe infection.

Ultrasound screening can begin to differentiate septic arthritis from inflammatory causes such as juvenile idiopathic arthritis and transient synovitis, and the contralateral and surrounding joints can be examined for comparison.

MRI is an excellent tool to delineate osteomyelitis and infections of the soft tissues but should be used judiciously. A child under 4 years of age may require a general anaesthetic for an MRI, and the risk needs to be balanced with the diagnostic gain. If septic arthritis is suspected, joint fluid should be aspirated as an emergency, and if the child is septic antibiotics should be commenced immediately. The joint should undergo urgent irrigation and debridement, and repeated washout may be necessary.

## Treatment

If the limp is resolving, the child can often be safely discharged with analgesia and advice. It is suggested that the following criteria should be met before considering discharge:

- Well child

- Normal investigations

- No concerns about abuse or neglect

- Reliable caregivers who comprehend advice to return if the situation deteriorates

If septic arthritis is suspected, joint fluid should be aspirated as an emergency before antibiotics are commenced. The joint should undergo urgent irrigation and debridement, and repeated washouts may be required.

## Hip Aspiration

This procedure is a surgical emergency and should be performed in the operating theatre under sterile conditions. Fluoroscopy is used to confirm placement of the needle in the hip joint.

- Palpate the adductor longus tendon in the joint crease (**Fig. 10.16A**).

- Insert the needle under the tendon and direct towards the hip joint (**Fig. 10.16B**).

- Confirm placement with fluoroscopy (**Fig. 10.16C**).

- Aspirate hip. If fluid is clear and clinical suspicion is low, washout is not required. If fluid is not clear, proceed to washout.

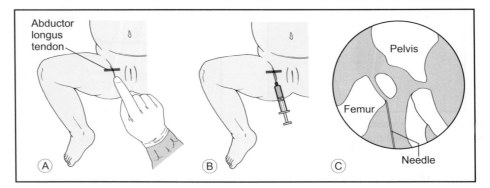

Fig. 10.16 Hip aspiration A) palpate adductor longus tendon B) insert needle under tendon and direct towards the hip C) confirm placement with fluoroscopy.

## Hip Washout

This technique uses a modified anterior (Smith–Peterson) approach and is the most commonly used open approach for hip irrigation in a child.

- Palpate the anterior superior iliac spine (ASIS) (**Fig. 10.17A**).

- Perform a bikini line incision centred 1 cm below the ASIS.

- Identify the interval between the tensor fascia lata (TFL) and sartorius (**Fig. 10.17B**).

- Protect the lateral femoral cutaneous nerve.

- In the deeper layer, identify the interval between the TFL and rectus femoris. The reflected head can be removed to expose the capsule. (**Fig. 10.17C**).

- Perform a capsulotomy and excise the capsule (approximately 5mm squared) (**Fig. 10.17D**).

- Irrigate the hip.

Treatment for osteomyelitis involves commencing empirical antibiotics after blood cultures have been obtained and tailoring antibiotics if an organism and its sensitivities are known. Unlike adults, definitive treatment with antibiotics is usually achieved without surgery. Discussion with microbiologists and local hospital

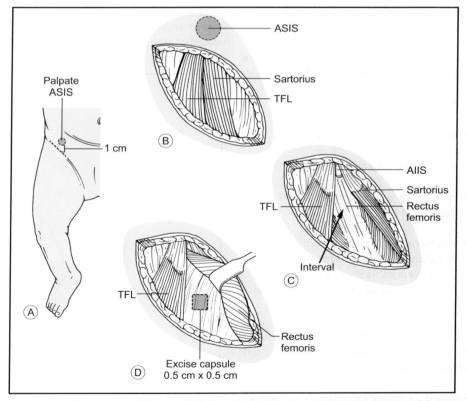

Fig. 10.17 Open hip washout A) Palpate ASIS B) make incision in groin crease inferior to ASIS C) identify interval between TFL and sartorius D) excise portion of capsule to allow for ongoing drainage.

protocol should guide the antibiotic choice and duration, but it typically involves a minimum of 2 weeks of intravenous therapy, followed by an additional 4 weeks of oral therapy.

*Staphylococcus aureus* is a common causative organism in all age groups. Neonates, particularly preterm, are susceptible to a range of organisms including *Streptococcus* species and may be multifocal. *Kingella kingae* should be considered in children less than 5 years old and may only be grown on extended culture from blood or an aspirate in blood culture bottles. Chicken pox may precede bone or joint infection, and its immune-lowering capabilities and the presence of skin lesions can predispose a child to severe infection. *Pseudomonas* is a possible organism when there is a puncture wound through the sole of a shoe or from dirty water.

If a child with osteomyelitis is not responding to antibiotic treatment, consider the following:

- Are the antibiotics the correct ones?

- Are the doses sufficiently high?

- Is there another source of infection?

- Is there a subperiosteal or soft tissue collection?

- Has the infection spread into the joint? This is particularly likely in joints with an intraarticular metaphysis such as the hip, proximal humerus, proximal radius and distal lateral tibia.

If there is a collection, worsening osteomyelitis or joint involvement, surgery is required to decompress and debride the infection.

Treatment of chronic osteomyelitis involves antibiotics, debridement and occasionally reconstructive procedures. Long-term sequelae of infection include growth arrest, avascular necrosis and deformity, and long-term follow-up is frequently required to ensure normal growth ensues.

## PAEDIATRIC FOOT CONDITIONS

## CLUBFOOT: CONGENITAL TALIPES EQUINOVARUS

### Clinical Summary

Clubfoot refers to a typical deformity of the foot or feet in the newborn. The hind foot is in equinovarus, the midfoot is adducted and the forefoot supinated and in cavus (**Fig. 10.18**). The severity of the condition is reflected by the rigidity of the deformities. In the most mildly affected children, the foot can passively be reduced into the normal position. This is termed

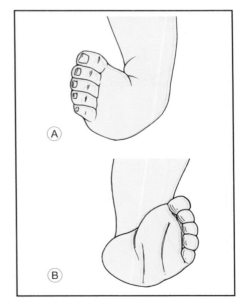

Fig. 10.18 Diagram showing typical features of clubfoot. A) Hindfoot equinus and varus, forefoot adduction. B) Medial skin crease and midfoot cavus. This position is not passively correctable.

flexible clubfoot and may represent intrauterine moulding and be unrelated to congenital talipes equinovarus (CTEV). It has a benign outlook. Fixed or rigid CTEV is pathological and resistant to immediate passive correction.

Approximately 1 in 1000 children are born with CTEV, with 50% having both feet affected. It is twice as common in boys as it is in girls. The cause is unknown, with no clear inheritance pattern, but incidence varies with race, and the condition does occur more frequently in some families.

Clubfoot deformity can be nonidiopathic in conditions such as CP, spina bifida or arthrogryposis.

## Symptoms

CTEV causes no symptoms in the nonambulatory infant but without treatment will ultimately significantly impair the ability to stand and walk on the affected side.

When an infant is identified as having the typical foot deformity as described above, the clinician should carry out a full examination from head to toe. Features of any condition associated with an acquired type of clubfoot should be sought. The head and spine should be inspected for abnormalities and generalized muscle tone assessed. The passive position and range of motion of all four limbs may indicate a systemic condition such as arthrogryposis. The lower limbs should be inspected for any skin dimpling or suggestion of tibial shortening, which suggests tibial dysplasia which can mimic CTEV.

The feet should then be examined to ensure that the typical features of CTEV are present. Adduction of the midfoot may be present in the absence of hindfoot deformity, in which case the diagnosis is metatarsus adductus, not CTEV. All the deformities present should be assessed for the degree of passive correctability. The Pirani score can be used to measure severity and predict success of treatment and is subdivided into midfoot and hindfoot sections (**Table 10.4**).

## Investigation

There are no specific tests to diagnose CTEV. Radiographs of the lower limb may be indicated if the features are atypical or the diagnosis is in doubt clinically, e.g., concern about possible tibial dysplasia. Similarly, genetic testing may have a role when more systemic abnormalities are observed.

## Treatment

The mainstay of treatment is serial manipulation with casting as described by Dr Ponseti. For the best results, treatment is commenced

| Table 10.4 Pirani Score for CTEV | | | |
|---|---|---|---|
| **Parameters** | **Mild** | **Moderate** | **Severe** |
| **Midfoot** | | | |
| Curved lateral border | 0 | 0.5 | 1 |
| Medial foot crease | 0 | 0.5 | 1 |
| Talar head coverage | 0 | 0.5 | 1 |
| **Hindfoot** | | | |
| Posterior heel crease | 0 | 0.5 | 1 |
| Rigid equinus | 0 | 0.5 | 1 |
| Palpable heel | 0 | 0.5 | 1 |

within the first few weeks of life. A weekly casting regime is implemented during which the foot is manipulated into a specific position and cast (**Fig. 10.19**). In the interim period between casts, stress–relaxation occurs, in which the ligaments relax into their new position, allowing further manipulation at the following stage.

---

### ✓ Key Points: Correction Stages of CTEV

The order for CTEV correction can be remembered using the **CAVE** mnemonic:

**C**avus
**A**dduction
**V**arus
**E**quinus

---

Stage 1 is correction of the forefoot cavus with manipulation and then application of a long-leg cast to hold the position. Stage 2 occurs a week later, and the cast is removed and gentle manipulation of the forefoot into abduction using the head of the talus as the fulcrum is performed. The forefoot is kept in supination and never pronated. A series of weekly manipulations and casts may be needed to bring the

forefoot into alignment with the midfoot on the head of the talus, but once this is achieved the hindfoot will then come out of varus.

In approximately 25% of children, the hindfoot can then be manipulated out of equinus aiming for 20 degrees of dorsiflexion. For the other 75%, a percutaneous tenotomy of the Achilles tendon is required to bring the heel down. Once the final corrected position is achieved, the child is placed in boots and bar (**Fig. 10.20**)

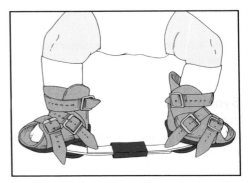

Fig. 10.20 Boots boots and bar orthosis with feet in 60 degrees external rotation and 20 degrees of dorsiflexion. Maintained full-time for 3 months, then during sleep/nap time until school age.

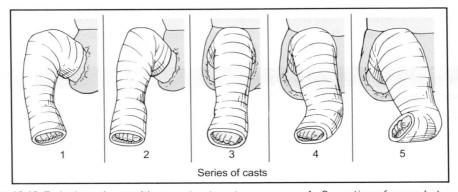

Fig. 10.19 Typical casting positions as treatment progresses. 1. Correction of cavus but supinating the midfoot to line up with hind foot (note, this position typically makes the deformity look worse). 2. Correction of adduction. 3. Correction of hindfoot varus. 4. Correction of equinus. 5. Maintenance of dorsiflexion (usually following percutaneous tenotomy).

for 3 months 23 hours a day, then 12 hours overnight for up to 4 years.

Success relies on the family's ability to comply with maintaining the casts and orthosis. Up to 80% of children treated this way end up with flexible, painless feet and normal function for many years.

## Ongoing Management

Some children relapse during or after treatment. A minor degree of relapse can respond well to further manipulation and casting, particularly if due to relative tightening of the gastrosoleus with growth. As CTEV is a condition which causes abnormalities of lower leg muscle balance (irrespective of treatment), some children develop dynamic supination, in which they display obligate excessive supination of the forefoot in gait. This can be treated with transfer of the tibialis anterior tendon lateral to the cuneiform to rebalance the foot. This works well and has minimal adverse long-term effects and is best carried out from about the age of 3.

More significant relapse occurring later and associated with stiffness may need correction of bony deformity. Fixed heel varus can be treated with calcaneal osteotomy to lateralize the Achilles insertion. Recurrent, fixed midfoot adductus can be addressed with lateral column shortening plus possible medial column lengthening. This can be achieved by osteotomy of the cuboid or anterior process of the calcaneum and opening wedge osteotomy of the medial cuneiform. These procedures can realign the foot for improved shoe wear and plantar contact but can lead to longer term issues with stiffness.

## THE CALCANEOVALGUS FOOT

## Clinical Summary

Calcaneovalgus foot describes the foot which is held with the heel down and the foot in maximal

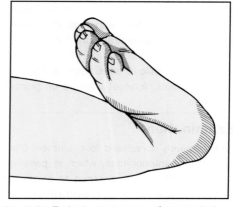

Fig. 10.21 Typical appearance of congenital calcaneovalgus foot in extreme dorsiflexion.

dorsiflexion. The typical appearance is seen at birth and can appear quite dramatic. It is important to establish if the diagnosis is that of typical, congenital calcaneovalgus (**Fig. 10.21**) or another more problematic pathology. The former condition is benign and self-corrects over the first few months of life. Alternative conditions with similar appearances are outlined in the Key Point box below. The cause of typical benign congenital calcaneovalgus is not known, but it is associated with other conditions representative of intrauterine crowding. The most important associated condition is DDH, and the hips of an infant with calcaneovalgus foot deformity must have their hips closely examined or imaged.

---

### ✓ Key Points: Differential Diagnosis of Congenital Dorsiflexed Foot

---

- Calcaneovalgus foot: valgus heel, dorsiflexion deformity within foot

- Fibular hemimelia (partial or complete absence of the fibula, no palpable lateral malleolus, anteromedial bow of tibia)

- Posteromedial tibial bowing: apex of deformity lies midtibia, not at ankle

- Congenital vertical talus: rocker bottom appearance to foot with heel in equinus. Vertical talus on lateral X-ray

- Congenital oblique talus: less severe than vertical talus, forefoot lines up on plantarflexion

## Examination

An excessively dorsiflexed foot is noted, often against the anterior tibia, which is passively correctable. This is in contrast to congenital vertical talus, which is not correctable. No palpable talar head is present, and a supple midfoot is noted.

## Treatment

The mainstay of treatment for calcaneovalgus is home stretching by parents for 3–6 months. Serial casting may be performed in the rare refractory cases in which the foot cannot plantar flex beyond neutral.

## TARSAL COALITION

### Clinical Summary

A failure of separation between the tarsal bones during development is thought to be relatively common, with most cases remaining asymptomatic and undiscovered. The coalitions most frequently encountered are between the calcaneum and talus (subtalar) and/or the calcaneum and navicular **Fig. 10.22**). It is important to note that more than one coalition can coexist.

### Symptoms

Patients tend to present from about the age of 10 years with chronic mid- or hindfoot pain and a stiff, flat foot appearance.

### Clinical Examination

In stance, it will be seen that the affected foot has a planovalgus appearance with no correction on tiptoe standing. Passive movement of the hindfoot will show marked stiffness or absence of subtalar movement, and passive rotation of the midfoot will also be restricted.

## Investigation

AP and oblique radiographs of the foot will show a calcaneonavicular coalition with either no separation of the bones or a long anterior calcaneal process (Anteater sign **Fig. 10.22**). Subtalar coalition can be more subtle to spot on a plain radiograph, and computed tomography scanning is a much more reliable investigation when this is suspected. MRI can be helpful to see nonossified coalitions and to rule out alternative causes of pain. Bone coalitions are called synostosis cartilaginous coalitions are synchondrosis, and fibrous coalitions are syndesmosis.

## Treatment

Pain from a coalition can settle spontaneously, and conservative symptomatic management with analgesia and cast immobilization is appropriate in all cases initially. This can be accomplished by accommodating insoles or a period

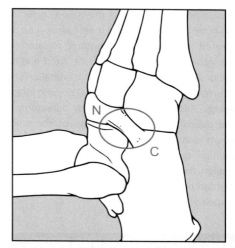

Fig. 10.22 Diagram of radiographic appearance of a calcaneonavicular coalition. The coalition if fibrous or bony, between the navicular (N) and calcaneus (C). Note the long anterior process of the calcaneum ('anteater sign').

of immobilization in a cast. It is important to note that the pes planus deformity does not improve. For those who continue to be in pain despite a trial of several months of conservative measures, surgery can be considered.

For calcaneonavicular coalitions, the bar can be accessed and excised via a dorsolateral incision (Ollier approach) distal to the lateral malleolus. Fat or muscle (extensor digitorum brevis) may be interposed in the resulting gap to try and prevent recurrence.

Subtalar coalitions of less than 30% of the width of the joint can be excised via a medial approach distal to the tip of the medial malleolus. Larger subtalar coalitions have a high recurrence rate when treated with excision, and completion of the subtalar arthrodesis is considered a more reliable treatment in that circumstance.

As none of these surgical procedures address the planovalgus deformity, some surgeons advocate calcaneal osteotomy with lateral column lengthening in addition to excision of the coalition.

## METATARSUS ADDUCTUS

### Clinical Summary

Children are born with adduction of the forefoot affecting one or both feet, although it may not become apparent for a few months. The deformity arises at the junction of the mid- and forefoot, and importantly, the hindfoot is completely normal. The cause is unknown, but it is included in the spectrum of conditions associated with intrauterine crowding, and there is a slightly increased risk of hip dysplasia in children with this foot deformity.

### Symptoms

The condition is painless, and function is normal.

## Clinical Examination

The examiner will find the forefoot to be in adduction, which may be partially passively correctable. The heel will be in a normal position. The presence of a normal heel differentiates this condition from CTEV. There may be associated femoral anteversion and internal tibial torsion.

## Investigations

No imaging of the foot is required if the clinical features are typical.

## Treatment

The majority (80%) will spontaneously correct over the first 2–3 years of life. Casting may be helpful in the most rigid or slowly resolving cases. As there is no functional impairment from residual metatarsus, adductus in life surgery rarely has any role in treatment.

## PAINFUL HEEL: CALCANEAL APOPHYSITIS (SEVER'S)

### Clinical Summary

One of most common presentations of calcaneal apophysitis is that of pain at the insertion of the tendo Achilles in children from 8 to 12 years. Boys are more commonly affected, and the symptoms are often unilateral or, if bilateral, asynchronous. The reason why this condition develops at this age is not understood, but it is hypothesised that the increasing power and tension in the gastrosoleus overloads the less mature insertion of the tendoachilles on the calcaneal apophysis.

### Symptoms

Pain is felt at the back of the heel during and after exercise or on initial movement after rest. Occasionally, the pain can extend under the heel. Constant rest pain or marked nocturnal pain are not normally seen in simple apophysitis.

## Clinical Examination

There should be no visible abnormality. Any swelling or erythema suggests an alternative diagnosis. The patient will be tender to fingertip pressure at the insertion of the tendoachilles. There may be some tightness of the gastrocsoleus, but this is not a consistent finding.

## Investigation

No imaging is required if the clinical features are typical. In atypical cases a plain radiograph or MRI of the calcaneum can be useful to exclude alternative diagnoses.

## Treatment

No specific treatment has been shown to be helpful. Advice on avoiding aggravating activities, application of ice and use of anti-inflammatory drugs is usually given. Physiotherapy to stretch the calf muscles is sometimes advocated, and in severe intractable cases, a short period in a walking cast can alleviate the pain. The most important element of treatment, however, is reassuring the child and family of the benign diagnosis and the fact that the symptoms always settle, leaving no lasting impairment.

## CEREBRAL PALSY

CP is a neurological disorder caused by a non-progressive brain injury or malformation occurring while the child's brain is developing. It is the most common chronic disability in childhood, and while the underlying damage to the brain is nonprogressive, the effects on the child's neuromuscular system are progressive due to persisting tone, paresis and skeletal growth. The prevalence is about 2 per 1000 live births, and prematurity is a well-known risk factor. The musculoskeletal aspects of CP may not be the dominant clinical problem as children with CP often have multiple impairments (**Table 10.5**).

## Classifications

Classification of CP is based on subtypes. The classification system provided by the Surveillance of Cerebral Palsy in Europe (SCPE) group is widely used (**Table 10.6**), but clinicians may still use topographical descriptions: hemiplegia (one side of the body affected), diplegia (predominantly affecting both lower limbs but can include some upper limb involvement) and total body involvement (all four limbs, trunk and head control affected).

The Gross Motor Function Classification System (GMFCS) is widely used as a functional classification to describe motor levels in children with CP and is summarized in **Fig. 10.23**.

## Diagnosis

Consider CP as a diagnosis with adverse events in the perinatal period, particularly prematurity and intraventricular haemorrhages. It may take several months for problematic muscle tone to develop, and walking is often delayed.

### Table 10.5  Impairments Associated with CP

| | |
|---|---|
| Communication | Increased tone* |
| | Muscle weakness* |
| Learning difficulties | Impaired mobility* |
| Epilepsy | Hip displacement* |
| Vision | Joint contracture* |
| Hearing | Spinal deformity* |
| Pain – tone/gastric/chip | |
| Continence | |
| Eating and drinking | |
| Saliva control | |
| Sleep | |
| Behaviour | |

*managed by physiotherapists and orthopaedic surgeons

## Table 10.6    SCPE Collaborative Group

| SCPE Subtypes | | Additional Features by Subtype |
|---|---|---|
| **SPASTIC CP** | Bilateral spastic (BS-CP) Unilateral spastic (hemiplegia) | Increased tone Pathological reflexes <br> * increased reflexes, e.g., hyperreflexia <br> * pyramidal signs, e.g., Babinski response <br> Resulting in abnormal pattern of movement and posture |
| **DYSKINETIC CP** | Dystonic Choreo athetotic | Involuntary, uncontrolled, recurring, occasionally stereotyped movements; primitive reflex patterns predominate; muscle tone varies |
| **ATAXIC CP** | | Loss of orderly muscular coordination, so that movements are performed with abnormal force, rhythm and accuracy |

Surveillance of cerebral palsy in Europe: a collaboration of cerebral palsy surveys and registers. *Developmental Medicine and Child Neurology. 2000; 42: 816–24*. https://onlinelibrary.wiley.com/doi/abs/10.1111/j.1469-8749.2000. tb00695.x?sid=nlm%3Apubmed.

## Assessment

A multidisciplinary approach is employed including physiotherapists, neurologists, orthotists, occupational therapists, community paediatrician and orthopaedic surgeons. This approach will help focus on what is important to the patient rather than focussing on less relevant functional limitations.

It can be time-consuming to prepare a child for examination in the clinic, and a rushed examination will be flawed if it causes the child distress or insufficient time to allow relaxation of abnormal muscle tone.

## Examination

Typically in CP, there is spasticity and muscle weakness and increased muscle tone, often coupled with immobility. This leads to muscle shortening, joint contractures and limb deformity. An imbalance of agonist and antagonistic muscle groups occurs. A common example is seen in the evolution of a fixed equinus (plantarflexion) deformity at the ankle due to persisting spasticity and subsequent shortening of the ankle plantar flexors and relative weakness of the antagonists and the dorsiflexors. Gravity may also contribute to the equinus deformity.

**Gait:** It is essential to assess gait (coronal and sagittal planes) in a child who can walk as part of the examination of their musculoskeletal system (**Fig. 10.24**). The prerequisites for efficient gait are summarized in **Table 10.7**. Focus, in turn, on foot, knee and hip and then upper body. It may be possible to identify, for example, that toe clearance is problematic or that the hip or knee are held in flexion throughout.

Gait is too complex to relies solely on visual observations, and it is now standard practice to obtain a laboratory-based gait analysis. The

# GMFCS E and R between 6th and 12th birthday:
## Descriptors and illustrations

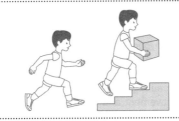

### GMFCS level I

Children walk at home, school, outdoors and in the community. They can climb stairs without the use of a railing. Children perform gross motor skills such as running and jumping, but speed, balance and coordination are limited.

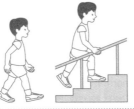

### GMFCS level II

Children walk in most settings and climb stairs holding onto a railing. They may experience difficulty walking long distances and balancing on uneven terrain, inclines, in crowded areas or confined spaces. Children may walk with physical assistance, a hand-held mobility device or use wheeled mobility over long distances. Children have only minimal ability to perform gross motor skills such as running and jumping.

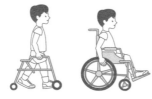

### GMFCS level III

Children walk using a hand-held mobility device in most indoor settings. They may climb stairs holding onto a railing with supervision or assistance. Children use wheeled mobility when traveling long distances and may self-propel for shorter distances.

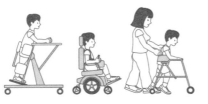

### GMFCS level IV

Children use methods of mobility that require physical assistance or powered mobility in most settings. They may walk for short distances at home with physical assistance or use powered mobility or a body support walker when positioned. At school, outdoors and in the community, children are transported in a manual wheelchair or use powered mobility.

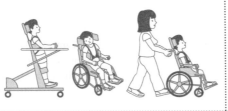

### GMFCS level V

Children are transported in a manual wheelchair in all settings. Children are limited in their ability to maintain antigravity head and trunk postures and control leg and arm movements.

**Fig. 10.23** The Gross Motor Function Classification System (GMFCS) level is practical method of communicating functional level between healthcare professionals.

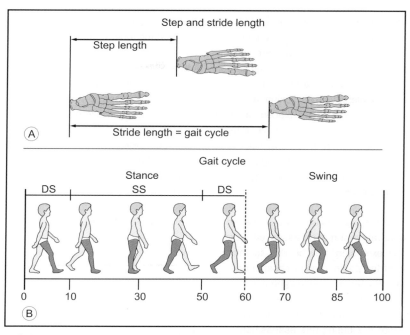

Fig. 10.24 Gait considerations. A) Step and stride length. B) The timing of the cycle is expressed in percentages, and in normal gait the stance phase lasts for 60% of the cycle and swing 40%. In stance there, are two periods of double support (DS) when both feet are on the ground and one of single support (SS) when the opposite limb is in swing phase.

| Table 10.7  Prerequisites for Efficient Gait |
| --- |
| Stability in stance phase |
| Foot clearance in swing |
| Optimal positioning of the foot in terminal swing |
| Sufficient step length |
| Energy conservation |

analysis provides details of a patient's walking ability based on video assessment, joint ranges of movement (kinematics), forces acting on the limbs (kinetics), muscle activity (electromyography), foot pressure and energy consumption.

**Static assessment:** Apply gentle, continual stretch to muscle groups to overcome the increased muscle tone and allow an accurate assessment. Passive movement of affected limbs can be painful, and patients with communication difficulties may not be able to alert the examiner that they are in pain.

**Spine**: The spine is best assessed with the patient sitting to identify head control and scoliosis. Helping to support the patient's trunk can help differentiate between fixed and flexible spinal deformity. Pelvic obliquity should be noted as it will influence apparent leg length difference and may be a sign of hip displacement.

**Upper limbs**: While the patient remains sitting, the upper limbs can be examined for range of motion, muscle tone and fixed deformity of the joints.

**Hips**: The hips are best assessed with the patient lying supine with their pelvis near the end of the couch. Inspection can identify the resting position of the hips and suggest leg length inequality, which may indicate hip displacement. Full passive range of motion should be checked with hips in extension and flexion, taking care to identify fixed flexion using the Thomas test. The patient is placed prone to check rectus femoris length and hip rotation and to allow estimation of femoral neck anteversion by palpating when the greater trochanter is maximally prominent during internal rotation (**Fig. 10.25**).

**Knees**: The resting position should be noted and passive range of motion assessed. Restriction of full extension may be due to intrinsic tightness of the posterior joint capsule or short hamstrings. Posterior capsule tightness is quantified with the hips in extension (hamstrings relaxed). It is important to ensure the opposite hip does not flex during this assessment as it allows pelvic movement and an overestimation of hamstring length on the examined side.

**Ankle**: The range of plantar and dorsiflexion should be checked with the heel held in varus to prevent escape of the heel into valgus which can give an overestimation of hindfoot dorsiflexion. Restriction of dorsiflexion with the knee flexed is predominantly due to shortening of the soleus while the additional influence of the gastrocnemius whose origin is above the knee can be assessed when the knee is brought into its position of maximal extension (**Fig. 10.26**).

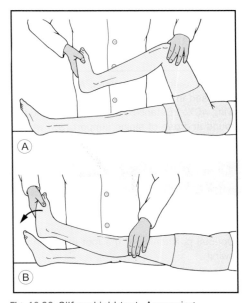

Fig. 10.26 Silfverskiold test. Assessing gastrocnemius length. With the knee extended, fixed ankle plantarflexion ('equinus contracture') can arise from the soleus and/or gastrocnemius. As gastrocnemius originates above the knee, flexing the knee would improve a gastrocnemius contracture. If it does not, the contracture is due to combined tightness of both muscles. This can guide the level of planned surgical release: combined at the level of the Achilles tendon or gastrocnemius alone at the musculotendinous junction.

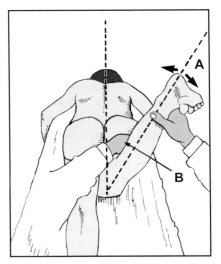

Fig. 10.25 Femoral anteversion. To examine anteversion by palpation, the patient lies prone, and the examiner places one hand on the greater trochanter (GT) and rotates the hip until the GT is most prominent laterally (A). At this point the angle of the shin compared to vertical is appreciated from the end of the bed (B). This is the femoral anteversion angle.

**Foot**: The passive position of the feet when in weight-bearing and non-weight-bearing positions is appreciated. Hindfoot equinus can be present with varus and supination of the midfoot, which leads to the patient weight bearing on the dorsolateral aspect of the forefoot. Alternatively, the hindfoot may be in an equinovalgus position with flattening of the midfoot and weight bearing on the medial aspect. If deformity is present, the position of maximum correction should be identified.

## Management of Musculoskeletal Problems in CP

**Physiotherapy:** The primary role of a physiotherapist is to reduce pain and restore and maintain physical function. Weakness and persisting spasticity are often causes of deteriorating mobility as children get older, and physiotherapists have a key role in optimizing a patient's function and posture. Preventing or slowing the development of muscle shortening is important in trying to maintain muscle strength. Patients' mobility may be helped by using a mobility aid, and postural support may include the use of a standing frame, sleep system or wheelchair adaptations.

**Orthoses**: Orthoses are externally applied devices which support or enhance function via control of joint alignment/movement, altering load, redistribution of pressure and accommodation/correction of deformity.

An ankle foot orthosis is commonly used to support the foot and ankle in a functional position, to slow or prevent evolving deformity and to improve the biomechanics of gait. An orthosis which extends above the knee is termed a knee–ankle–foot orthosis, but this device is rarely used in CP because of the risk of impeding knee motion. A thoraco lumbar sacral orthosis (TLSO) may be provided for a patient who does not have control of spinal posture to improve their posture for feeding and sitting. Scoliosis is common in GMFCS IV and V patients, and while a TLSO may help posture, it does not prevent curve progression.

**Tone management**: Improvement in muscle spasticity can be achieved with medical therapies.

Oral antispasmodics such as baclofen can reduce muscle tone globally. Its use is limited by undesirable side effects such as sedation or drooling. A more effective dose can be given when the drug is delivered intrathecally via a surgically implanted programmable pump. This approach has proven to be very useful for spasticity management in GMFCS level IV and V patients. Disadvantages include risk of infection and the need to replace the pump battery about every 5 years.

Botulinum toxin blocks transmission at the neuromuscular junction and, when injected directly, can reduce muscle tone. This can reduce spasticity, but the effect is not permanent and only lasts a few months, but injections can be repeated. It should be noted that botulinum is useful for spasticity but not for muscle shortening.

Selective dorsal rhizotomy (SDR) involves sectioning a proportion of the dorsal L2 to S1 nerve roots. When successful, the procedure can provide a lasting reduction in muscle tone and improved lower limb function. SDR is mostly used in GMFCS level I and II patients when spasticity is impeding gait. Prospective patients should undergo a rigorous preoperative assessment to ensure that tone reduction is highly likely to improve their walking efficiency as the procedure is irreversible and potentially disastrous due to irreversible muscle weakness and possible incontinence.

**Surgical management:** Surgery for children with CP should be performed in a specialist children's centre as these children often have comorbidities that may require postoperative support in a high-dependency ward for the more complex procedures. Surgery may be considered for children who walk (GMFCS I–III) to improve gait and for those who do not (GMFCS IV–V) to improve conditions such as spinal deformity, hip displacement and painful posture due to limb deformity.

**Spine**: GMFCS level IV and V (**Fig. 10.23**) patients are at a high risk of developing scoliosis. If the deformity reaches a point where it prevents the child from sitting comfortably, causes pain from rib impingement or threatens respiratory function, a spinal fusion should be considered. This entails spinal fusion over a long segment from high thoracic vertebrae to L5 or sacrum.

**Hip**: Hip problems are found both in walkers and nonwalkers. In the former, excessive femoral anteversion can affect gait adversely, whereas in the latter there is a well-recognized increased risk of hip displacement in higher GMFCS levels (1% in GMFCS I and 90% in GMFCS V).

Excessive femoral anteversion is a common problem in the walker, as it persists in children with CP, whereas it usually resolves by about 6–7 years of age in typically developing children. The consequence for children with CP with excess femoral anteversion is an internally rotated knee in gait with or without a compensatory external tibial torsion. When gait is adversely affected, the patient should have a gait analysis, and, if confirmed, the excessive femoral anteversion can be treated with derotation osteotomy of the proximal femur to a give an anteversion angle of about 15 degrees.

In the nonwalker, clinical examination to detect a displaced hip is unreliable because of pelvic obliquity, muscle contractures and excess tone. For this reason, X-ray surveillance of children with CP is recommended, and by identifying children at risk, early surgery for displacing hips

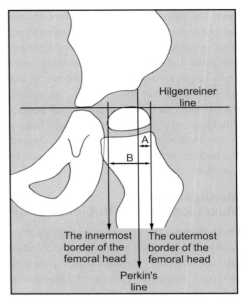

Fig. 10.27 Reimer's migration index. A is divided by B. This represents the proportion of the upper femoral epiphysis that is uncovered by the acetabulum.

has reduced the incidence of hip dislocation in the CP population in recent years. Hip displacement is measured using the Reimer migration percentage (MP) (**Fig. 10.27**).

When a hip is considered at risk of progressive displacement (MP >40), surgical stabilization with a shortening, varising, derotation proximal femoral osteotomy may be considered (**Fig. 10.28**).

If there is acetabular dysplasia, an acetabuloplasty should be added to optimize recentration of the hip.

Once dislocated, a symptomatic hip would need femoral and pelvic osteotomies, but if the femoral head and acetabular deformities are so severe and beyond reconstruction, a proximal femoral excision may be considered. Contralateral femoral varus osteotomy may be performed concurrently to maintain balance of used. Management of crouch gait will depend on the underlying cause(s) but may be a combination of the following principles: restore knee extension, unload the painful patellofemoral joint, restore the length–tension curve of the quadriceps, balance agonist and antagonist muscles at the knee, manage excess tone and use ankle foot orthoses to stabilize the ankle joint and realign ground reaction forces in gait postoperatively.

**Foot and ankle**: A mild to moderate equinus contracture of the hindfoot can be tolerated and compensated with heel wedges. It can be managed with a combination of physiotherapy with or without serial casting to stretch short muscles and an ankle foot orthosis to accommodate or maintain the improved position of the ankle and tone management. Severe equinus prevents shoe wear or splintage, may cause flexion at the knee and hip and interferes with foot prepositioning in terminal swing and foot contact in stance.

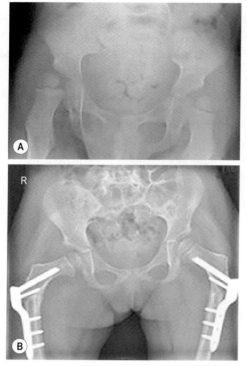

Fig. 10.28 Management of displacing hips with proximal varus derotation femoral osteotomies A) radiographic with bilateral valgus proximal femoral necks and displacing heads. B) following varus derotation osteotomy.

femoral lengths and rotation to optimize seating and pelvic alignment.

**Knee**: The walker's flexed-knee (crouch) gait is common, and the underlying reasons are complex and require an assessment in a gait lab. Crouch gait may result from flexion contractures at the hip, knee and ankle and weakness of the quadriceps, which may progress to patella alta and a long patellar tendon; short hamstrings; and excess tone in the hip, knee and ankle flexors without contracture or a combination thereof. Tenotomies should be avoided to conserve muscle strength, but if musculotendinous lengthening is required, an intramuscular or fractional lengthening technique is

Varus deformity of the hindfoot can be due to excess tone/shortening in the gastrocnemius, soleus and tibialis posterior. Midfoot adduction/supination is caused by excess tone/shortening of tibialis anterior. The tibialis posterior can be lengthened intramuscularly at the same time as gastrocnemius lengthening, or both muscles can be split with the lateral portions transferred laterally to achieve better dynamic balance. When deformities are fixed, muscle balancing procedures need to be combined with osteotomy to realign the calcaneus or midfoot. Fusion may be required to prevent recurrent deformity.

For the foot with hindfoot valgus and associated pes planus, there are often multiple factors to consider. The most important consideration is to ensure correction of malrotation of the entire lower limb. The gastrocnemius and soleus are often short, as are the peroneal muscles. If this cannot be controlled in a splint, then gastrocnemius lengthening can be combined with lateral column lengthening if the foot is still flexible. If rigid, then fusion of the talo-calcaneal, talonavicular and calcaneo cuboid joints (triple fusion) may be required.

**Upper limb:** The surgical principles for the lower limb also apply to orthopaedic management of the upper limb. A careful assessment of joint ranges of motion, tone, functional impairments and a record of patient/carer aims of management are standard. A video recording of upper limb function using standard activities-orientated tasks is made. Only a small number of patients are suitable for upper-limb surgery. Important criteria for surgery include intelligence, motor function, sensibility, age and motivation.

There are procedures designed to improve function and posture. These include release of contracture, musculotendinous lengthening, tendon transfer and joint stabilization. This surgery may be carried out by hand surgeons, plastic surgeons and orthopaedic surgeons specializing in CP and depend on local arrangements.

While surgery to improve arm posture and hand function is usually indicated in hemiplegics, some procedures are indicated in patients who have no useful upper limb function. For example, in hemiplegia, the clinical problem may be excessive wrist flexion putting finger and thumb function out of a functional range. One solution might be to fuse the wrist to place the fingers and thumb in a more functional position. Adduction deformity of the thumb and 'thumb in palm' deformity are amenable to surgical improvement.

Skin hygiene problems may occur in children who have no useful upper limb function. These problems are typically seen at the elbow, hand and wrist where severe contractures may result in skin maceration or even ulceration. An anterior release of the elbow, even if modest, may improve hygiene significantly. Musculotendinous lengthening of the wrist,

finger and thumb flexors and wrist fusion are reliable procedures to alleviate skin hygiene problems and may have the added benefit that the hand can rest on the tray of a wheelchair or seating device.

---

## Clinical Pearls

---

1. Multidisciplinary approach to assessment and treatment in CP is essential.

2. Focus on how to manage pain and improve function that is relevant to the patient/caregiver.

3. The risk of hip displacement increases with severity of spastic CP.

4. The success of surgery relies upon careful assessment and planning.

5. Recovery after surgery may be prolonged.

---

## PAEDIATRIC KNEE

### Clinical Summary

Knee pain, instability and deformity are very common presentations in the child and adolescent. One of the most important differential diagnoses in the presentation of knee pain is referred pain from the hip. Do not miss a diagnosis such as Perthes or SCFE because the focus has remained on the knee. Infection and malignancy are also two important diagnoses to exclude (**Fig. 10.29**).

### Knee Pain Related to Growth and Overuse

Anterior knee pain is very common with growth and, in the younger child, may be the manifestation of the benign leg pains of childhood: growing pains. This typically presents as nocturnal pain in both legs, and the child is

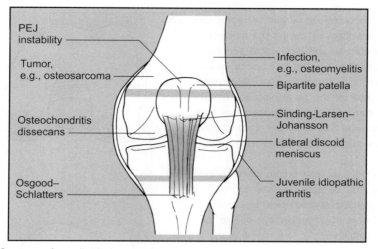

PEJ instability

Tumor, e.g., osteosarcoma

Osteochondritis dissecans

Osgood–Schlatters

Infection, e.g., osteomyelitis

Bipartite patella

Sinding-Larsen–Johansson

Lateral discoid meniscus

Juvenile idiopathic arthritis

Fig. 10.29 Sources of paediatric knee pain.

generally unaffected during the day. Growing pains is a diagnosis of exclusion, and pathology must be actively ruled out.

In the older child and adolescent, the effect of growth, often combined with sporting overuse, can present at the tibial tuberosity (tibial tubercle apophysitis or Osgood–Schlatter disease), the inferior pole of the patella (Sinding-Larsen–Johansson disease) or the patella tendon (patellar tendinitis). These conditions represent traction-induced inflammation, which is self-limiting and resolves with maturity. Furthermore, the rapid increase in bone length with relative delay in soft tissues 'catching up' can give rise to muscle/tendon tension and pain.

Examination findings include tenderness, swelling of the tibial tuberosity in Osgood–Schlatter disease and decreased quadriceps flexibility.

Management is symptomatic and includes physiotherapy and activity modification. For more severe cases, nonsteroidal anti-inflammatory drugs (NSAIDs) may be required, combined with a period of rest from intense sporting activities.

## Bipartite Patella

The patella normally forms from a single ossification centre, but if there are two or more centres which then fail to fuse, a bi- or tripartite patella forms. This is the case for 2%–3% of the normal population, and the vast majority are asymptomatic. Symptoms may develop following trauma, with separation of the fragment and fibrous union.

Examination reveals tenderness around the accessory patellar portion, which is typically superolateral. Treatment of the painful bipartite patella involves rest and NSAIDs and, if necessary, immobilization for a few weeks. Occasionally, surgery is required to excise the fragment arthroscopically or via a direct lateral approach, with or without a lateral release.

## Discoid Meniscus

A discoid meniscus is a common anatomical variant, affecting the lateral compartment almost exclusively. The cause is unknown, although discoid menisci have been found in infants of a few months of age, suggesting an early causal event. There are three types according to the Watanabe classification.

Type I is the complete variant, whereby the meniscus is thickened, covers the majority of the lateral plateau and has stable peripheral attachments. Type II is the incomplete variant, which is similarly stable to type I, but covers less than 80% of the tibial plateau. Type III (Wrisberg variant) has normal meniscal morphology, however has no posterior attachment to the tibial plateau so is abnormally mobile.

A discoid meniscus may remain asymptomatic indefinitely, may be found incidentally, or may present with instability and tears. Type I menisci tend to present at an earlier age due to their inherent instability.

The child may present with a popping or snapping sensation, which is usually nonpainful and does not interfere with activities. The diagnosis is suspected from radiographs revealing a flattened lateral femoral condyle and widening of the joint space and confirmed with MRI.

Mild symptoms can be managed nonoperatively with observation. Children may present with a loss of terminal knee extension, and pain may develop in the older child due to meniscal instability or tearing. In these cases, surgery is required to partially resect or 'saucerize' the meniscus to leave a stable, normally shaped remnant.

## Osteochondritis Dissecans

Osteochondritis dissecans (OCD) is characterised by the dissection of a soft, loose or detached portion of cartilage and bone from the surrounding joint (**Fig. 10.30**). It is normally located on the posterolateral aspect of the medial femoral condyle, and although the aetiology is unclear, a mechanical cause is the most likely. As loads are applied to the distal femur, the stresses on the subchondral bone are greatest at the medial femoral condyle. Other aetiologies include direct trauma, impingement from a tall tibial spine and a genetic predisposition. Pathologically, OCD is characterised by avascular necrosis of the

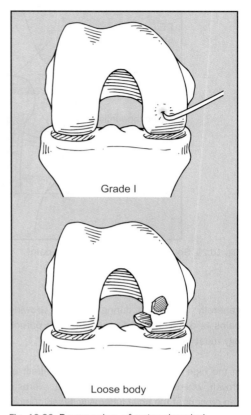

Grade I

Loose body

Fig. 10.30 Progression of osteochondral disease from softening of a discrete region of articular cartilage, progressing to full thickness loss, or 'osteochondral dissecans', where a loose body *dissects or* detaches with a fragment of underlying subchondral bone.

subchondral bone, with ischaemia and fibrosis of the overlying hyaline cartilage.

The natural history is influenced by the age of the patient and size and location of the lesion. The prognosis is favourable in children before physeal closure, those with smaller lesions and those with lesions on the medial femoral condyle, with healing occurring within 6 months for more than two-thirds of patients.

Patients present with anterior knee pain, and if the fragment has become detached, mechanical

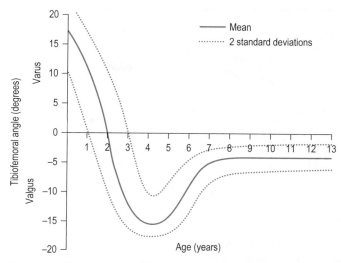

Fig. 10.31 Salenius curve. Development of the coronal tibiofemoral angle during growth.

symptoms such as locking, swelling and giving way are observed. With a nondetached OCD, there may only be tenderness over the medial femoral condyle with the knee in flexion. With detachment, there may be quadriceps wasting, an effusion, crepitus or a loss of extension.

Radiographs should include an AP, lateral and a flexed or 'notch' AP, and lesions can be further examined with MRI.

Nonoperative management is advised for minimally symptomatic and stable lesions and typically involves restricting sporting activities.

If there are mechanical symptoms, or signs on the MRI that the lesion is unstable or detached, or if after 6 months of nonoperative management the symptoms fail to settle or imaging does not show signs of healing, arthroscopic treatment is advised. This may involve drilling an intact lesion, in situ fixation of a loose fragment, microfracture of the subchondral bone or osteochondral grafting.

## Genu Varum

Genu varum or bowed legs is an extremely common presentation in paediatric orthopaedics. In the majority of cases, the appearance represents normal physiology, and families can be reassured. Babies are born with 15–20 degrees of varus which spontaneously resolves with growth, such that the tibiofemoral angle is neutral by 2 years old and, in maximal valgus, by 3–4 years old (**Fig. 10.31**).

The varus can be accentuated by concomitant internal tibial torsion, which is also common in this age group.

If children have symptoms such as pain or a limp, or if the deformity is unilateral, asymmetrical, severe or worsening, then consideration should be given to other diagnoses (**Table 10.8**).

AP, lateral and long-leg alignment radiographs (or hip, knee and ankle views) and blood tests should be performed.

In skeletally immature patients, pathological varus can be treated with growth modulation, whereby a plate and screw construct is placed extraperiosteally, acting as a tension band to tether the growth of the lateral physes until correction is achieved (**Fig. 10.32**). If the physes are nearing closure or have closed, the deformity may require correction with internal or external fixation.

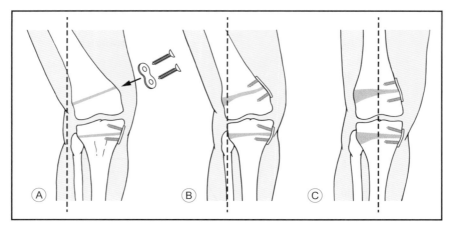

Fig. 10.32 Surgical correction can be achieved by "guided growth". A) Temporary application of an 'eight-plate' on one side of the epiphysis results in B) gradual angular correction of deformity. C) Dotted lines denote the mechanical axis of the lower limb.

| Table 10.8   Causes of Genu Varum | |
|---|---|
| Physiological (age 0–4) | |
| Pathological | Infantile tibia vara (Blount's disease) |
| | Adolescent tibia vara |
| | Physeal disturbance secondary to trauma or infection |
| | Metabolic bone disease, e.g., hypophosphataemic rickets |
| | Generalized skeletal dysplasia |
| | Focal fibrocartilaginous dysplasia |

## Genu Valgum

Genu valgum or knock knees is normal between the ages of 2 and 8 and is maximal at age 4. In addition to the coronal alignment, leg lengths and the rotational profile should be assessed, (**Fig. 10.25**) as the appearance can be accentuated by a leg length discrepancy, increased femoral anteversion, or the combination of femoral retroversion and adduction, as seen in SCFE.

Other causes include valgus following infection or trauma. This may be due to a physeal fracture leading to a partial growth arrest, malunion or the Cozen phenomenon.

Cozen is described as a valgus following proximal tibial fracture without an associated fracture of the fibula. The cause is unknown but may be due to tethering of the lateral physis, stimulation of the medial physis or soft tissue interposition. The deformity is maximal at a year postinjury and spontaneously resolves with time.

Valgus is also seen with tumour-like conditions, including fibrous dysplasia and enchondromatosis, and with metabolic bone disease. Renal osteodystrophy rickets classically produces valgus, as renal failure is acquired in the physiological valgus age range, whereas patients with familial hypophosphataemic rickets develop varus, as the disease is active during early infancy, coinciding with physiological varus.

Severe pathological valgus may require surgical growth modulation with plates applied to the medial aspect of the physes (**Fig. 10.32**).

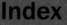

Page numbers followed by *b, t,* and *f* indicate boxes, tables, and figures, respectively.

Enneking staging system, 247, 247*t*
Enteropathic arthritis (EnA), 15–16, 225
European Bone and Joint Infection Society, 51, 52*f*
Ewing's sarcoma, 243–244, 246*f*
Excisional arthroplasty, 5, 31, 113
External tibial torsion, 90
Extraarticular hip pathology, 55, 55*t*
Extracorporeal irradiation, 251

**F**
Fascia lata, 65
Fasciectomy, 201
Fasciotomy, 201
Fat pad impingement, 88
Feet *see* Foot
Femoral anteversion, 277–278, 278*f*
Femoral neck anteversion, 90
Femoral osteotomy, 45*f*, 45
Femoral preparation, 65
Femoroacetabular impingement (FAI), 41, 59
Fibrillation, 3
Fibroblast growth factor (FGF), 2
Fibular hemimelia, 271
Fingers
    deformities, 202, 202*f*
    trigger, 198
First metatarsal osteotomy, 109, 110*f*, 111*b*
First ray, anatomy of, 105–106, 108*f*
First ray disorders, 105
Fixed or mobile bearing, 80
Flat foot, 130
Flexor carpi ulnaris, 181*f*, 182
Flexor tendon pulley system, 198*f*, 198
Fluid sweep test, 101, 102*f*
Foot
    club *see* Club foot
    deformity, 130
    flat *see* Flat foot
    osteology, 106*f*–107*f*
    pes planus *see* Flat foot
Foot & ankle, 105
    Achilles tendinopathy, 136
    ankle arthritis, 124
    Charcot arthropathy, 140
    chronic ankle instability, 119, 120*t*
    clinical examination, 143
    diabetic foot, 139
        screening, 139
        ulcers, 140
    differential diagnosis, 144*t*
    first ray, 105–106, 108*f*
    foot deformity, 130
    Freiberg disease, 116, 117*f*
    hallux rigidus, 113, 114*f*–115*f*
    hallux valgus, 106, 108*f*
    hallux varus, 111, 112*f*

Foot & ankle *(Continued)*
    hindfoot arthritis, 126
    history-taking, 144
    lesser toe deformity, 115, 116*f*
    midfoot arthritis, 128
    Morton's neuroma, 117, 119*f*
    osteochondral defects, 122
    pes cavovarus, 133
    pes planovalgus, 130
    plantar fasciitis, 137
Foot conditions, 268
Foraminal stenosis, 214
Forearm rotation, 191, 192*f*
Forefoot, 105
Freiberg disease, 116
    investigation, 116, 117*f*
    management, 116*f*, 117
    signs, 116
    symptoms, 116
Froment's sign, 183*f*, 183
Froment test, 193
Frozen shoulder, 156, 156*f*
    investigations, 157
    symptoms, 157
    treatment, 157
Fusion (arthrodesis), 5, 31

**G**
Gait, 46, 104*f*, 104
    types, 264, 264*t*
Ganz osteotomy, 45*f*, 45
    surgical technique, 46
Gap balancing (GB), 84
Gartner classification, 153*f*, 153
Genu valgum or knock knees, 286
Genu varum or bowed legs, 285, 286*f*, 286*t*
Giant cell tumour, 242, 243*f*
Glasgow prognostic score, 236, 236*t*
Glenohumeral joint
    corticosteroid injection, 157, 158*b*
    osteoarthritis, 160
        investigation, 159*f*, 160
        signs, 160
        symptoms, 160
        treatment, 160
Glenoid dysplasia, 155
Glenolabral articular disruption (GLAD), 155
Glucosamine or chondroitin sulphate supplements, 76
Greater trochanter, 59
Great toe, 105–106
    hallux rigidus, 113, 114*f*–115*f*
    hallux valgus, 106, 108*f*
    hallux varus, 111, 112*f*
'Grip and grind' pain, 187*f*, 191
Gross motor function classification system (GMFCS), 274, 276*f*